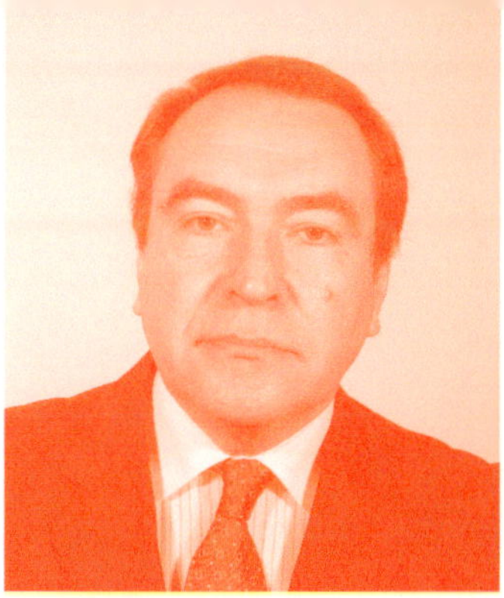

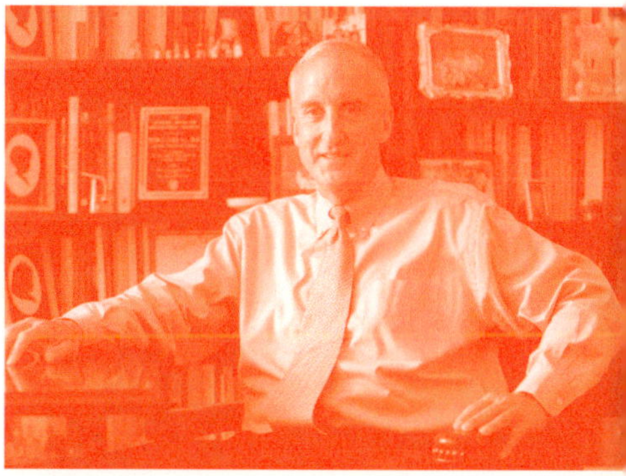

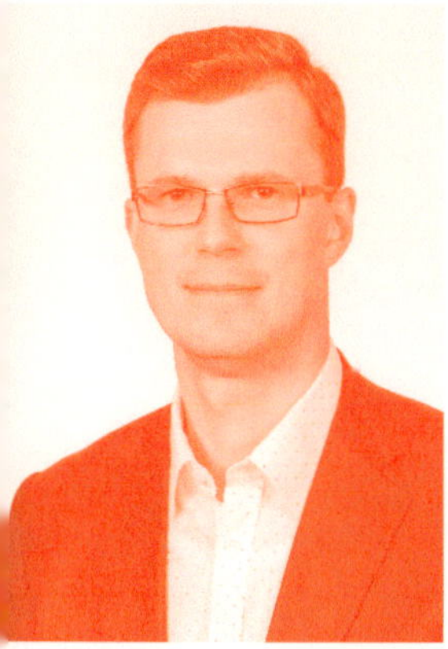

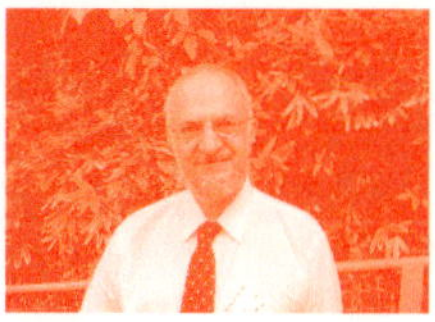

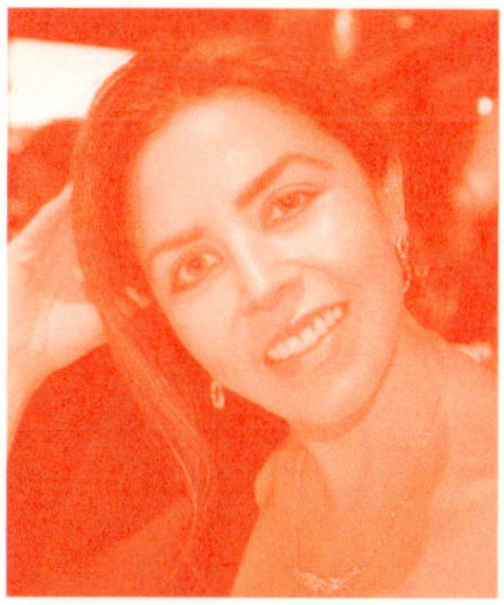

Supporting open minds since 2005

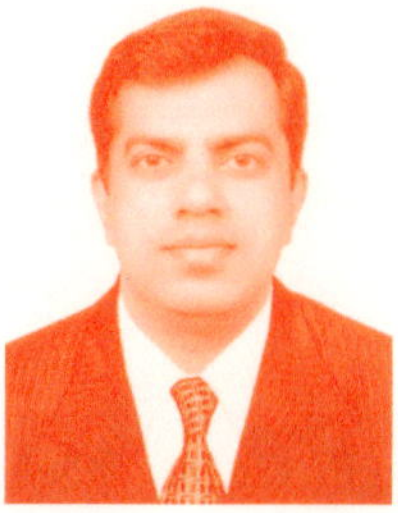

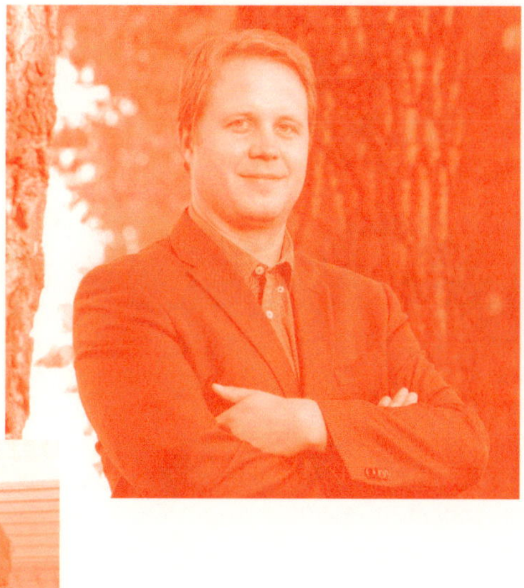

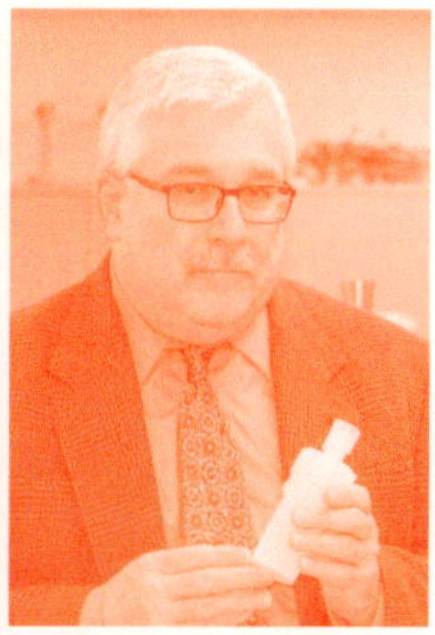

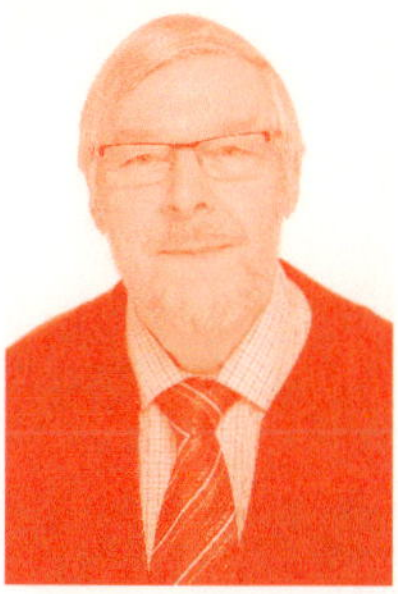

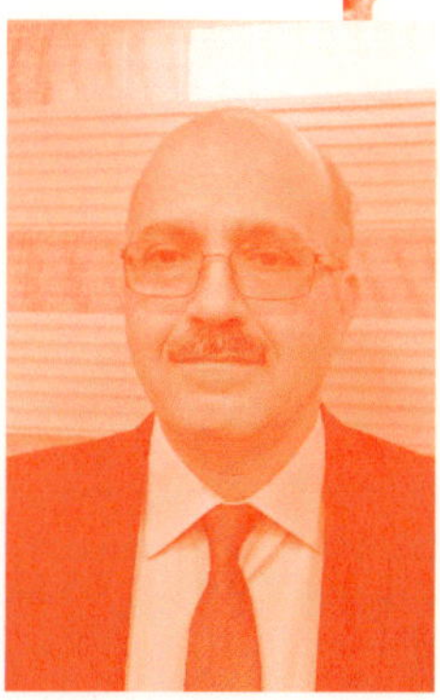

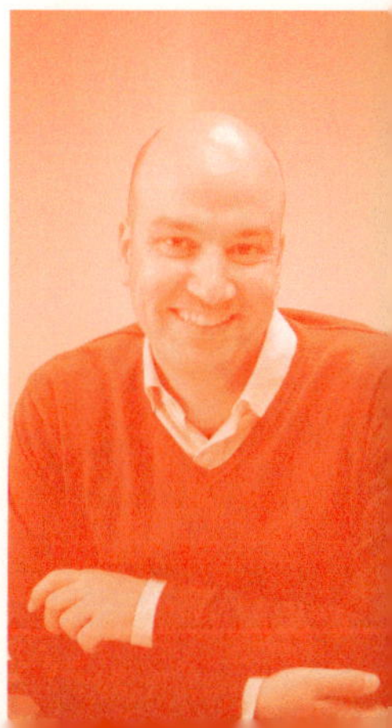

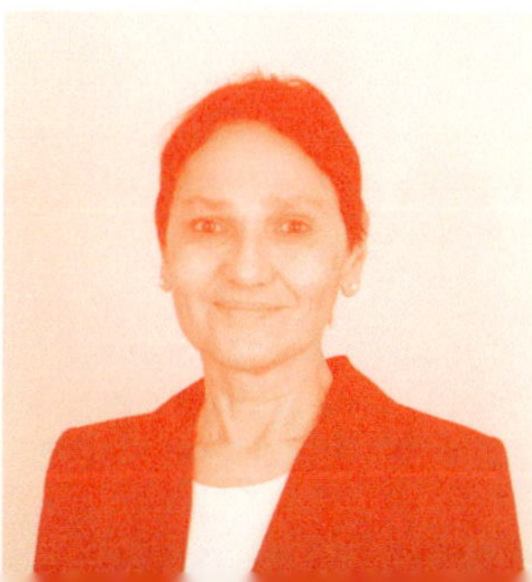

Leishmaniasis - General Aspects of a Stigmatized Disease
http://dx.doi.org/10.5772/intechopen.95200
Edited by Leonardo de Azevedo Calderon

Contributors
Huseyin Istanbullu, Gulsah Bayraktar, R. Sivayogana, Aishwarya Krishnakumar, S. Kumaravel, Rajesh Rajagopal, P. Ravikanth, Mohammed Hassan Flaih, Tatiane Aranha da Penha-Silva, Sandra Alves de Araújo, Ana Lucia Abreu-Silva, Jaqueline Diniz Pinho, Marcelo de Souza Andrade, Karim Abdulkadim Muftin Al Zadawi, Samuel K. Kwofie, Gabriel B. Kwarko, Emmanuel Broni, Michael B. Buenor Adinortey, Michael D. Wilson, Nargis Shaheen, Chaitenya Verma, Naveeda Akhter Qureshi, Juliany Cola Fernandes Rodrigues, Brunno Renato Farias Verçoza, Alisson Amaral Da Rocha, Joseane Lima Prado Godinho, Sara Teixeira de Macedo-Silva, Gabrielle dos Santos da Silva e Miranda, Milena Barenco Pires De Abreu Sodré, Victor Feliciano Dos Santos Ramos, Patricia Xander, Andrey Sladkevicius Vidal, Talita Vieira Dupin, Aline Correia Costa de Morais, Rogéria Cristina Zauli, Wagner Luiz Batista, Medhavi Sudarshan, Sumit Sharan, Lara J. Herrero, Elina Panahi, Christopher S. Peacock, Danielle I. Stanisic, Leonardo de Azevedo Calderon, Natanael Endrew Souto Maior Torres Bonfim, Ana Lígia Barbour Scott

First published in London, United Kingdom, 2022 by IntechOpen
IntechOpen is the global imprint of INTECHOPEN LIMITED, registered in England and Wales, registration number: 11086078, 5 Princes Gate Court, London, SW7 2QJ, United Kingdom
Printed in Croatia

British Library Cataloguing-in-Publication Data
A catalogue record for this book is available from the British Library

Additional hard and PDF copies can be obtained from orders@intechopen.com

Leishmaniasis - General Aspects of a Stigmatized Disease
Edited by Leonardo de Azevedo Calderon
p. cm.
Print ISBN 978-1-83968-081-6
Online ISBN 978-1-83968-082-3
eBook (PDF) ISBN 978-1-83968-092-2

For EU product safety concerns:
IN TECH d.o.o., Prolaz Marije Krucifikse Kozulić 3, 51000 Rijeka, Croatia, info@intechopen.com or visit our website at intechopen.com.

Meet the editor

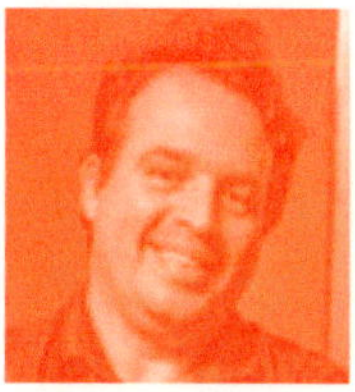

Leonardo de Azevedo Calderon obtained a bachelor's degree and a doctorate in Biological Sciences from the University of Brasília (UnB), Brazil, in 2000 and 2004, respectively. He is a researcher in public health at the Oswaldo Cruz Foundation, lecturer in the Medicine Department, Federal University of Rondônia, Brazil, and head of the Center for the Study of Biomolecules Applied to Health. He has experience in the fields of biochemistry, molecular biophysics, and bioinformatics, working mainly in the prospection and development of new chemical entities with potentially useful activities in future therapies for leishmaniasis and malaria.

Contents

Preface

According to the World Health Organization, leishmaniasis is a neglected tropical disease caused by more than twenty different species of obligate protozoan parasites from the genus *Leishmania* that are transmitted by the bites of infected female sandflies. It is a major global public health problem that has shown an increasing burden over the last decade [1]. It is a disease of poverty, with 350 million people affected by poverty, malnutrition, displacement, and poor housing conditions at major risk of infection in approximately 100 endemic countries in large areas of the tropics, subtropics, and the Mediterranean basin [2]. An estimated 700,000 to 1 million new cases occur each year. *Leishmania* parasites cause two main clinical forms of the disease: visceral and cutaneous leishmaniasis. Visceral leishmaniasis is the most severe, systemic form that is usually fatal unless treated [3]. Cutaneous leishmaniasis is usually limited to an ulcer that self-heals, but can also lead to scarring, disfigurement, and stigmatization as disability outcomes [3]. Therapies for leishmaniasis are numerically restricted, which makes the treatment vulnerable to the emergence of pharmacoresistance. Therefore, efforts to develop new efficient therapies for this disease is imperative, demanding the sum of efforts of researchers and students from all over the globe in the incessant search for new knowledge that leads to the elimination of leishmaniasis. This book is a useful resource for health professionals as well as students in fields related to leishmaniases, such as biochemistry, molecular and cell biology, biotechnology, medicine, pharmacology, epidemiology, and treatment, as well as a reference for health professionals.

Leonardo de Azevedo Calderon
Fiocruz Rondônia,
Oswaldo Cruz Foundation,
Medicine Department,
Federal University of Rondônia,
Porto Velho, Brasil

References

[1] World Health Organization (WHO). Leishmaniais. [Available from: https://www.who.int/health-topics/leishmaniasis#tab=tab_1].

[2] Akhoundi M, Kuhls K, Cannet A, Votýpka J, Marty P, Delaunay P, Sereno D. A Historical Overview of the Classification, Evolution, and Dispersion of Leishmania Parasites and Sandflies. PLoS neglected tropical diseases. 2016;**10**(3):e0004349.

[3] Burza S, Croft SL, Boelaert M. Leishmaniasis. Lancet. 2018; 392: 951-970.

Section 1

Biology

Chapter 1

Leishmaniasis: Molecular Aspects of Parasite Dimorphic Forms Life Cycle

Natanael Endrew Souto Maior Torres Bonfim, Ana Lígia Barbour Scott and Leonardo de Azevedo Calderon

Abstract

According to WHO, Leishmaniasis is a complex neglected disease caused by a protozoa parasite from over 20 Leishmania species transmitted by more than 90 sandfly species, showing three main forms: visceral, cutaneous, and mucocutaneous. The efficient prevention and control of leishmaniasis are very difficult to achieve, depending on the combination of different intervention strategies, usually resulting in failure. Additionally, the correct diagnostics require the combination of clinical signs with laboratory tests, and only a few therapeutical options are available for patients. To improve this scenario, greater efforts in research for control and treatment are needed. For this purpose, the study and understanding of the life cycle of Leishmania are mandatory for all researchers who intend to dedicate their careers to the different aspects of this important disease. In order to support beginning researchers in the study of leishmaniasis, we propose in this review an update in the current knowledge about the major molecular aspects involved in the development of dimorphic forms of Leishmania parasites that replicate in the gut of sandflies (promastigotes) and in mammalian cells (amastigotes) and the relationship with host's immune system.

Keywords: neglected disease, protozoan, leishmania, amastigote, promastigote

1. Introduction

The vectors of leishmaniasis are dipterans belonging to the Psychodidae family, belonging to the genera Phlebotomus (Old World), and Lutzomyia (New World), with wide distribution in warm and temperate climates [1]. Only female sandflies are hematophagous and when infected become vectors [2], they can contaminate, in addition to humans, other mammals such as domestic dogs and cats, making them important reservoirs of the protozoan [3]. These vectors have been more active in the twilight and post-dusk, sheltering during the day in humid, shaded places and well protected from the winds, for example, wild animal burrows, wood holes, bamboo cavities [4].

Protozoan parasites of the genus Leishmania are the causative agents of leishmaniasis, a group of neglected tropical diseases whose clinical manifestations vary depending on the infectious species of Leishmania and weakness of the host [5]. Leishmaniasis presents an unstable epidemiological pattern, presenting unpredictable fluctuations in the number of cases in each region. In the Old World, it was initially described as a dermal condition known as Rish-e-Balkhi (Balkh Wound) as well as "kala-azar". In the New World, leishmaniasis parasites were first described in 1909 by Adolpho Carlos Lindenberg, Antonio Carini, and Ulysses de Freitas Paranhos in skin lesions of patients with 'Bauru's ulcers' in the state of São Paulo, Brazil [6]. Currently, there are three groups of parasites of the genus Leishmania classified into different subgenera and these vary depending on which parts of the vector's gut are colonized by the parasites [7].

It is now known that leishmaniasis can present different characteristics that vary from skin lesions (such as erythematous or hypopigmented macules, papules, nodules, and patches) to visceralization, depending on the species of infecting parasite and the immune response developed by the host (**Figure 1**). However, it is known that cultural, environmental, and socioeconomic factors play an important role. Furthermore, due to the outbreak of tegumentary leishmaniasis in conflict zones in the Middle East, it reveals that war, ecological disasters, and forced migration are other factors associated with leishmaniasis risk factors [6]. Leishmaniasis-causing protozoa have two main life cycle morphologies: the amastigote phase [without apparent flagellum], which is intracellular in the mammalian host, and the promastigote phase [presence of flagellum in the anterior position of the cell] in the fly. The promastigote phase presents five main forms: procyclic, nectomonad, leptomonad, haptomonad, and metacyclic [7]. The growth of the flagellum in the promastigote occurs in several cell cycles. There are clear implications for the mechanisms of regulation of flagellum length, life cycle stage differentiation, and trypanosomatid division in general, and post-genomic analyzes of Leishmania cell biology have contributed to a better understanding of these mechanisms, not only regarding cell differentiation but also to the molecular mechanisms behind the protozoan infection, both in the vector and in the hosts [8].

Studies indicate that leishmaniasis parasites have adaptation mechanisms that allow the optimal activity of each life stage at its corresponding environmental pH [9]. For example, at pH 7.0 it produces morphologically mixed populations of promastigotes in the stationary phase, but it also includes a subpopulation with similar morphology to the metacyclic (**Figure 2**) [18, 19].

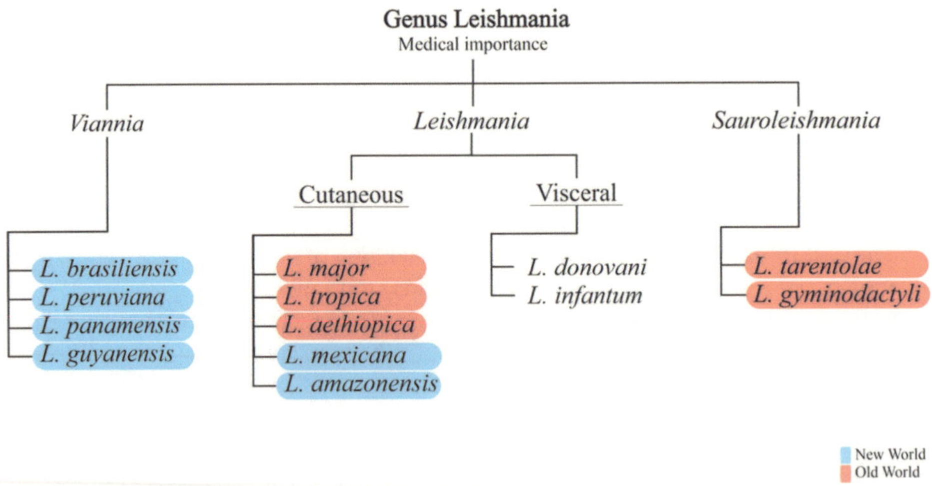

Figure 1.
Representative scheme of the genus Leishmania classification illustrating three subgenres. The species presented include some of the more investigated that are the focus of biomedical research. They were colored by occurrences in the old world (blue boxes) and new world (red boxes), and the without colors occur in both regions. Parasites of the Leishmania and Viannia subgenus infect mammals, while Sauroleishmania infects reptiles as vertebrate hosts. Adapted from [1, 7].

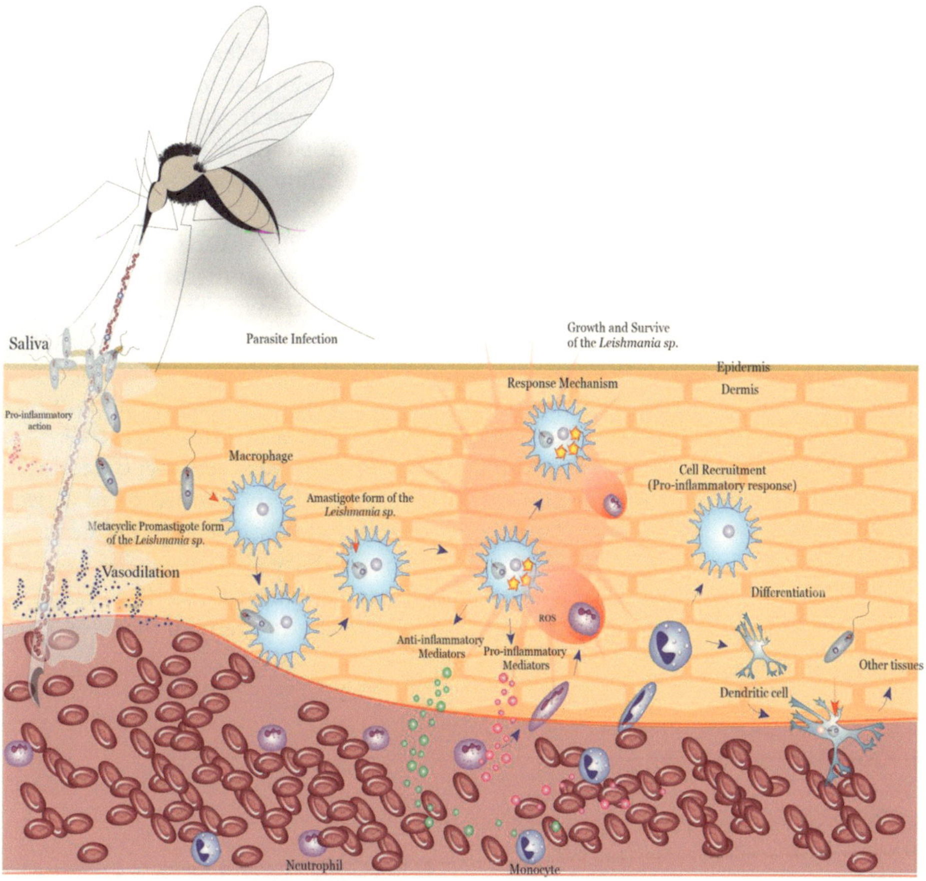

Figure 2.
Representative scheme of Leishmania differentiation process inside the sand fly vector. AM = amastigote form, the decrease in temperature and an increase in pH is detected by the cell and stimulate cell differentiation [10, 11], through modulation of the expression of genes linked to cell functions [12]. PP = pro-cyclic promastigote form, the secretion of chitinol enzymes aids in the escape from peritrophic membrane allowing the fixation on the vector intestine wall [13], the decrease in pH linked to the increase in glucose in the medium stimulates differentiation and migration according to the gradient of glucose concentration [14] by modulating the expression of genes linked to different cellular functions [12]. NP = Nectomonad Promatigote form, migrate to the thoracic portion of the midgut and begin to secrete PSG [15], as well as a decrease in the expression of several genes [12]. LP = Leptomonad Promatigote form, PSG secretion and detection of decreased oxygenation and pH actives signals for cell differentiation [16] into HP = Haptomonad Promatigote which attaches to the thoracic midgut wall and produces the PSG gel [17], or differentiates into MP = Metacyclic Promatigote form, the infecting phase, which migrates to the anterior portion of the sand fly intestine and infects the host during the next meal [14]. The increase is represented as blue arrows and the decrease is represented as red arrows.

2. Amastigote form

Amastigote means "without apparent flagellum". The flagellum in amastigotes is internal and non-functional [7, 20]. This phase is a response to the phagocytation by its host's defense cells, presenting itself in an intracellular form inside the phagolysosome [21].

After the blood-feeding, digestive enzymes, including trypsin, chymotrypsin, aminopeptidase, carboxypeptidase, and alpha-glycosidase degrade ingested infected cells and expose amastigote forms to the peritrophic membrane. The change in conditions from the mammalian host to the vector's gut, active membrane receptors that detect the change in the environment as the pH increases, from ~4.0 to 5.5 in the phagolysosome to ~6.8 to 7.4 in the midgut vector [14, 21, 22] and temperature decrease, stimulate the development of the parasite into promastigote form [10, 11].

An important response of the parasite to this environmental change is the modulation of enzyme activity in the midgut, assigning different roles to these molecules than that suggested for the mucin-like structures, which appear to protect the parasite surface against the proteolytic enzymes [14]. The secretion of chitinase and N-acetylglucosaminidase enzymes protects from the intense enzymatic activity resulting from digestion, allowing the escape of peritrophic membrane towards the intestinal wall of the vector [13].

Several intracellular signals are triggered and are directly related to the transition from amastigote to promastigote. Relative expression studies revealed increased expression of several genes related to: (calmodulin binding; Cyclic nucleotide biosynthetic process; GTPase activity; GTP binding; DNA association; Nucleosome activity; Nucleosome assembly; Synthesis-coupled proton transport ATP; Mitochondrial proton transporter ATP synthase; Intracellular signal transduction; Dinein complex; Protein complex; Protein heterodimerization activity; Protein polymerization; Proteolysis; Phosphorus-oxygen lyase activity; Calcium-dependent cysteine-type endopeptidase] and a decrease in the expression of genes related to: (Antioxidant activity; Peroxiredoxin activity; Cysteine-type peptidase activity; DNA catabolic process; Triglyceride lipase activity) [12].

Transformation of amastigotes to promastigotes occurs within 12–18 h. These initially transformed promastigotes are termed procyclic and remain short, ovoid, and only slightly mobile [14].

3. Promastigote forms

3.1 Procyclic form

A procyclic promastigote is similar to a cell in G1 or post-S phase that has inherited the new short flagellum [23]. Its morphological characteristic is a body length of 6.5–11.5 μm and the flagellum is shorter than the body length and can have variable body width [20]. The intense multiplication of these forms starts at approximately 18–24 h [14], the divisor promastigotes are found in rosettes with flagella directed towards the center. In promastigotes, the flagellum extends from the cell body, hits and moves the organism, emerging from the anterior end of the cell [7].

Membrane protein classes of the parasite enable the attachment of the procyclic promastigote to the midgut wall of the vector and compatibility between Leishmania species with the vector species. The main membrane glycoconjugates, including their unique and common structures, are lipophosphoglycans–LPG, glycophosphatidylinositol lipids–GIPLs, glycoprotein 63–gp63, secreted acid phosphatases–sAP, secreted proteophosphoglycans–sPPG [14].

The fact that significant differences in LPG-mediated binding were observed when different vector species were compared suggest that the molecules that serve as parasite attachment sites can vary between different species of sandflies.

Serum digestion products destroy incompatible Leishmania species, furthermore, studies suggest that inter- and intraspecies-specific polymorphisms in the LPG phosphoglycan domains may result in species- and strain-restricted intestinal binding and thus determine vector competence. Species- and strain-specific and may therefore provide the evolutionary pressure for structural LPG polymorphisms [14, 24]. Developmental-regulated modifications in LPG structure control the specificity of the midgut adhesion stage [25, 26]. Recent findings indicate that non-LPG-mediated fixation is used by some other species of Leishmania [27–31].

The gp63, also known as leishmanolysin, is a 63 kDa zinc metalloproteinase containing a GPI anchor and is expressed on the surface of promastigotes of several Leishmania species. It plays an important role in the annexation of the leishmaniasis protozoan and has stood out in several studies related to the understanding of the development and virulence of the parasite [31–36].

Gut-associated lectins or lectin-like molecules, which have been described for sandflies and presented as signaling sites conducive to parasite fixation [37–39].

Alternatively, lower affinity and less specific interactions, mediated by shared covering structures and/or flagellar proteins, may be sufficient for the parasite to resist the expulsive force it is exposed to in the vectors. Directing the anterior migration of unattached promastigotes to the thoracic midgut and stomodeal valve has generally been attributed to a glucose concentration gradient [14].

3.2 Nectomonad form

During 36–60 h, rapid multiplication continues, accompanied by the transformation of promastigotes into a long, slender, highly mobile form called nectomonads [14]. Nektós, comes from the Greek and means: "who swims". Its morphological characteristic is the body length greater than or equal to 12 μm with variable body width and flagellar length [20]. A nectomonad promastigote is like an S-phase cell [23]. The cell differentiation signals triggered, in comparison to the procyclic ones, a significant decrease in the expression of genes related to: Nucleosome activity and assembly; protein heterodimerization; DNA association; core; kinetochore; administration of calmodulin [12].

3.3 Leptomonad form

By 60–72 h, an enormous number of nectomonads are found bundled up in the anterior portion of the abdominal midgut, with many attached via their flagella to the microvilli of the epithelial cells. The anterior migration of promastigotes to the region of the cardia [middle thoracic intestine] and stomodeal valve proceeds until a large accumulation of parasites behind the valve is reached. A leptomonad promastigote is similar to a cell in the same stages of the cell cycle as a procyclic promastigote, but which has inherited the older, longer flagellum [23]. Leptos, comes from the Greek and means: "slender, thin, small". Its morphological characteristic is body length 6.5–11.5 μm, with flagellum greater than body length and variable body width [20]. Found lining the surface of the stomodeal valve and there can be differentiated haptomonad and metacyclic promastigotes [40].

3.4 Haptomonad form

It is the transformation of leptomonads into short, broad forms called haptomonads, which are occasionally seen to divide [7]. It comes from the Greek haptein, and means: "to hold, denoting contact or combination", the morphological characteristic of haptomonads is the discoid expansion of the tip of the flagellum, with body shape and variable flagellar length [20]. The haptomonad forms bind through hemidesmosomes to the thin cuticular layer called the intima of the stomodeal valve or to each other through the secretion of a viscous gel-like matrix that restricts its motility [17].

The main component of the gel secreted by promastigotes (PSG) is a high molecular weight glycoprotein called filamentous proteophosphoglycan [15]. The identification of PSG strengthened the hypothesis of vector valve blockage, because the gel-forming properties of the filamentous proteophosphoglycan–fPPG may provide the physical obstruction necessary to cause regurgitation in the vector during repast [7].

The gelatinous nature of PSG, together with its high cell density, can cause local oxygen depletion, and anaerobiosis is also known to stimulate metacyclogenesis [16]. Furthermore, after differentiating leptomonad promastigotes in the middle of the PSG plug, metacyclic promastigotes can migrate to either pole, concentrating on the former in response to a chemotactic suggestion. The possibility of Leishmania responding to sugars or saliva released from the culture that could form a gradient in the midgut remains to be addressed [20].

3.5 Metacyclic form

The name "metacyclic" comes from the Greek Meta and means: "Between". They are morphologically classified as short, slender, body length less than or equal to 8 μm, body width less than or equal to 1 μm, and highly active with a flagellum at least twice the length of the cell body and are generally not seen in the division [7, 20].

When compared with the gene expression in the form of neptomonads, we can observe the regulation of several cellular activities, with the negative expression of genes related to rRNA processing and the small subunit process (SSU) [12].

Metacyclic promastigotes, originating from the foregut or behind the stomodeal valve to the esophagus, pharynx, and proboscis, are inoculated during the meal, where they initiate the infection in the mammalian host [14]. However, there are at least three known components that lead to infection by the leishmaniasis protozoa: the metacyclic promastigotes themselves, which are obviously essential for transmission; sand fly saliva; and the gel secreted by promastigotes–PSG. Sandfly saliva is a well-established disease exacerbation factor [41], at least for tegumentary leishmaniasis. This is due to the fact that it contains potent compounds with vasodilatory and anti-hemostatic properties [42]. Co-inoculation of saliva with parasites has been shown to worsen the disease in several studies, and this is due to the modulatory capacity of the immune response to contribute to parasite survival and replication [43–45]. Likewise, PSG has also been shown to contribute to the worsening of the disease, being directly related to the increase in the number of metacyclic promastigote parasites co-inoculated with saliva [27]. The presence of parasites in the salivary glands of sandflies has already been reported by some studies and, therefore, it has been proposed as a fact of great relevance for transmission [46, 47].

4. Molecular aspects of the infection

The first interactions between Leishmania and the host's immune response are closely linked to the evolution of the disease or protection against the protozoan, and the vector's saliva directly contributes to these interactions [48]. Sandfly saliva is composed of active molecules that cause an imbalance in homeostasis at the host site, and aid repast [49]. The saliva of these arthropods contains a vast repertoire of pharmacologically active molecules that hinder the host's hemostatic, inflammatory, and immunological responses [48, 49]. When sand fly saliva is injected into the host's skin, it induces infiltration of inflammatory cells [50] and antibody production [51–53]. These disturbances in tissue physiology may also favor the release of Leishmania parasites, as the key to the success of Leishmania parasitism is the ability to evade host immune responses [48]. In this setting, immune complexes are formed [53] in the early stages of exposure. In addition, sand fly saliva also modulates costimulatory molecules and cytokine release by antigen-presenting cells [54–56].

Several active compounds with pharmaceutical properties have already been isolated from the saliva of sand flies such as the anticoagulant compound of Lufaxine (Inhibitor of Factor Xa from *Lutzomyia longipalpis*). This recombinant protein has potent and specific anticoagulant activity against factor Xa, a serine protease that cleaves prothrombin to generate thrombin and is involved in both the extrinsic and intrinsic coagulation pathway [57], preventing the activation of receptor 2 activated by protease and thereby inhibiting inflammation and thrombosis in C57BL/6 mice [58].

The action of the LuloHya compound, which acts as a hyaluronidase [55], has also been reported, and when co-inoculated with the parasites provides a more successful infection by Leishmania [59–61]. The Lundep protein, on the other hand, acts as an endonuclease and helps in the survival of parasites by inhibiting neutrophil traps (NET) in addition to preventing the activation by contact of FXIIa in human plasma [56, 60].

One of the most studied salivary peptides is a potent vasodilator known as maxadilan (MAX). In addition to vasodilation, this compound can also act as an immunomodulator in the host. It can up-regulate cytokines associated with a type 2 response (IL-10, IL-6, and TGF-β) and down-regulate type 1 cytokines (IL-12p70 and TNF-α), NO, and CCR7. This increased parasite survival in the vertebrate host in the early stages of infection [55, 56]. Studies involving the inhibition of human complement by the saliva of the sand fly *Lutzomyia longipalpis* showed the existence of inhibitors of the classical pathway in this species. As the anti-complement compound Salo [62] and is also considered as a potential transmission-blocking vaccine candidate against leishmaniasis [63].

Pharmacologically active molecules such as Maxadilan in *L. longipalpis* or PP-1 PP-2A inhibitors [Protein phosphorylation and dephosphorylation reactions, mediated by protein kinases and PPs, respectively, trigger signal transduction events that control diverse cellular responses to internal and external signals [64, 65] present in the saliva of *P. papatasi*, probably evolved to facilitate blood-feeding. However, as with many other biomolecules, salivary factors also exhibit other activities. In this case, Leishmania parasites benefit from the immunomodulatory effects of certain salivary factors to facilitate their establishment in the hostile environment of vertebrate skin [66].

Taken together, these data indicate that saliva is an endless issue, and several factors remain to be defined and how blocking these molecules is an open field for alternative tools against transmission [48, 49, 67]. **Figure 3** briefly illustrates the main aspects of how the infection of leishmaniasis parasites occurs in the host.

Recognition of the parasite by the host's immune system cells is the key to triggering effective Leishmania-specific immunity [5]. However, the parasite can persist in the host's myeloid cells, evading, delaying, and manipulating the host's immunity to escape host resistance and ensure its transmission [5].

Neutrophils are the first to infiltrate infection sites, where they generate an inflammatory response that restricts the parasite and acts to protect the organism, fighting infection through a series of mechanisms, being considered important modulators of leishmaniasis [68]. They are responsible for the formation of web-like structures called neutrophil extracellular traps (NETs) that can capture and/or kill microorganisms [68]. However, for some species of Leishmania, neutrophils can act as carriers that facilitate the silent infection of macrophages [69–71]. The 'Trojan Horse' model is based on the silent transmission of the parasite from neutrophils to macrophages and dendritic cells when macrophages and cells phagocyte from apoptotic neutrophils that are contaminated by Leishmania [70]. This model is evidenced in the reported ability of some Leishmania species, such as *L. major* and *L. braziliensis* [72, 73], to induce neutrophil apoptosis.

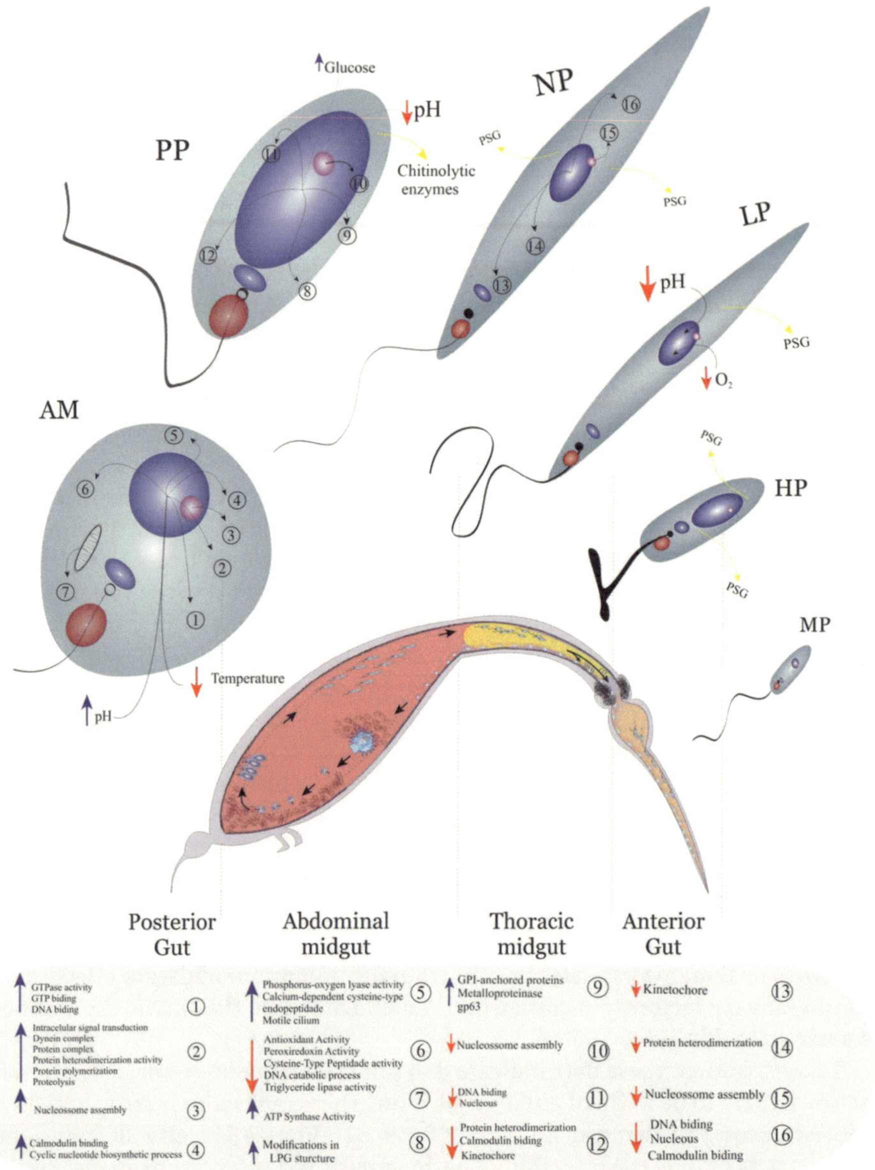

Figure 3.
Schematic representation of the leishmaniasis stages of infection. Parasite infection: Leishmania sp. enters through the lesion caused by the proboscis during the meal and infect local macrophages. Stimulated by compounds with vasodilating and anti-hemostatic properties present in the vector's saliva, an inflammatory reaction begins in the region where more immune cells are recruited to the site and can also be infected by protozoa in metacyclic form. Once phagocytosed, the protozoa become different in the amastigote form in the phagosome. Growth and survival of Leishmania sp.: Infected macrophages secrete anti-inflammatory and pro-inflammatory mediators, initiate immune response mechanisms, neutrophils release cytokines and reactive oxygen species–ROS in the region and monocytes, which differ into macrophages and dendritic cells, which become infected and migrate to other tissues. The increase is represented as blue arrows and decrease is represented as red arrows.

Macrophages are the main effector population involved in parasite elimination [5]. However, macrophages are the main host cells where the parasites grow and divide. The parasites infect, multiply gradually, and finally destroy macrophages releasing large numbers of viable amastigotes in the region [74]. Once inside the macrophage, and depending on the Leishmania species, the parasites delay the formation and maturation of phagosomes, preventing phagosome acidification and the action of proteases, while guaranteeing the nutrients necessary for its survival. Furthermore, the parasites modulate the cytokine secretion pattern and inhibit the generation of NO and ROS, while extending the survival of infected macrophages [5]. Genomic and transcriptomic analyzes have largely contributed to the understanding of the biology of Leishmania and revealed to us about the complex interactions that occur within the parasite–host-vector triangle, these interactions are responsible for the rapid activation and deactivation of various signaling pathways that lead to functions of macrophages [e.g., phagocytosis, chemokine secretion, and prostaglandin secretion] [75, 76]. Extracellular matrix interactions, metabolic changes, modulation of gene expression and several mechanisms that are still being studied have revealed how cell–cell interaction occurs and why leishmaniasis is such a complex disease as shown in **Figure 4**. The elimination of parasites by macrophages requires the preparation and development of an adaptive effector Th1 immunity driven by specific subtypes of dendritic cells [5].

Studies analyzing neutrophils infected by *L. major* parasites have shown that, when phagocytosed by cells in the skin tissue, they have the ability to inhibit the maturation and migration of dendritic cells, resulting in a delay in the development of adaptive immunity [72, 78, 79]. Dendritic cells are essential for the generation of a Th1-mediated immune response, fundamental for the control of leishmaniasis [80–82]. These parasites can act at different levels to inhibit dendritic cells, including modulation of the MAPK pathway, decreased antigen presentation capacity and IL-12 secretion, this inhibition being mediated by the activation of protein tyrosine phosphatase (PTPs) [83, 84]. In summary, the internalization of the opsonized protozoan by dendritic cells via FcγR (Fcγ receptor) promotes dendritic cell activation and IL-12 production. Furthermore, there is a down-regulation of costimulatory molecules, CD40 and CD86 after infection and gp63 cleaves the SNAREs protein (soluble NSF binding protein receptor), preventing the assembly of the NADPH oxidase complex [5]. An analysis of the gene expression of lesions with Cutaneous Leishmaniasis showed increased P27 [85] and decreased expression of the A2 gene [86]. IL-10 is important for the persistence of the parasite in the lesion, preventing its complete elimination from the lesion, despite the presence of a protective immune response [87]. Furthermore, circulating antibody is crucial for susceptibility to the development of tegumentary leishmaniasis [88] and a progressive increase in tissue IL-10 expression during infection suggests a role in susceptibility [89]. The amastigotes from the cutaneous leishmaniasis lesion are coated with IgG, and the internalization of opsonized amastigotes by macrophages induces the production of IL-10 and a consequent increase in the intracellular growth of the parasite [90].

Tissue damage is promoted by inappropriate epidermal signals driven by dendritic cells. Furthermore, studies indicate that nTregs are essential for the development and maintenance of persistent skin infection and reactivation of infections caused by the Leishmania parasite [91]. Understanding which dendritic cell populations are critical to triggering and achieving immunity to Leishmania and how parasites inhibit its activation and migration will help to improve a rational design of vaccines aimed at neutralizing the parasite's virulence factors, along with the use of the most appropriate adjuvants [5]. These recurrent injuries may result from the Koebner phenomenon [92] which refers to skin lesions appearing in lines of mechanical trauma, seen in some skin diseases such as psoriasis.

Antimicrobial peptides are innate immunity mechanisms that contribute to host defense. LL-37 is a peptide derived from human cathelicidin (CAP180, a multifunctional regulator of the innate and adaptive immune response, having a leishmanicidal activity, increasing phagocytosis in dendritic cells and macrophages, and acting as an activator or suppressor of the adaptive immune response depending on the concentration [91].

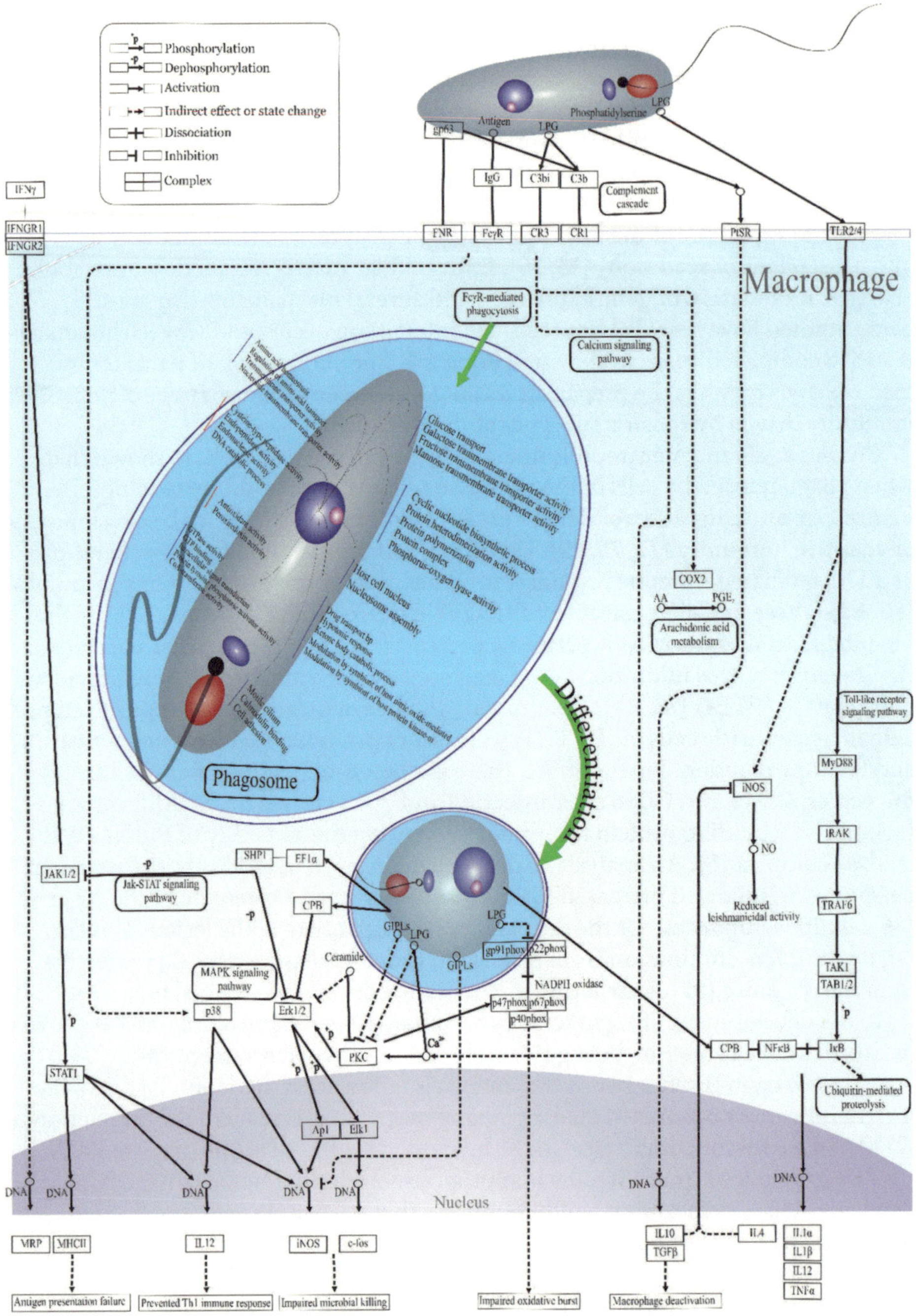

Figure 4.

Diagram representing the major reports about modulation of internal reactions in macrophages infected by the parasite causing leishmaniasis. Leishmania sp. internalization and cell differentiation is successfully achieved, mediated by modulating the expression of genes linked to various cellular functions [12] and by the alteration of signaling events in the host cell, leading to increased production of autoinhibitory molecules such as TGF-beta and decreased induction of cytokines such as IL12 for protective immunity. The production of nitric oxide is also inhibited. furthermore, defective expression of major histocompatibility complex (MHC) genes silences subsequent macrophage-mediated T cell activation, resulting in abnormal immune responses [77]. SHP-1 down-regulates JAK2, Erk1/Erk2 MAP, NF-B, IRF-1, and AP-1 kinases, thereby inhibiting IFN-inducible macrophage functions (e.g., nitric oxide, IL-12 production, and immunoproteasome formation), STAT1 degradation by the proteasome is dependent on PKC and other phosphatases (eg, phosphatase IP3 and calcineurin) and surface parasite molecules such as LPGs play a key role in altering several secondary pathways, for example, PKC, Ca^{+2} and phosphatidyl inositol), regulating important phagocyte functions such as NO and superoxide production [75]. The increase is represented as blue arrows and the decrease is represented as red arrows.

Natural regulatory T cells rapidly accumulate in the dermis, where they suppress, both through IL-10 dependent and independent mechanisms, the capacity of CD4 + CD25 effector T cells to eliminate the parasite from the site [91]. One of the immunopathological consequences of active visceral leishmaniasis in humans is the suppression of T cell responses mainly to the Leishmania antigen [93]. The immune responses induced during visceral leishmaniasis in experimental data are markedly different from those induced in cutaneous leishmaniasis [94]. Furthermore, gene expression studies of tissues infected with visceral leishmaniasis reveal the modulation of the expression of genes P27, Ufm1 [85] and A2 [95]. A spectrum of clinical manifestations occurs in visceral leishmaniasis, ranging from asymptomatic or oligosymptomatic disease to progressive disease with severe manifestations such as hepatosplenomegaly, fever, pancytopenia, and hypergammaglobulinemia [96].

These particularities must have to be studied in order to permit the understanding of how different Leishmania species could promote different forms of the disease can generate such different immune responses [94].

5. Conclusion

The morphological development of the parasite has been regulated by the environment in which it is found, being perceived by chemotactic receptors that identify these environmental changes (e.g. pH and oxygenation), modulating several genes and thus triggering various intracellular processes, processes that depend on the stage of development that the parasite is at when receiving such stimuli. About the molecular aspects involved in the infection, we can say that current research has indicated a strong relationship between the immune response and the way in which leishmaniasis will manifest itself.

In order to benefit the socio-economically vulnerable individuals affected by leishmaniasis, many young researchers start their studies in leishmaniasis from an early age in scientific initiation programs, often conducting their studies well beyond the PhD. These young researchers are the audience that this book chapter is dedicated. Because we believe that the study and understanding of the life cycle of Leishmania are mandatory for all researchers who intend to dedicate their careers to the different aspects of this important disease. From epidemiological studies to the development of new therapies, a good understanding of the parasite's life cycle is essential for the success of all initiatives.

Author details

Natanael Endrew Souto Maior Torres Bonfim[1,2], Ana Lígia Barbour Scott[2] and Leonardo de Azevedo Calderon[1,3*]

1 Center for the Study of Biomolecules Applied to Health, Oswaldo Cruz Foundation (Fiocruz), Fiocruz Rondônia, Porto Velho, Brazil

2 Laboratory of Computational Biophysical and Biology, Center for Mathematics, Computing and Cognition, Federal University of ABC, São Paulo, Brazil

3 Medicine Department, Federal University of Rondônia (UNIR), Porto Velho, Brazil

*Address all correspondence to: leonardo.calderon@fiocruz.br

References

[1] Akhoundi M, Kuhls K, Cannet A, et al. A historical overview of the classification, evolution, and dispersion of Leishmania parasites and Sandflies. PLoS Neglected Tropical Diseases. 2016;**10**(3):e0004349. DOI: 10.1371/journal.pntd.0004349

[2] Pimenta PFP, Saraiva EMB, Rowton E, et al. Evidence that the vectorial competence of phlebotomine sand flies for different species of Leishmania is controlled by structural polymorphisms in the surface lipophosphoglycan. Proceedings of the National Academy of Sciences of the United States of America. 1994;**91**(19):9155-9159. DOI: 10.1073/pnas.91.19.9155

[3] De Almeida MC, Vilhena V, Barral A, et al. Leishmanial infection: Analysis of its first steps. A review. Memórias do Instituto Oswaldo Cruz. 2003;**98**(7): 861-870. DOI: 10.1590/s0074-02762003000700001

[4] Forattini OP. Nota sobre criadouros naturais de flebôtomos em dependências peri-domiciliares, no estado de São Paulo. Arquivos da Faculdade de Higiene e Saúde Pública. 1953;7(2):157-168. DOI: 10.11606/issn.2358-792x.v7i2p157-168

[5] Martínez-López M, Soto M, Iborra S, et al. Leishmania hijacks myeloid cells for immune escape. Frontiers in Microbiology. 2018;**9**:883. DOI: 10.3389/fmicb.2018.00883

[6] Steverding D. The history of leishmaniasis. Parasites & Vectors. 2017;**10**:82. DOI: 10.1186/s13071-017-2028-5

[7] Bates PA. Transmission of Leishmania metacyclic promastigotes by phlebotomine sand flies. International Journal for Parasitology. 2007;**37**(10): 1097-1106. DOI: 10.1016/j.ijpara.2007.04.003

[8] Wheeler RJ, Gluenz E, Gull K. The cell cycle of Leishmania: Morphogenetic events and their implications for parasite biology. Molecular Microbiology. 2011;**79**:647-662. DOI: 10.1111/j.1365-2958.2010.07479.x

[9] Zilberstein D, Shapira M. The role of pH and temperature in the development of Leishmania parasites. Annual Review of Microbiology. 1994;**48**:449-470. DOI: 10.1146/annurev.mi.48.100194.002313

[10] Bates P, Rogers M. New insights into the developmental biology and transmission mechanisms of Leishmania. Current Molecular Medicine. 2004;**4**:601-609. DOI: 10.2174/1566524043360285

[11] Kamhawi S. Phlebotomine sand flies and Leishmania parasites: Friends or foes? Trends in Parasitology. 2006;**22**(9):439-445. DOI: 10.1016/j.pt.2006.06.012

[12] Inbar E, Hughitt VK, Dillon LAL, et al. The transcriptome of Leishmania major developmental stages in their natural sand fly vector. MBio. 2017;**8**(2):e00029-e00017. DOI: 10.1128/mBio.00029-17

[13] Schlein Y, Jacobson RL, Shlomai J. Chitinase secreted by Leishmania functions in the sandfly vector. Proceedings of the Royal Society B: Biological Sciences. 1991;**245**:21-126. DOI: 10.1098/rspb.1991.0097

[14] Sacks D, Kamhawi S. Molecular aspects of parasite-vector and vector-host interactions in Leishmaniasis. Annual Review of Microbiology. 2001;**55**:453-483. DOI: 10.1146/annurev.micro.55.1.453

[15] Ilg T, Stierhof YD, Craik D, et al. Purification and structural characterization of a filamentous, mucin- like proteophosphoglycan secreted by Leishmania parasites. The Journal of Biological Chemistry.

1996;**271**(35):21583-21598. DOI: 10.1074/jbc.271.35.21583

[16] Méndez S, Fernández-Pérez FJ, de la Fuente C, et al. Partial anaerobiosis induces infectivity of Leishmania infantum promastigotes. Parasitology Research. 1999;**85**:507-509. DOI: 10.1007/s004360050587

[17] Dostálová A, Volf P. Leishmania development in sand flies: Parasite-vector interactions overview. Parasites & Vectors. 2012;**5**:276. DOI: 10.1186/1756-3305-5-276

[18] Bates PA, Tetley L. *Leishmania mexicana*: Induction of Metacyclogenesis by cultivation of promastigotes at acidic pH. Experimental Parasitology. 1993;**76**: 412-423. DOI: 10.1006/expr.1993.1050

[19] Zakai HA, Chance ML, Bates PA. In vitro stimulation of metacyclogenesis in *Leishmania braziliensis*, *L. donovani*, *L. major* and *L. mexicana*. Parasitology. 1998;**116**(4):305-309. DOI: 10.1017/s0031182097002382

[20] Rogers ME, Chance ML, Bates PA. The role of promastigote secretory gel in the origin and transmission of the infective stage of *Leishmania mexicana* by the sandfly Lutzomyia longipalpis. Parasitology. 2002;**124**:495-507. DOI: 10.1017/s0031182002001439

[21] Mukkada A, Meade J, Glaser T, et al. Enhanced metabolism of Leishmania donovani amastigotes at acid pH: An adaptation for intracellular growth. Science. 1985;**229**:1099-1101. DOI: 10.1126/science.4035350

[22] Telleria EL, Araújo APO de, Secundino NF, et al. Trypsin-like serine proteases in Lutzomyia longipalpis – Expression, activity and possible modulation by Leishmania infantum chagasi, PLoS One 2010;5: e10697. DOI: 10.1371/journal.pone.0010697

[23] Sunter J, Gull K. Shape, form, function and Leishmania pathogenicity: From textbook descriptions to biological understanding. Open Biology. 2017;7: 170165. DOI: 10.1098/rsob.170165

[24] Adler S. Factors determining the behaviour of Leishmania sp. in Sandflies. Harefuah. 1938;**14**:4-8

[25] Pimenta PFP, Turco SJ, McConville MJ, et al. Stage-specific adhesion of Leishmania promastigotes to the sandfly midgut. Science. 1992;**256**(5065):1812-1815. DOI: 10.1126/science.1615326

[26] Kamhawi S, Ramalho-Ortigao M, Van MP, et al. A role for insect galectins in parasite survival. Cell. 2004;**119**(3):329-341. DOI: 10.1016/j.cell.2004.10.009

[27] Rogers ME, Ilg T, Nikolaev AV, et al. Transmission of cutaneous leishmaniasis by sand flies is enhanced by regurgitation of fPPG. Nature. 2004;**430**:463-467. DOI: 10.1038/nature02675

[28] Svobodova M, Votypka J, Peckova J, et al. Distinct transmission cycles of *Leishmania tropica* in 2 adjacent foci, northern Israel. Emerging Infectious Diseases. 2006;**12**(12):1860-1868. DOI: 10.3201/eid1212.060497

[29] Volf P, Myskova J. Sand flies and Leishmania: Specific versus permissive vectors. Trends in Parasitology. 2007;**23**:91-92. DOI: 10.1016/j.pt.2006.12.010

[30] Myskova J, Svobodova M, Beverley SM, et al. A lipophosphoglycan-independent development of Leishmania in permissive sand flies. Microbes and Infection. 2007;**9**(3):317-324. DOI: 10.1016/j.micinf.2006.12.010

[31] Jecna L, Dostalova A, Wilson R, et al. The role of surface glycoconjugates in Leishmania midgut attachment examined by competitive binding assays and experimental development in sand flies. Parasitology. 2013;**140**:1026-1032. DOI: 10.1017/S0031182013000358

[32] Button LL, Robert MW. Molecular cloning of the major surface antigen of leishmania. The Journal of Experimental Medicine. 1988;**167**(2):724-729. DOI: 10.1084/jem.167.2.724

[33] Etges R, Bouvier J, Bordier C. The major surface protein of Leishmania promastigotes is a protease. The Journal of Biological Chemistry. 1986;**261**(20): P9098-P9101. DOI: 10.1016/s0021-9258(18)67621-5

[34] Bouvier J, Schneider P, Etges R. Leishmanolysin: Surface metallo-proteinase of Leishmania. Methods in Enzymology. 1995;**248**:614-633. DOI: 10.1016/0076-6879(95)48039-0

[35] Ilg T, Montgomery J, Stierhof Y-D, et al. Molecular cloning and characterization of a novel repeat-containing Leishmania major gene, ppg1, that encodes a membrane-associated form of Proteophosphoglycan with a putative glycosylphosphatidylinositol anchor. The Journal of Biological Chemistry. 1999;**274**:31410-31420. DOI: 10.1074/jbc.274.44.31410

[36] Elhay MJ, McConville MJ, Handman E. Immunochemical characterization of a glyco-inositol-phospholipid membrane antigen of *Leishmania major*. Journal of Immunology. 1988;**141**:1326-1331

[37] Volf P, Kiewegová A, Svobodová M. Sandfly midgut lectin: Effect of galactosamine on Leishmania major infections. Medical and Veterinary Entomology. 1998;**12**:151-154. DOI: 10.1046/j.1365-2915.1998.00089.x

[38] Volf P, Killick-Kendrick R, Bates PA, et al. Comparison of the haemag-glutination activities in gut and head extracts of various species and geographical populations of phlebotomine sandflies. Annals of Tropical Medicine and Parasitology. 1994;**88**:337-340. DOI: 10.1080/00034983.1994.11812874

[39] Wallbanks KR, Ingram GA, Molyneux DH. The agglutination of erythrocytes and Leishmania parasites by sandfly gut extracts: Evidence for lectin activity. Tropical Medicine and Parasitology. 1986;**37**:409-413

[40] Killick Kendrick R, Molyneux DH, Ashford RW. Leishmania in phlebotomid sandflies I. modifications of the flagellum associated with attachment to the mid-gut and oesophageal valve of the sandfly. Proceedings of the Royal Society B: Biological Sciences. 1974;**187**:409-419. DOI: 10.1098/rspb.1974.0085

[41] Titus RG, Ribeiro JMC. Salivary gland lysates from the sand fly lutzomyia longipalpis enhance leishmania infectivity. Science. 1988;**239**(4845): 1306-1308. DOI: 10.1126/science.3344436

[42] Ribeiro JMC. Role of saliva In blood-feeding by arthropods. Annual Review of Entomology. 1987;**32**:463-478. DOI: 10.1146/annurev.en.32.010187.002335

[43] Kamhawi S. The biological and immunomodulatory properties of sand fly saliva and its role in the establishment of Leishmania infections. Microbes and Infection. 2000;**2**:1765-1773. DOI: 10.1016/s1286-4579(00)01331-9

[44] Rohousová I, Volf P. Sand fly saliva: Effects on host immune response and Leishmania transmission. Folia Parasitologica. 2006;**53**:161-171. DOI: 10.14411/fp.2006.022

[45] Sumova P, Polanska N, Lestinova T, et al. Phlebotomus perniciosus recombinant salivary proteins polarize murine macrophages toward the anti-inflammatory phenotype. Frontiers in Cellular and Infection Microbiology. 2020;**10**:427. DOI: 10.3389/fcimb.2020.00427

[46] Killick-Kendrick R, Killick-Kendrick M, Tang Y, et al. Metacyclic promastigotes of Leishmania in the salivary glands of experimentally

infected phlebotomine sandflies. Parasite. 1996;**3**(1):55-60. DOI: 10.1051/parasite/1996031055

[47] Freitas RA, Naiff RD, Barrett TV. Species diversity and flagellate infections in the sand Fly Fauna near Porto Grande, state of Amapá, Brazil (Diptera: Psychodidae. Kinetoplastida: Trypanosomatidae). Memórias do Instituto Oswaldo Cruz. 2002;**97**:53-59. DOI: 10.1590/s0074-02762002000100008

[48] Andrade BB, de Oliveira CI, Brodskyn CI, et al. Role of sand fly saliva in human and experimental leishmaniasis: Current insights. Scandinavian Journal of Immunology. 2007;**66**:122-127. DOI: 10.1111/j.1365-3083.2007.01964.x

[49] Afonso MMDS, Duarte R, Miranda JC, et al. Studies on the feeding habits of Lutzomyia (Lutzomyia) longipalpis (Lutz & Neiva, 1912) (Diptera: Psychodidae: Phlebotominae) populations from endemic areas of American visceral Leishmaniasis in Northeastern Brazil. Journal of Tropical Medicine. 2012;**2012**:1-5. DOI: 10.1155/2012/858657

[50] Anjili CO, Mbati PA, Mwangi RW, et al. The chemotactic effect of Phlebotomus duboscqi (Diptera: Psychodidae) salivary gland lysates to murine monocytes. Acta Tropica. 1995;**60**:97-100. DOI: 10.1016/0001-706x(95)00112-r

[51] Andrade BB, Teixeira CR, Barral A, Barral-Netto M. Haematophagous arthropod saliva and host defense system: A tale of tear and blood. Anais da Academia Brasileira de Ciências. 2005;**77**(4):665-693. DOI: 10.1590/S0001-37652005000400008

[52] Valenzuela JG, Belkaid Y, Garfield MK, Mendez S, Kamhawi S, Rowton ED, et al. Toward a defined anti-Leishmania vaccine targeting vector antigens: Characterization of a protective salivary protein. The Journal of Experimental Medicine. 2001;**194**(3):331-342. DOI: 10.1084/jem.194.3.331

[53] Belkaid Y, Kamhawi S, Modi G, Valenzuela J, Noben-Trauth N, Rowton E, et al. Development of a natural model of cutaneous leishmaniasis: Powerful effects of vector saliva and saliva preexposure on the long-term outcome of Leishmania major infection in the mouse ear dermis. The Journal of Experimental Medicine. 1998;**188**(10):1941-1953. DOI: 10.1084/jem.188.10.1941

[54] Barral A, Honda E, Caldas A, Costa J, Vinhas V, Rowton ED, et al. Human immune response to sand fly salivary gland antigens: A useful epidemiological marker? The American Journal of Tropical Medicine and Hygiene. 2000;**62**(6):740-745. DOI: 10.4269/ajtmh.2000.62.740

[55] Brodie TM, Smith MC, Morris RV, Titus RG. Immunomodulatory effects of the Lutzomyia longipalpis salivary gland protein maxadilan on mouse macrophages. Infection and Immunity. 2007;**75**(5):2359-2365. DOI: 10.1128/IAI.01812-06

[56] Wheat WH, Pauken KE, Morris RV, Titus RG. Lutzomyia longipalpis salivary peptide maxadilan alters murine dendritic cell expression of CD80/86, CCR7, and cytokine secretion and reprograms dendritic cell-mediated cytokine release from cultures containing allogeneic T cells. Journal of Immunology. 2008;**180**(12):8286-8298. DOI: 10.4049/jimmunol.180.12.8286

[57] Ruf W. Roles of factor Xa beyond coagulation. Journal of Thrombosis and Thrombolysis. 2021;**52**:391-396. DOI: 10.1007/s11239-021-02458-8

[58] Collin N, Assumpção TCF, Mizurini DM, Gilmore DC, Dutra-Oliveira A, Kotsyfakis M, et al. Lufaxin, a novel factor Xa inhibitor from the salivary gland of the sand fly *Lutzomyia longipalpis* blocks

protease-activated receptor 2 activation and inhibits inflammation and thrombosis in vivo. Arteriosclerosis, Thrombosis, and Vascular Biology. 2012;**32**(9):2185-2198. DOI: 10.1161/ATVBAHA.112.253906

[59] Chagas AC, Oliveira F, Debrabant A, Valenzuela JG, Ribeiro JMC, Calvo E. Lundep, a sand fly salivary endonuclease increases Leishmania parasite survival in neutrophils and inhibits XIIa contact activation in human plasma. PLoS Pathogens. 2014;**10**(2):e1003923. DOI: 10.1371/journal.ppat.1003923

[60] Martin-Martin I, Chagas AC, Guimaraes-Costa AB, Amo L, Oliveira F, Moore IN, et al. Immunity to LuloHya and Lundep, the salivary spreading factors from *Lutzomyia longipalpis*, protects against Leishmania major infection. PLoS Pathogens. 2018;**14**(5):e1007006. DOI: 10.1371/journal.ppat.1007006

[61] Volfova V, Hostomska J, Cerny M, Votypka J, Volf P. Hyaluronidase of bloodsucking insects and its enhancing effect on leishmania infection in mice. PLoS Neglected Tropical Diseases. 2008;**2**(9):e294. DOI: 10.1371/journal.pntd.0000294

[62] Ferreira VP, Fazito Vale V, Pangburn MK, Abdeladhim M, Mendes-Sousa AF, Coutinho-Abreu IV, et al. SALO, a novel classical pathway complement inhibitor from saliva of the sand fly Lutzomyia longipalpis. Scientific Reports. 2016;**6**:19300. DOI: 10.1038/srep19300

[63] Asojo OA, Kelleher A, Liu Z, Pollet J, Hudspeth EM, Rezende WC, et al. Structure of SALO, a leishmaniasis vaccine candidate from the sand fly Lutzomyia longipalpis. PLoS Neglected Tropical Diseases. 2017;**11**(3):e0005374. DOI: 10.1371/journal.pntd.0005374

[64] Cohen P. The structure and regulation of protein phosphatases. Vol. 58. Annual Review of Biochemistry. 1989;**58**:453-508. DOI: 10.1146/annurev.bi.58.070189.002321

[65] Haystead TAJ, Sim ATR, Carling D, Honnor RC, Tsukitani Y, Cohen P, et al. Effects of the tumour promoter okadaic acid on intracellular protein phosphorylation and metabolism. Nature. 1989;**337**(6202):78-81. DOI: 10.1038/337078a0

[66] Waitumbi J, Warburg A. Phlebotomus papatasi saliva inhibits protein phosphatase activity and nitric oxide production by murine macrophages. Infection and Immunity. 1998;**66**(4):1534-1537. DOI: 10.1128/IAI.66.4.1534-1537.1998

[67] Rêgo FD, Soares RP. *Lutzomyia longipalpis*: An update on this sand fly vector. Anais da Academia Brasileira de Ciências. 2021;**93**(3):1-29. DOI: 10.1590/0001-3765202120200254

[68] Hurrell BP, Regli IB, Tacchini-Cottier F. Different Leishmania species drive distinct neutrophil functions. Trends in Parasitology. 2016;**32**(5):392-401. DOI: 10.1016/j.pt.2016.02.003

[69] Laskay T, van Zandbergen G, Solbach W. Neutrophil granulocytes-Trojan horses for Leishmania major and other intracellular microbes? Trends in Microbiology. 2003;**11**(5):210-214. DOI: 10.1016/s0966-842x(03)00075-1

[70] Laskay T, van Zandbergen G, Solbach W. Neutrophil granulocytes as host cells and transport vehicles for intracellular pathogens: Apoptosis as infection-promoting factor. Immunobiology. 2008;**213**(3-4):183-191. DOI: 10.1016/j.imbio.2007.11.010

[71] John B, Hunter CA. Neutrophil soldiers or Trojan horses? Science. 2008;**321**(5891):917-918. DOI: 10.1126/science.1162914

[72] Ribeiro-Gomes FL, Peters NC, Debrabant A, Sacks DL. Efficient capture of infected neutrophils by dendritic cells in the skin inhibits the early anti-Leishmania response. PLoS Pathogens. 2012;**8**(2):e1002536. DOI: 10.1371/journal.ppat.1002536

[73] Falcão SAC, Weinkopff T, Hurrell BP, Celes FS, Curvelo RP, Prates DB, et al. Exposure to *Leishmania braziliensis* triggers neutrophil activation and apoptosis. PLoS Neglected Tropical Diseases. 2015;**9**(3):e0003601. DOI: 10.1371/journal.pntd.0003601

[74] Handman E, Spira DT. Growth of Leishmania amastigotes in macrophages from normal and immune mice. Zeitschrift für Parasitenkunde. 1977;**53**(1):75-81. DOI: 10.1007/BF00383117

[75] Olivier M, Gregory DJ, Forget G. Subversion mechanisms by which Leishmania parasites can escape the host immune response: A Signaling point of view. Clinical Microbiology Reviews. 2005;**18**(2):293-305. DOI: 10.1128/CMR.18.2.293-305.2005

[76] Cantacessi C, Dantas-Torres F, Nolan MJ, Otranto D. The past, present, and future of Leishmania genomics and transcriptomics. Trends in Parasitology. 2015;**31**(3):100-108. DOI: 10.1016/j.pt.2014.12.012

[77] Kanehisa Lanboratories. Leishmaniasis – Reference pathway. 2020. Available from: https://www.kegg.jp/kegg-bin/show_pathway?map05140

[78] Ribeiro-Gomes FL, Romano A, Lee S, Roffê E, Peters NC, Debrabant A, et al. Apoptotic cell clearance of Leishmania major-infected neutrophils by dendritic cells inhibits CD8+ T-cell priming in vitro by Mer tyrosine kinase-dependent signaling. Cell Death & Disease. 2015;**6**(12):e2018-e2018. DOI: 10.1038/cddis.2015.351

[79] Peters NC, Pagán AJ, Lawyer PG, Hand TW, Henrique Roma E, Stamper LW, et al. Chronic parasitic infection maintains high frequencies of short-lived Ly6C+CD4+ effector T cells that are required for protection against Re-infection. PLoS Pathogens. 2014;**10**(12):e1994538. DOI: 10.1371/journal.ppat.1004538

[80] León B, López-Bravo M, Ardavín C. Monocyte-derived dendritic cells formed at the infection site control the induction of protective T helper 1 responses against Leishmania. Immunity. 2007;**26**(4):519-531. DOI: 10.1016/j.immuni.2007.01.017

[81] Ashok D, Schuster S, Ronet C, Rosa M, Mack V, Lavanchy C, et al. Cross-presenting dendritic cells are required for control of Leishmania major infection. European Journal of Immunology. 2014;**44**(5):1422-1432. DOI: 10.1002/eji.201344242

[82] Martínez-López M, Iborra S, Conde-Garrosa R, Sancho D. Batf3-dependent CD103 + dendritic cells are major producers of IL-12 that drive local Th1 immunity against *Leishmania major* infection in mice. European Journal of Immunology. 2015;**45**(1):119-129. DOI: 10.1002/eji.201444651

[83] Contreras I, Gómez MA, Nguyen O, Shio MT, McMaster RW, Olivier M. Leishmania-induced inactivation of the macrophage transcription factor AP-1 is mediated by the parasite metallo-protease GP63. PLoS Pathogens. 2010;**6**(10):e1001148. DOI: 10.1371/journal.ppat.1001148

[84] Iborra S, Martínez-López M, Cueto FJ, Conde-Garrosa R, Del Fresno C, Izquierdo HM, et al. Leishmania uses Mincle to target an inhibitory ITAM Signaling pathway in dendritic cells that dampens adaptive immunity to infection. Immunity. 2016;**45**(4):788-801. DOI: 10.1016/j.immuni.2016.09.012

[85] Sharma P, Gurumurthy S, Duncan R, Nakhasi HL, Salotra P. Comparative in vivo expression of amastigote up regulated Leishmania genes in three different forms of Leishmaniasis. Parasitology International. 2010;**59**(2): 262-264. DOI: 10.1016/j.parint. 2009.11.003

[86] Zhang WW, Mendez S, Ghosh A, Myler P, Ivens A, Clos J, et al. Comparison of the A2 gene locus in *Leishmania donovani* and *Leishmania major* and its control over cutaneous infection. The Journal of Biological Chemistry. 2003;**278**(37):35508-35515. DOI: 10.1074/jbc.M305030200

[87] Belkaid Y, Hoffmann KF, Mendez S, Kamhawi S, Udey MC, Wynn TA, et al. The role of interleukin [IL]-10 in the persistence of Leishmania major in the skin after healing and the therapeutic potential of anti–IL-10 receptor antibody for sterile cure. The Journal of Experimental Medicine. 2001; **194**(10):1497-1506. DOI: 10.1084/ jem.194.10.1497

[88] Kima PE, Constant SL, Hannum L, Colmenares M, Lee KS, Haberman AM, et al. Internalization *of Leishmania mexicana* complex amastigotes via the fc receptor is required to sustain infection in murine cutaneous Leishmaniasis. The Journal of Experimental Medicine. 2000;**191**(6):1063-1068. DOI: 10.1084/ jem.191.6.1063

[89] Melby PC, Yang Y-Z, Cheng J, Zhao W. Regional differences in the cellular immune response to experimental cutaneous or visceral infection with *Leishmania donovani*. Infection and Immunity. 1998;**66**(1): 18-27. DOI: 10.1128/IAI.66.1.18-27.1998

[90] Kane MM, Mosser DM. The role of IL-10 in promoting disease progression in Leishmaniasis. Journal of Immunology. 2001;**166**(2):1141-1147. DOI: 10.4049/jimmunol.166.2.1141

[91] Tapia FJ, Díaz NL, Rodríguez OL, Sánchez M. Tegumentary Leishmaniasis: Immunology and molecular biology. Gazeta Médica da Bahia. 2009;**79**(3): 84-90

[92] Yaghoobi R, Maraghi S, Bagherani N, Rafiei A. Cutaneous leishmaniasis of the lid: A report of nine cases. Korean Journal of Ophthalmology. 2010;**24**(1):40-43. DOI: 10.3341%2Fkjo.2010.24.1.40

[93] Carvalho EM, Teixeira RS, Johnson WD. Cell-mediated immunity in American visceral leishmaniasis: Reversible immunosuppression during acute infection. Infection and Immunity. 1981;**33**(2):498-500. DOI: 10.1128/ iai.33.2.498-500.1981

[94] Goto H, Lindoso JAL. Immunity and immunosuppression in experimental visceral leishmaniasis. Brazilian Journal of Medical and Biological Research. 2004;**37**(4):615-623. DOI: 10.1590/ S0100-879X2004000400020

[95] Zhang W-W, Matlashewski G. Characterization of the A2-A2rel gene cluster in *Leishmania donovani*: Involvement of A2 in visceralization during infection. Molecular Microbiology. 2001;**39**(4):935-948. DOI: 10.1046/j.1365-2958.2001.02286.x

[96] Badaro R, Jones TC, Carvalho EM, Sampaio D, Reed SG, Barral A, et al. New perspectives on a subclinical form of visceral Leishmaniasis. The Journal of Infectious Diseases. 1986;**154**(6):1003-1011. DOI: 10.1093/infdis/154.6.1003

Chapter 2

Protective and Pathogenic Immune Responses to Cutaneous Leishmaniasis

Elina Panahi, Danielle I. Stanisic, Christopher S. Peacock and Lara J. Herrero

Abstract

Leishmania (Kinetoplastida: Trypanosomatidae) parasites are known to cause a broad spectrum of clinical diseases in humans, collectively known as the leishmaniases. Cutaneous leishmaniasis is the most common clinical presentation with varying degrees of severity largely driven by host immune responses, specifically the interplay between innate and adaptive immune response. The establishment of a T lymphocyte driven cell-mediated immune response, leading to activated phagocytic cells, leading to *Leishmania* parasite killing and control of infection. Alternatively, the *Leishmania* parasite manipulates the host immune system, enabling parasite proliferation and clinical disease. Here we review how the cumulative interactions of different aspects of the host immune response determines disease outcome, severity, and immunity to re-infection.

Keywords: *Leishmania*, innate immunity, adaptive immunity, cytokine, T-cell response, immunopathology

1. Introduction

The leishmaniases are a diverse group of vector-borne diseases resulting from infection with parasites of the genus *Leishmania* (*L.*) (Kinetoplastida: Trypanosomatidae). More than 20 species of *Leishmania* parasites are considered public health threats with the *Leishmania* (*Leishmania*) and *Leishmania* (*Viannia*) subgenera encompassing the medically important human pathogenic *Leishmania* parasites (reviewed in [1]). Leishmaniasis is acquired through the bite of an infected phlebotomine sandfly, with the genera *Phlebotomus* (Old World; OW) and *Lutzomyia* (New World; NW) responsible for human transmission. The *Leishmania* life-cycle (**Figure 1**) is complex as the parasites alternate between a flagellated promastigote form within the insect vector (reviewed in [2]) and an intracellular amastigote form that resides within phagolysosomes of mammalian phagocytic cells (reviewed in [3]). Clinical manifestations of infection with *L.* (*Leishmania*) and *L.* (*Viannia*) species vary from spontaneous self-healing localized lesions (cutaneous leishmaniasis; CL) to life-threatening systemic multi-organ disease (visceral leishmaniasis; VL, also known as kala-azar). Nearly all *Leishmania* parasites can cause CL of varying severity ranging from sub-clinical (also referred to as asymptomatic;

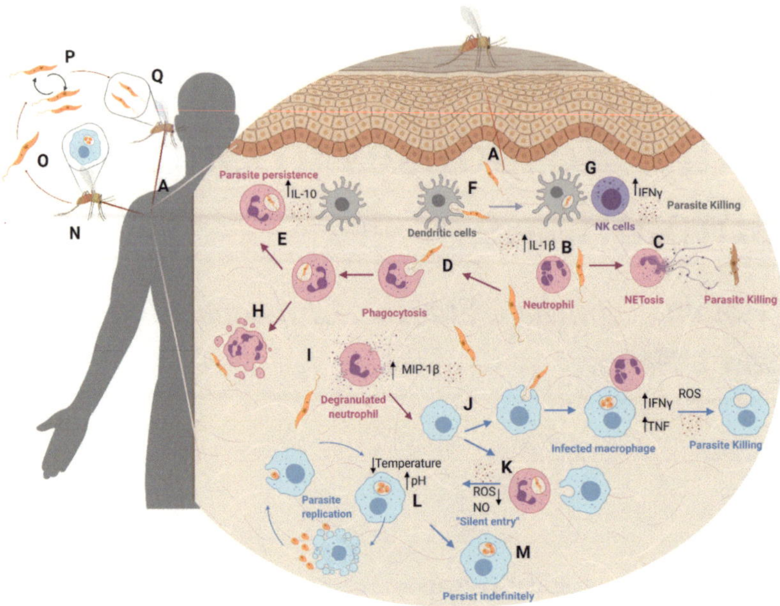

Figure 1.

The development of Leishmania parasites and their interaction with cells of the immune system. (A) During blood feeding, promastigotes are injected into the skin. (B) Neutrophils are the first phagocytic cells to arrive at the site of inoculation and play several roles. They arrive rapidly and release interleukin-1β (IL-1β), which is triggered by sandfly gut microbiota and promotes phagocytosis. (C) Neutrophils release neutrophil extracellular traps (NETs) and kill promastigotes through NETosis. (D) Neutrophils phagocytose promastigotes and (E) infected neutrophils interact with dendritic cells (DCs) inducing IL-10 which favors parasite survival. (F) DCs also phagocytose promastigotes and (G) interact with natural killer cells, resulting in the production of IFNγ. (H) Leishmania can escape apoptotic neutrophils. (I) Neutrophils degranulate and release mediators, such as macrophage inflammatory protein (MIP-1β), which recruits monocytes and macrophages. (J) Macrophages phagocytose promastigotes and neutrophils can then activate infected macrophages to induce intracellular parasite killing by releasing reactive oxygen species (ROS). (K) Apoptotic infected-neutrophils are engulfed by macrophages providing a silent entry for the parasite by downregulating ROS and nitric oxide (NO). (L) Within the macrophage, the promastigotes undergo significant biochemical and metabolic changes by transforming into their intracellular amastigote form to proliferate and infect more cells and/or (M) persist indefinitely. The life cycle is continued when (N) a female phlebotomine sandfly ingests a blood meal containing Leishmania infected phagocytes. (O) Within the vector, the amastigotes develop into the promastigote stage, (P) replicate and undergo further development (not shown here) (Q) concluding in a migration to the stomodeal valve to enable transmission to a mammalian host. Created with BioRender.com

reviewed in [4]) and self-resolving lesions to persistent chronic infections that result in severe tissue destruction and disfigurement (**Table 1**) [1].

The interaction between the parasite and the host immune response is complex and varied leading to a range of possible different disease outcomes. While the species of *Leishmania* parasite plays a large role in determining disease manifestations, host immunity and genetics largely influence the severity of infection. The classic T helper 1/T helper 2 (T_H1/T_H2) model has been applied for many years to explain the disease severity and outcome, with $CD4^+$ T_H1 cells mediating resistance to *Leishmania* and $CD4^+$ T_H2 cells promoting host susceptibility [12]. However, this assumption is based primarily on an experimental *Leishmania* (*L.*) *major* model of infection in congenic mouse strains, which are not entirely relevant to human infections. The model fails to explain the different immune responses and clinical presentations observed in the range of CL phenotypes caused by the various *Leishmania* species. Similar to the immunological spectrum observed in humans, the combination of mouse strain (reviewed in [13]), mode of challenge [14], infectious dose [15] and infecting parasite species or strain (reviewed in [16]), influences clinical presentation. With a focus on innate and adaptive immunity and subsequent immunopathology, here we describe

Clinical form	*Leishmania* parasite	Clinical manifestations in humans	References
Old world cutaneous leishmaniasis			
LCL	**Subgenus** *Leishmania*	Characterized by a single localized skin lesion that develops over a period of weeks to months at the site of the phlebotomine sandfly bite. Erythema first appears before developing into a papule. This further advances into a nodule, which progressively becomes ulcerated with a well-demarcated, raised border. Depending on the infective parasite, LCL may present in various forms (see below). Following resolution of disease, permanent scarring is common	[1, 5–9]
	Leishmania aethiopica	Rather than having a classic ulcer, patients present with crusty lesions with a patchy distribution, local oedema, and color changes often persisting for several years	
	Leishmania major	Multiple ulcero-crusted nodules and wet sores; necrosis and severe inflammation	
	Leishmania infantum *Leishmania donovani*	Manifests as papules and nodules with minimal ulceration that recovers slowly. More commonly causes systemic infection	
	Leishmania tropica	Dry ulcerating lesions, frequently presenting in multiple sites which may persist for several years	
MCL	*Leishmania aethiopica*	Mucosal lesions present simultaneously with lesions on the skin; primarily on the skin with spread to mucosa afterwards	
DCL	*Leishmania aethiopica*	Chronic and progressive condition affecting large areas of the skin with multiple nodules across the skin that often lack ulceration. Parasites grow uncontrollably in lesions and lesion growth can persist for decades	
New world cutaneous leishmaniasis, collectively grouped as American tegumentary leishmaniasis (ATL)			
LCL	**Subgenus** *Viannia* *Leishmania braziliensis* *Leishmania guyanensis* *Leishmania panamensis* **Subgenus** *Leishmania* *Leishmania mexicana* *Leishmania amazonensis*	Presents with severe, ulcerating lesions that may later manifest as MCL (see below). Characterized by single or multiple ulcerated lesions with elevated borders. The self-healing time of lesions can range from a few months (*L. mexicana*) to several years (e.g., *L. braziliensis*).	[1, 10]
MCL	*Leishmania braziliensis* *Leishmania guyanensis* *Leishmania panamensis*	Healed LCL can progress to destruction of the mucosa affecting predominately the nasopharyngeal mucosa (90% have had a previous history of CL). Characterized by the destruction of tissues of the nasal septum, lips, and palate. The excessive immune response seen with MCL has been attributed to the presence of *Leishmania* double-stranded RNA (dsRNA) virus (LVR), which is unique to the NW *L.* (*Viannia*) subgenus [11]	
DCL	**Subgenus** *Leishmania* *Leishmania amazonensis* *Leishmania mexicana*	Multiple non-healing cutaneous lesions, erythematous nodules and papules with various types of eruptions. DCL manifests as multiple widespread papules and non-ulcerating nodules with large numbers of viable parasites	
DsCL	*Leishmania braziliensis*	Characterized by multiple pleomorphic lesions in two or more non-contiguous areas of the body. Lymphatic spread is common for *L. braziliensis* DsCL is characterized by various lesions located on the body with few detectable parasites	

**Abbreviations: NW, New World; OW, Old World; LCL, localized cutaneous leishmaniasis; MCL, mucocutaneous leishmaniasis; DCL, diffuse cutaneous leishmaniasis; DsCL, disseminated cutaneous leishmaniasis.*

Table 1.
*Clinical manifestations of cutaneous leishmaniasis caused by medically important Old World and New World Leishmania parasites.**

the key immune responses induced by cutaneous *Leishmania* infection. We further discuss the coordination between innate and adaptive immune responses in parasite control and how persistent parasites play an important role in protective immunity.

2. The innate immune system in *Leishmania* infection and disease

The innate immune response is the host's first line of defense against invading pathogens and consists of physical (e.g., skin), chemical (e.g., nitric oxide and reactive oxygen species), soluble factors (e.g., complement, chemokines and cytokines) and cellular defenses (e.g., neutrophils and macrophages), all of which play a vital role in determining the course of infection.

2.1 Complement activation

Inoculated *Leishmania* promastigotes rapidly interact with the host's complement system. All three complement pathways (alternative, classical and lectin) are involved to varying degrees in *Leishmania* parasite killing and result in the activation of complement (C) protein C3 convertase cleaving C3 to generate C3b (**Figure 2**; reviewed in [17]). C3b facilitates the deposition of the C5b-C9 membrane attack complex (MAC) onto the surface of culture-derived stationary phase *Leishmania* promastigotes (a stage predominately found in the sandfly midgut), resulting in lysis of the parasite and subsequent uptake by phagocytic cells [17, 18]. C3b also acts as an opsonin, promoting direct phagocytosis and destruction by immune cells. *In vitro* experiments demonstrated killing of up to 90% of culture-derived procyclics *Leishmania* promastigotes (including *L. donovani*, *L. amazonensis*, *L. infantum* and *L. major* species) via complement-mediated lysis within the first few minutes of serum contact [19]. The remaining resistant parasites used the surface bound C3b to enter immune cells and cause infection. Contrary to culture-derived procyclics promastigotes, metacyclic promastigotes (the infective stage that is deposited into the skin by blood-feeding phlebotomine sandflies) are able to subvert phagocytosis to promote their survival and mediate host pathogenesis [17–19]. The glycocalyx component, known as lipophosphoglycan (LPG), and metalloproteinase glycoprotein 63 (GP63), is distinct to the surface of the infective metacyclic promastigotes, preventing the formation of MAC and complement lysis by cleaving the C3b into an inactive form of C3b (iC3b) [18, 20, 21], thereby subverting the complement system. The MAC can also be physically inhibited by elongated LPG on the surface of metacyclic promastigotes [17]. Moreover, iC3b serves as an opsonin that facilitates the parasite's uptake by binding to complement receptor 1 (CR1) and CR3 on macrophages and neutrophils. Binding via CR3 inhibits the production of interleukin 12 (IL-12) and oxidative burst, which provides safe parasite entry into macrophages [22].

2.2 Pattern recognition receptors on innate immune cells

Pathogen recognition receptors (PRRs) expressed on innate immune cells are critical for recognizing invading pathogens via pathogen-associated molecular patterns (PAMPs) and initiating the host immune response (**Figure 3**). Toll-like receptors (TLRs) and Nod-like receptors (NLRs) are the most studied PRRs in leishmaniasis and play a dual role in promoting protection or resistance depending on the infecting *Leishmania* species, which receptor the parasite interacts with first and the model used [23–25].

Both TLR2 and TLR4 (extracellular receptors) are found on the surface of host macrophages and neutrophils and recognize *Leishmania* promastigote LPG and GP63

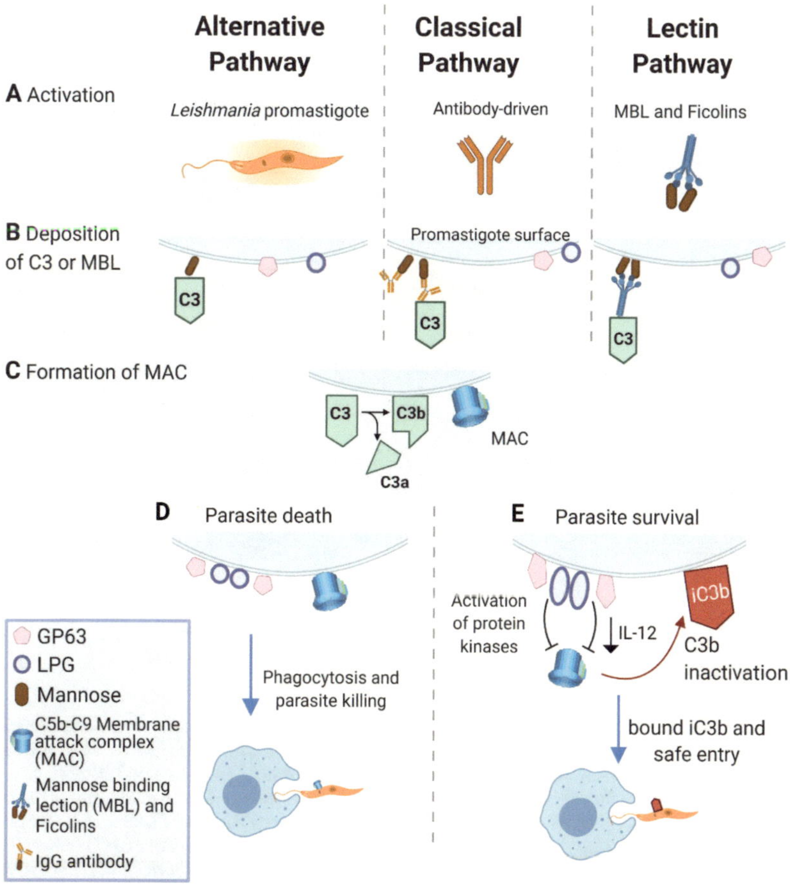

Figure 2.
Activation of complement by Leishmania parasites. (A) All three complement pathways are activated by the Leishmania parasite. (B) The alternative pathway is activated directly by the Leishmania parasite and is considered to be the main complement pathway involved in Leishmania clearance. The classical pathway is antibody-driven, while the lectin pathway is activated by the binding of mannose-binding lectin and ficolin on the parasite [16]. (C) Following activation of all pathways, the complement protein C3 convertase cleaves C3 to generate C3b. C3b facilitates the deposition of the C5b-C9 membrane attack complex (MAC) onto the surface of the Leishmania parasite, (D) ultimately resulting in uptake by neutrophils and macrophages following lysis of the parasite. (E) However, the lipophosphoglycan (LPG) metalloproteinase glycoprotein (GP63) on the parasite's surface inhibits MAC formation through its virulence factor, such as activating protein kinase and inducing interleukin-12 (IL-12) [16]. LPG and GP63 resist complement lysis by cleaving the C3b into inactive C3b (iC3b) to inhibit MAC convertase leading to safe entry into host cells and protection from complement-mediated attack. Created with Biorender.

[23–25] and *Leishmania* amastigote LPG (*L. major* specific) and proteophosphoglycan (PPG), which are expressed on the amastigote and promastigote surface [26, 27].

TLRs are activated and use the adaptor protein myeloid differentiation primary response 88 (MyD88) or TIR-domain-containing adapter-inducing interferon-β (TRIF) for signal transduction. The MyD88 adapter was shown to be required for the clearance of *L. major* infection in C57BL/6 mice, with MyD88-null C57BL/6 mice showing a greater susceptibility to infection than WT mice [23]. Furthermore knocking out TLR2 in C57BL/6 mice [$TLR2^{-/-}$] resulted in mice displaying higher resistance to *Leishmania* (*V.*) *braziliensis* infection compared to WT and this resistance was associated with increased enhanced IFN-γ production [24]. Similarly, C57BL/6 $TLR2^{-/-}$ mice infected with *Leishmania* (*L.*) *amazonensis* showed a reduced parasite burden compared to infected WT C57BL/6 mice [25]. It has been proposed that LPG on the surface of *Leishmania* promastigotes may explain why TLRs promote

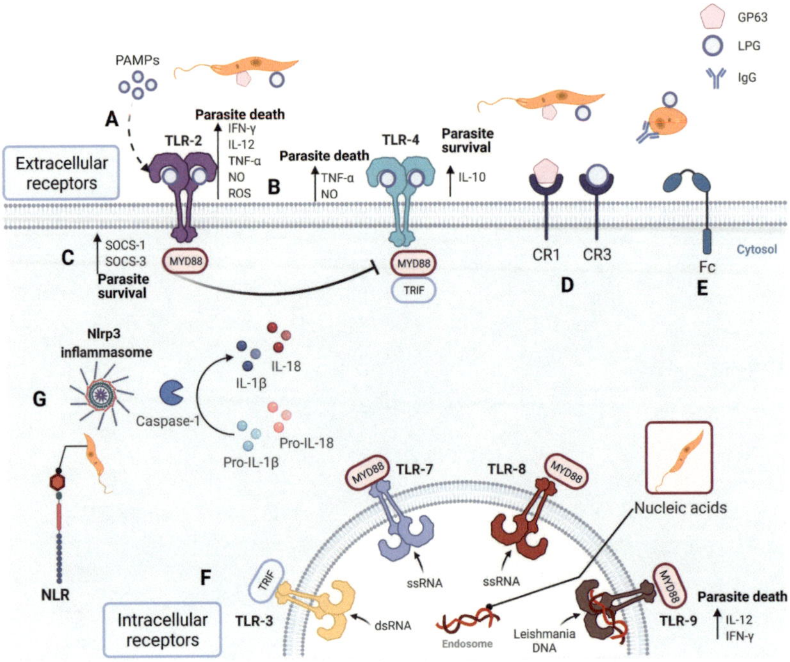

Figure 3.
Macrophage recognition of Leishmania parasites. Toll-like receptors (TLR) are categorized as extracellular receptors (TLR2 and TLR 4) and intracellular receptors (TLR3, TLR7, TLR8 and TLR9). TLRs are activated and use the adaptor proteins (myeloid differentiation primary response 88 (MyD88) or TIR-domain-containing adapter-inducing interferon-β (TRIF)) for signal transduction, which is important for Leishmania clearance. TLR2, TLR4, TLR7, TLR8 and TLR9 use MyD88, TLR3 uses TRIF and TLR4 uses both MyD88 and TRIF. (A) On the macrophage surface, TLR2 and TLR4 recognize lipophosphoglycan (LPG) molecules found on the surface of Leishmania promastigotes and amastigotes (L. major). (B) Upon recognition of Leishmania, macrophages release cytokines and nitric oxide (NO) that promote either parasite death or survival. (C) TLR2 activation by LPG can also induce the release of suppressor of cytokine signaling 1 (SOCS-1) and SOCS-3, which inhibits TLR4 signaling. (D) Complement receptors 1 (CR1) and CR3 are also categorized as extracellular receptors and can recognize LPG and metalloproteinase glycoprotein 63 (GP63) both expressed on the promastigote surface. (E) Fc receptors, located on the extracellular surface of macrophages, can also recognize immunoglobulin G (IgG) on the surface of amastigotes. (F) Intracellular TLRs recognize Leishmania RNA (TLR3, TLR7 and TLR8) and DNA (TLR 9). In the cytoplasm, (G) the NLRP3 inflammasome activates caspase-1, which cleaves pro-interleukin-1β (IL-1β) and pro-IL-18 to generate mature IL-1β and IL-18. Created with Biorender.com.

both protection and resistance, as the density and diversity of surface polysaccharide extensions to the LPG molecules varies between *Leishmania* species and between their morphological stages [24]. Similarly, TLR4 has a dual role that depends on the time of stimulation [28]. When TLR4 on mouse macrophages is primed *in vitro* with interferon-γ (IFNγ) prior to *L. major* infection, host protective TNF-α and NO are induced, promoting parasite killing. However, when IFNγ is added at the time of infection without sufficient priming time, macrophages increase IL-10 production, favoring parasite persistence [28, 29]. Interestingly, *ex vivo* studies using human monocytes from CL patients revealed that infection with *L. braziliensis* up-regulated TLR2 and TLR4 expression on inflammatory monocytes subsets [30, 31]. Moreover, a correlation with detrimental outcomes of CL was linked to the TLR up-regulation and production of TNF-α and IL-10 in infected monocytes [31]. These results using monocytes from human CL patients infected with *L. braziliensis* suggest that TLR2 and TLR4 expression triggers an inflammatory response and pathology.

TLR3, TLR7 and TLR9 are intracellular receptors recognizing *Leishmania* parasites in the endosomes of macrophages and are activated by *Leishmania* nucleic acids [17]. TLR9 is the most studied intracellular receptor and is associated with disease outcome having an important role in the early events of lesion development and parasite burden. A direct correlation was seen between TLR9 expression and lesion size in mice infected with *L. braziliensis* [32, 33]. Similarly *ex vivo* human monocytes from CL patients presenting with larger lesion size, were found to express higher levels of TLR9 [33]. Little is still known about the role of TLR3 in CL. TLR3 promotes immune protection against *L.* (*Leishmania*) *donovani* (visceral *Leishmania* species) through the production of TNF-α and NO [34]. Recent studies identified TLR7 as having an essential role in early *L. major* infection control by neutrophils. In TLR7^{-}/$^{-}$ C57BL/6 mice infection with *L. major* leads to long-term exacerbation of CL [35].

In contrast to TLRs, NLRs are cytoplasmic pattern recognition receptors. The NLRP3 inflammasome is a major regulator of IL-1β and IL-18 in *Leishmania* infection [36]. Similar to TLRs, the involvement and role of NLRs is dependent on the infecting *Leishmania* species. In murine models, activation of the inflammasome and IL-1β production have been shown to be associated with a protective role in parasite control during infection with *L. amazonensis* and *L. braziliensis* [37–39]. In contrast, they have no involvement in resistance to *L. major* infection. Moreover, the NLRP3 inflammasome promotes the development of TH2 cells resulting in non-healing lesions during *L. major* infection in BALB/c mice [40].

2.3 Innate cellular immunity

The recruitment and activation of innate immune cells are critical for the killing of invading pathogens by phagocytosis. However, these cells can also facilitate the survival of *Leishmania* parasites (**Figure 1**). *Leishmania* has evolved mechanisms to subvert host killing by modulating the response of specific immune cells. Macrophages and monocytes are the primary host cell for *Leishmania* parasites; however, a variety of immune cells are recruited to the inoculation site and play critical roles in determining the course of infection and disease outcome.

2.3.1 Neutrophils

Neutrophils are the first phagocytic cells to arrive at the site of the phlebotomine sandfly bite [41]. These cells are capable of clearing *Leishmania* parasites early in infection through phagocytosis and via the production of an array of microbicidal factors that target *Leishmania* parasites (recently reviewed in [42]). Neutrophils release neutrophil extracellular traps (NETs) to capture and kill *Leishmania* promastigotes through a cell death mechanism (NETosis) [43]. Infected neutrophils degranulate and secrete inflammatory mediators, such as the chemokine macrophage inflammatory protein 1β (MIP-1β) and CC-chemokine ligend-3 (CCL3), aiding in the migration of macrophages, and recruitment of monocytes and dendritic cells [44, 45]. Under normal circumstances, compromised neutrophils undergo spontaneous apoptosis, however prevention of neutrophil apoptosis is an important mechanism that *Leishmania* uses to subvert death [41, 44]. For example, infected apoptotic neutrophils can act as silent vectors by providing a safe entry for *Leishmania* promastigotes into macrophages without triggering mechanisms to kill *Leishmania* [44, 46]. This silent entry into macrophages has been likened to the Trojan horse scenario [41, 47], as the promastigotes suppress neutrophil apoptosis until macrophages arrive at the site of infection and then downregulate the microbicidal responses (ROS and NO) [44, 48]. Infected neutrophils are engulfed by macrophages allowing promastigotes to transform into amastigotes and proliferate. *L. major* is able to delay neutrophil apoptosis for up to two days by inducing the secretion of the anti-apoptotic cytokines IL-8 and granulocyte macrophage colony-stimulating factor (GM-CSF) [48]. Infected neutrophils undergoing apoptosis have also been reported to release higher levels of MIP-1β to attract macrophages to the site of infection thereby ensuring a safe entry for the parasite [44].

The ability of neutrophils to promote parasite killing or parasite survival [35, 49] appears to be *Leishmania* species-specific, impacted by the route of infection [35, 50], and influenced by the genetic background of the host [41, 44, 49, 51–53]. Studies investigating the role of neutrophils in the development of CL utilized two mouse models namely the susceptible (BALB/c) and resistant (C57BL/6) mice and found differences in the number of neutrophils recruited at the site of *L. major* inoculation. Interestingly, only lesions of susceptible mice demonstrated a sustained presence of neutrophils and this was associated with early IL-4 activation and the development of aT_H2 response [51]. These observations suggest that in susceptible BALB/c mice the early events of the immune response are important in initiating a subsequent T_H differentiation following infection with *L. major*.

In vitro studies with human neutrophils suggest that they play either protective or pathogenic roles depending on the infecting *Leishmania* species. A study comparing neutrophils from CL and healthy subjects, which were then infected with *L. braziliensis ex vivo*, observed that neutrophils from CL patients produced more ROS and higher levels of the chemokines CXCL8 and CXCL9 which are both associated with the recruitment of neutrophils and T_H1-type cells [54]. Neutrophils from both groups were equally competent to phagocytose *L. braziliensis*, however the cells from CL patients exhibited a pro-inflammatory profile necessary for parasite clearance [54]. The protective role of neutrophils depends on the infecting *Leishmania* species. *In vitro* infection of human neutrophils with *L. amazonensis* resulted in neutrophil production of ROS and leukotriene B4 (an inflammatory mediator) leading to neutrophil degranulation and the killing of *L. amazonensis* [55, 56]. In contrast, human neutrophils infected with *L. major* have been shown to contribute to pathogenesis through the secretion of high levels of MIP-1β, which attracts macrophages to the site of infection. These macrophages then engulf apoptotic infected-neutrophils, thereby providing a silent and safe parasite transmission into macrophages [44].

2.3.2 Macrophages and monocytes

Macrophages and monocytes are recruited to the inoculation site by degranulating, infected neutrophils releasing inflammatory mediators, such as MIP-1β and CCL2 [44, 57]. These cells become infected either by phagocytosing apoptotic *Leishmania*-infected neutrophils, by free *Leishmania* promastigotes that have escaped neutrophils, or by amastigotes that have previously ruptured their host cell [41]. Cells of the monocyte lineage are the main host cells of *Leishmania* parasites and once inside, *Leishmania* promastigotes differentiate into amastigotes, where they survive and replicate.

Both macrophages and monocytes are efficient in controlling *Leishmania* in the early stages of infection (reviewed in [3]). During phagocytosis, these cells release ROS, through a mechanism known as the respiratory burst, which kills *Leishmania* rapidly leading to early parasite control [30]. These cells also produce NO, which is generated by inducible NO synthase (iNOS) [58]. NO diffuses across cell membranes to initiate parasite killing within both the NO-producing cells and bystander cells [58]. For macrophages to release ROS that is sufficient in parasite killing, the cells need to first be activated by IFNγ and TNF-α, which enhance the respiratory burst [59]. Though non-activated macrophages will still release ROS through the respiratory burst following infection, it is insufficient to kill *Leishmania*. In a mouse model, the respiratory burst and subsequent release of ROS that occurs in *Leishmania*-infected macrophages were found to be insufficient to kill the parasites if the host cell was not previously activated by IFNγ [59]. During infection, the main producers of IFNγ are CD4+ T_H1 cells. Prior to the differentiation and activation of CD4+ T_H1 cells, natural killer (NK) cells are the primary producers of IFNγ [60]. In contrast, *in vitro studies* with human and mouse monocytes infected with *Leishmania* species showed competence in parasite killing through the secretion of ROS and without the need for prior activation [30, 47, 59].

The majority of studies investigating the role of NO have used rodent models, where NO is considered necessary to control *Leishmania* [58, 61, 62], however it is not yet clear if NO is required for *Leishmania* control in humans as activated human macrophages have not been shown to produce NO upon *Leishmania* infection [59, 63], It has been suggested that inhibiting NO promotes *Leishmania* infection in phagocytes [63]. Similar, the exact role of ROS in human *Leishmania* infection is yet to be elucidated, although it is believed that the production of ROS is an important mechanism in eradicating *Leishmania* parasites throughout the course of disease [59].

2.3.3 Dendritic cells

DCs play an important role as a bridge between the innate and adaptive immune systems (reviewed in [64]). In addition to phagocytosing *Leishmania* parasites and infected apoptotic neutrophils [45], DCs are important in the maintenance of immunity and in rapid stimulation of the adaptive immune response during the early stage of infection. DCs present *Leishmania*-specific antigen to naïve T cells and promoting their differentiation. The migration of DCs to the lymph node (where they activate T cells) is vital to establish an efficient adaptive immune response. *Leishmania* has evolved strategies to inhibit interaction between DCs and T cells by reducing DC migration [64, 65]. It was demonstrated that *Leishmania* was capable of blocking CCR2 (expressed on DC surface) thereby impairing the cells' ability to migrate, however the mechanisms used by the parasite remain elusive [65].

3. Adaptive immune system in *Leishmania* infection and disease

Following the involvement of innate immune cells in targeting *Leishmania* parasites and antigen presentation, immune cells of the adaptive immune system are activated to induce a *Leishmania*-specific response. The adaptive immune system plays a pivotal role in *Leishmania* infection through the interplay between T cell-mediated and antibody-mediated immune responses and the induction of immune memory. The complexity of these immune responses, which facilitate the resolution of CL is also reflected by the various phenotypes of clinical CL presentations observed in individuals [66]. On one end of the immune spectrum, a strong T cell response is observed. Although the high levels of IFNγ lead to parasite control, an exacerbated T helper (T_H) type-1 response and increased number of CD8+ cytotoxic T cells may also lead to the development of MCL. In contrast, the other end of the immune spectrum is characterized by a high level of *Leishmania*-specific antibodies and a limited T cell-mediated response. Individuals have an uncontrolled parasite load (as parasites are not neutralized by antibodies), which is a consequence of low levels of T_H1 cytokines and this results in DCL manifestations [16, 67, 68]. An intermediate level of both T cell and antibody responses will lead to a form of CL that will normally self-heal over time.

3.1 $CD4^+$ T cells

The generation of *Leishmania*-specific $CD4^+$ T cells is required for protective immunity, and they play a major role in shaping the adaptive immune response. $CD4^+$ T_H cells are essential in determining disease outcome by driving the differentiation and activation of different $CD4^+$ T_H cell subsets through the production of cytokines, which either mediate host protection or promote disease pathogenesis (**Figure 4**).

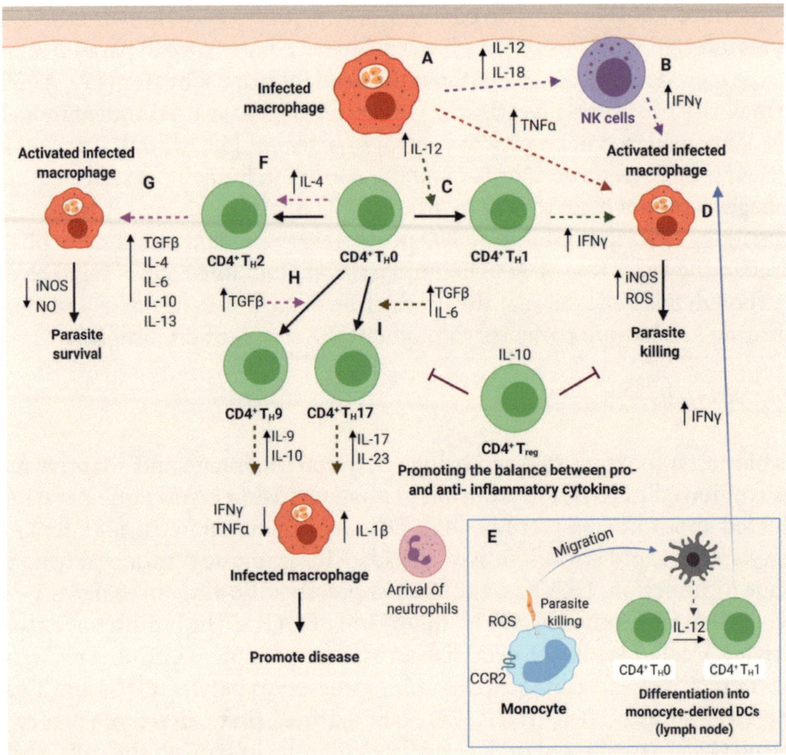

Figure 4.
Interaction between immune cells and Leishmania parasites. (A) Infected macrophages produce pro-inflammatory cytokines such as interleukin-12 (IL-12), IL-18 and tumor necrosis factor-α (TNF-α). These cytokines (B) recruit natural killer (NK) cells to the infection site and (C) promote CD4+ TH cell differentiation into CD4⁺ T_H1. (B) NK cells and (C) CD4⁺ T_H1 cells activate infected macrophages by producing interferon-γ (IFNγ). (D) Activated infected macrophages then release reactive oxygen species (ROS) and inducible nitric oxide synthase (iNOS), which results in parasite killing. (E) Infected monocytes kill Leishmania parasites through the release of ROS and migrate to the lymph node. Here they promote CD4⁺ T_H1 differentiation by producing IL-12. CD4+ TH1 migrates to the skin where they (D) activate infected macrophages. In contrast (F) CD4⁺ T_H cells produce IL-4 (an anti-inflammatory cytokine) which drives the differentiation of CD4+ TH2 cells. (G) Secretion of anti-inflammatory cytokines (such as transforming growth factor-β; TGFβ) by CD4⁺ T_H2 suppresses the production of iNOS and NO by macrophages leading to parasite survival. (H) TGFβ drives the differentiation into CD4⁺ T_H9 cells, which downregulates the release of IFNγ and TNF-α from infected macrophages, thereby promoting disease. (I) TGFβ and IL-6 drives differentiation into CD4⁺ T_H17 cells that stimulates the secretion of IL-1β and infiltration of neutrophils that are believed to aggravate the disease. Adapted from [69]. Created with Biorender.com

Previously, it was widely believed that the induction of either a CD4⁺ T_H1 or T_H2 response determined the outcome of infection i.e., induction of protection versus pathology. Subsequent studies have shown that there are a multitude of factors that contribute to the outcome of *Leishmania* infection, thus the T_H1/T_H2 model oversimplifies a complex interaction between host and parasite. Factors such as the genetic background of the model (or host) and the *Leishmania* parasite (species and strain) studied, contribute to differential disease outcomes. It is acknowledged that several CD4⁺ T cell subsets are implicated in disease outcome, such as CD4⁺ regulatory T (T_{reg}) cells, CD4⁺ T helper populations (T_H1, T_H2, T_H9 and T_H17 effector) and T follicular helper (TF_H) cells [58, 70–72].

Cytokines produced by CD4⁺ T cell subsets and other infected immune cells are generally classified as pro-inflammatory or anti-inflammatory and have been shown to be differentially associated with disease protection or progression, respectively (**Table 2**). Their role in activating and recruiting immune cells to the infection site shapes the adaptive immune response.

Immune mediators	Cell association/expressed by	General function	Role in cutaneous leishmaniasis
IL-1	• Secreted by epithelial cells, endothelial cells, activated macrophages, DCs, neutrophils and lymphocytes	• Pro-inflammatory cytokine • Critical regulator for early differentiation of T_H17 cells • Supports the generation of IFNγ secreting T cells (similar to IL-12) • Prolonged high levels of IL-1α induces T_H2 differentiation and increases pathology severity • IL-1β promotes (with IL-23) development of T_H17 cells	• Maintains cytokine secretions in T_H17 effector cells (together with IL-6 and IL-23) • Can be both protective by secretion of IL-1α and promotion of TNF-α production, and pathogenic during *Leishmania* infection • Secretion of IL-1α mediates disease resolution, reduction in parasite burden and enhancement of T_H1 response (via higher secretion of IFNγ and lower production of IL-4) • Continuous treatment with IL-1α in *L. major* infected C57BL/6 mice induced T_H2 responses and promoted disease susceptibility [69] • IL-1β treatment during early phases in *L. major* infected C57BL/6 mice mediates protection by promoting T_H1 responses [69] • Conversely, during the chronic phase, IL-1β can contribute to pathogenesis and worsen clinical symptoms of CL in *L. major* infected C57BL/6 mice through development of T_H17 cells and regulation of IL-17 levels [69] • IL-1β and IL-1α drive pathogenesis in *L. major* infected BALB/c mice. It was shown that IL-1α deficient and IL-1β deficient mice were resistant to infection and presented delayed nodule development and death [73]
IL-2	• $CD4^+$ T_H1 cells secrete IL-2 which promotes proliferation of T cells • Secreted in smaller amounts by $CD8^+$ T cells, NK cells and NKT cells [74]	• Pro-inflammatory and growth factor cytokine • Plays a dual role that may promote susceptibility to infection (by limiting secretion of IL-12 via T_H cells) and can also mediate resistance • Promotes immune responses by increasing proliferation and cytokine secretion (IFNγ by T_H1 cells), cytolytic activity ($CD4^+$, $CD8^+$ and NK cells; binding via IL-2 receptors on lymphocytes) • Can stimulate proliferation of T_H2 cells through generation of IL-4	• Involved in the protective immune response against CL and facilitates (along with IFNγ), macrophage activation and a T_H1 response and for parasite killing • Reduced IL-2 production has been associated with aggravated human CL [75]

Immune mediators	Cell association/expressed by	General function	Role in cutaneous leishmaniasis
IL-4	• Secreted by activated T cells, T_H2 cells and T_{FH} cells	• A signature anti-inflammatory cytokine of the T_H2-type immune response • Activates T_H2 cell differentiation from naïve $CD4^+$ T cells and production of T_H2-associated cytokines (IL-5, IL-10 and IL-13) • Powerful inhibitor of IFNγ-producing $CD4^+$ T cells and suppressor of T_H1 cells and pro-inflammatory cytokines	• Associated with non-healing forms of CL in mice (similar to IL-13) [76] • Induces T_H2 responses in *L. major* infected mice [77] • High levels of IL-4 in early stage of infection lead to the secretion of IL-12 by DCs and subsequent T_H1 proliferation [76] • Functions as a powerful inhibitor of IFNγ-producing $CD4^+$ T cells and suppressor of protective T_H1 immune responses
IL-6	• Secreted by T_H2 cells, macrophages, fibroblasts and endothelial cells	• Can act as a pro-inflammatory and anti-inflammatory cytokine • Together with TGFβ, IL-6 can stimulate production of T_H17 cells to secrete IL-17 and IL-10	• IL-6 deficient ($^{-/-}$) BALB/c mice showed no difference in pathology (parasite burden, lesion burden) when infected with *L. major* in comparison to BALB/c wild type (WT) mice. However, IL-$6^{-/-}$ mice did produce lower levels of T_H1 and T_H2 cytokines [78]
IL-8	• Secreted by tissue-resident macrophages in response to *Leishmania* infection	• Monocyte-derived neutrophil chemotactic factor; an activating cytokine • Plays a role in the initial recruitment and activation of neutrophils	• *L. major* infected neutrophils secrete high levels of IL-8 that leads to increased infiltration of neutrophils for parasite phagocytosis [79]
IL-10	• Secreted by Regulatory T (T_{reg}) cells, T_H2 and T_H9 cells, DCs, activated macrophages, NK cells and neutrophils	• Anti-inflammatory cytokine • Suppresses activity of T_H1 cells, NK cells and macrophages • Down-regulates expression of IFNγ, IL-2, IL-3 and TNF-α	• Important regulator of immunity in CL • Associated with CL susceptibility. High levels of IL-10 are strongly associated with non-healing forms of disease [16] • The absence of IL-10 in murine models is associated with the control of parasite replication and resolution of cutaneous infection. IL-$10^{-/-}$ mice express higher levels of IFNγ and produce more nitric oxide (NO) than IL-10 $^{+/+}$ mice [80]
IL-12	• Secreted by monocytes, macrophages, dendritic cells (DCs) and B lymphocytes	• Pro-inflammatory cytokine • Activates T helper type 1 (T_H1) differentiation; stimulates differentiation of naïve T cells into T_H1 effectors; inhibits T cell apoptosis • Together with IL-15, this cytokine facilitates IFNγ and TNF-α secretion by natural killer (NK) and T cells	• The absence of the IL-12, IL-23, and IL-27 promotes the development of a T_H2 response and increases susceptibility to *Leishmania* infection [81]

Immune mediators	Cell association/expressed by	General function	Role in cutaneous leishmaniasis
IL-13	• Secreted by T_H2 cells and NK cells	• Anti-inflammatory cytokine • Activates the differentiation of naïve T_H0 cells into T_H2 cells	• High levels are associated with chronic CL • BALB/c IL-$13^{-/-}$ mice were able to control *L. major* infection (production of T_H1 responses and effectively control parasite growth), whereas C57BL/6 mice became susceptible to disease pathology due to the increased T_H2 responses [82].
IL-17	• Secreted by T_H17 cells, DCs	• Pro-inflammatory cytokine and mediates tissue inflammation • IL-17 can both mediate protection and susceptibility • Stimulates secretion of cytokines and chemokines (e.g., TNF-α, IL-1β, CXCL1 and CXCL10)	• Increased levels of IL-17 (together with IL-23) and rapid neutrophil infiltration are associated with aggravated CL and ML diseases [83] • Increased IL-17-dependent neutrophil recruitment into lesions has been shown to significantly promote disease outcome (*L. major* infected BALB/c mice) [84] • BALB/c mice infected with L. major shows high levels of IL-17 in contrast to IL-$17^{-/-}$ BALB/c mice despite typical T_H2 development (reduction in recruitment of neutrophils in lesional tissue and CXCL2 levels in infected skin) [84]
IL-18	• Secreted by activated macrophages and DCs, $CD8^+$ memory T cells, neutrophils	• Pro-inflammatory cytokine • An IFNγ inducing factor (induces T_H1 responses via IFNγ production with IL-12) • Plays a role in early control of CL caused by *L. major*, but not critical for the development of protective T_H1 responses or resolution of infection	• IL-$18^{-/-}$ C57BL/6 mice had increased susceptibility to *L. major* infection in the early phase of infection but were able to resolve the infection similar to IL-$18^{+/+}$ mice due to an increased level of IL-12 and IFNγ secretion [85]
IL-22	• Secreted by T_H17, T_H1 cells and NKT cells	• Critical role in tissue repair during CL • Strengthens epithelial barrier functions; involved in tissue homeostasis, tissue repair and wound healing • Induces keratinocyte proliferation and hyperplasia resulting in thickening of the epidermis	• *L. major* infected IL-$22^{-/-}$ C57BL/6 mice developed increased pathology in contrast to WT mice due to deficient wound healing of keratinocytes in the absence of IL-22 [86] • IL-22 is associated with pathogenesis when secreted with cytokines such as IL-17 [70]
IL-27	• Secreted by macrophages and DCs	• Anti-inflammatory cytokine and pro-inflammatory • T_H17 cell suppressor • Promotes differentiation and production of IL-10 producing T_{reg} cells	• Promotes the differentiation and expansion of T_{reg} cells (main producers of IL-10) and suppresses T_H17 cells • IL-$27^{-/-}$ WSX-1 mice developed severe *L. major* infection, which correlated with the increased levels of IL-17 $CD4^+$ T_H17 cells, reduced levels of IL-10 and increased in IL-4 [87]

Immune mediators	Cell association/expressed by	General function	Role in cutaneous leishmaniasis
IFNγ	• Secreted by CD4⁺ T_H1 cells; CD8⁺ T_H1 cells, NK cells, and NKT cells	• Pro-inflammatory cytokine (involved in protection and pathology of CL) [88] • Stimulates iNOS expression and activity in infected cells, which promotes parasite killing • Stimulates NO secretion in activated macrophages and inhibits amastigote growth • Promotes differentiation of naïve CD4⁺ T_H cells into T_H1 cells and inhibits the development of T_H2 and T_H16 cells	• Compared to WT mice, C57BL/6, IFNγ $^{-/-}$ mice were more susceptible to *L. amazonensis* infection with large lesions, increased parasite burden and development of T_H2-type responses associated with increased IL-4 [89] • High levels of IFNγ can be detrimental and found in patients with MCL [7]
TNF-α	• Mostly produced by macrophages • Secreted by T_H1 cells, T_{FH} cells	• Pro-inflammatory cytokine (involved in protection and pathology of CL) • Plays a vital role in *Leishmania* clearance through increasing macrophage activity and NO synthesis	• Promotes T_H1/IFNγ responses against *L. major* infection • TNF-α $^{-/-}$ C57BL/6 mice infected with *L. major* manifested as fatal disease, a strong protective T_H1 response [90] • High levels of TNFα can promote disease pathogenesis leading to lesion chronicity [91]

–/–, deficient; DCs, dendritic cells; IL, interleukin; IFN, Interferon; MIP, macrophage inflammatory protein; NK, natural killer; NKT, natural killer T cells; NO, nitric oxide; TFH, T follicular helper cells; TGF, transforming growth factor; TH, T helper cell; TNF, tumor necrosis factor; Treg, T regulatory cell; WT, wild type.

Table 2.
Selection of cytokines and their role in cutaneous leishmaniasis.

It is recognized that the development of CD4⁺ T_H1 immune responses promotes host protection against CL and is associated with the production of pro-inflammatory cytokines (such as IFNγ and IL-12). CD4⁺ T_H1 cells are key producers of IFNγ, which has been shown in resistant and susceptible mouse models to be vital in controlling *L. major* parasites [92, 93]. In human and mice, the production of IFNγ activates infected macrophages to enhance the respiratory burst (as discussed above), which eliminates parasites residing and replicating within the phagolysosome, as explained earlier [59].

In contrast to the protective role of CD4⁺ T_H1 cells, susceptibility to *Leishmania* infection and CL progression is influenced by the induction of an IL-4-driven T_H2-type immune response as well as the production of the anti-inflammatory cytokines, IL-10, IL-13 and TGFβ [94]. Rodent studies have shown that IL-4-secreting CD4⁺ T_H2 cells and IL-10 secreting T_{reg} cells promote parasite growth and disease susceptibility [95]. For example, the CD4⁺ T_H2-secreting cytokines, IL-4 [96] and IL-10 [97], was identified as having important roles in BALB/c mice' susceptibility to infection. In the absence of IL-4 or IL-10, BALB/c mice, were able to control parasite growth and resolve lesions resulting in a protective CD4⁺ T_H1 response. Likewise, IL-10 likewise plays a role in disease self-healing C57BL/6 mice. When lacking IL-10, C57BL/6 mice exhibited a faster lesion healing time compared to WT [98]. The roles of IL-4 and IL-10 in promoting susceptibility in human patients with CL are less clear, although elevated IL-10 has been linked to uncontrolled parasite growth in VL [99].

Some cytokines are also considered to have a dual role in relation to disease outcome [100]. The production of the $CD4^+$ T_H1 cytokines IFNγ and TNF-α is critical in controlling *Leishmania* infection, however an aggravated production of these two cytokines have been affiliated with severe disease with lesion chronicity [91].

3.2 $CD8^+$ T cells

The role of $CD8^+$ T cells in *Leishmania* infection is still poorly understood. They have both a protective and a pathological role depending on whether the cells are producers of cytokines or are acting as cytolytic T cells, respectively (reviewed in [101]). The contribution and effectiveness of $CD8^+$ T cells in relation to parasite control is determined by the *Leishmania* species and experimental model (infective dose and host genetics).

RAG knockout (KO) mice (deficient in both B and T cells) developed lesions at a slower rate (*L. major* infection) compared to WT mice or not at all (*L. braziliensis* and *L. amazonensis* infection) [102–104]. When reconstituted with $CD8^+$ T cells, RAG KO mice developed severe pathology with lesions [102, 103]. In BALB/c mice infected with *L. braziliensis*, depletion of $CD8^+$ T cells resulted in reduced lesion size despite having a similar level of parasites in the skin compared with control mice [103].

Mimicking a natural low-dose infection with *L. major*, studies revealed that $CD8^+$ T cells play a role in protection, associated with high production of IFNγ, which activates macrophages leading to parasite control [102, 105]. Furthermore, IFNγ stimulates DCs to produce IL-12 which promote the development and differentiation of $CD4^+$ T_H1 cells. This suggests that $CD8^+$ T cells are important in skewing towards T_H1 response through the production of IFNγ and in eliminating the majority of parasites before lesion development. The role that $CD8^+$ T cells play in infection may be associated with their location in the host [106]. When located in the draining lymph node, $CD8^+$ T cells produce IFNγ and are protective [107]. In contrast, when migrating to the lesion site during infection, $CD8^+$ T cells produce lower levels of IFNγ and exhibit cytolytic activity, leading to cell death and an exaggerated inflammatory response that further promotes tissue damage [108]. This is supported by findings from a mouse model showing $CD8^+$ T cells that had migrated to the skin, produced lower levels of IFNγ and instead exhibited cytolytic activity promoting disease progression [103]. There is substantial evidence for a pathogenic role of $CD8^+$ T cells in patients infected with *L. braziliensis* [109–111]. As the disease progresses from small nodules to larger skin lesions, an increase in $CD8^+$ T cells and a decrease in CD4+ T cells was observed in the histopathological analysis of human skin lesions [112]. In CL patients a link between $CD8^+$ T cell mediated cytotoxicity and IL-1β inflammasome activation was observed [111]. This activation of NLRP3 inflammasome pathway and its promotion of disease inflammation is currently targeted for host-directed therapy [88, 106].

3.3 Regulatory T cells

The role of T_{reg} cells in *Leishmania* infection is still being elucidated, although though they have been shown in rodent models to be involved in disease pathology and parasite persistence depending on the experimental model used. $CD4^+$ $CD25^+$ T_{reg} cells have been shown to suppress $CD4^+$ T cell activity in *L. major*-infected C57BL/6 mice, thereby favoring parasite persistence [98, 113, 114]. T_{reg} cells influence both primary and secondary infections with *L. major*, as they render otherwise non-susceptible mice susceptible to infection [115]. However, their activity may also be dependent on the infecting *Leishmania* species. For example, T_{reg} cells play a protective role during infection with New World *Leishmania* species, such as *L. amazonensis* [95, 116]. Transferring T_{reg} cells from an *L. amazonensis*-infected mouse to a naïve mouse prior to infection with *L. amazonensis* reduced the development of lesions suggesting that they may also contribute to the control of immunopathogenic responses [116]. Understanding how T_{reg} cells are involved in human *Leishmania*-infections is still being explored, with evidence so far suggesting that these cells play a role at the infection site and contributing directly to parasite persistent as the main source of IL-10 production [95, 98].

3.4 B cells and antibodies

The function of B cells in CL has not conclusively been shown. During the initial *Leishmania* infection, antibody production by B cells themselves are not believed to play a role, in controlling parasites as *Leishmania* are intracellular. However, some studies indicate that B cells may regulate both protective and pathogenic immune responses during *Leishmania* infection, depending on the infecting species and model used. Production of *L. major* antibodies was shown to be important for DCs to phagocytose parasites, as the absence of antibodies by B cells resulted in larger lesions in B $cell^{-/-}$ mice, higher parasite load, low production of IFNγ and a decreased cell-mediated immune response [117]. Moreover, $IgG^{-/-}$ BALB/c mice infected with *L. major* resulted in larger lesions and higher parasite load compared to IgG^{+} BALB/c mice [118]. In contrast, a study using a BALB/c mice deficient in IgM transmembrane domain (μMT), thereby lacking mature B cells, observed that these mice were resistant to *L. major* infection [119]. Other studies using BALB/c mice lacking IL-4Rα expression specifically on B cells, mbicreIL-$4R\alpha^{-/lox}$ BALB/c mice, resulted in a protective host immunity [29, 119, 120].

There is still a lot of knowledge to gain on B cells' function and whether they play a part in protection or pathology during infection with *Leishmania* parasites.

4. Persistent *Leishmania* infection and emulating concomitant immunity

Naturally and experimental infection with cutaneous *Leishmania* species is controlled following the development of an adaptive T_H1 immune response. After induction of this response, parasite numbers decline in infected tissues, lesions heal and lifelong immunity against the infecting *Leishmania* species is gained [121]. Though recovery from cutaneous disease has been reached, a small number of *Leishmania* parasites normally remain indefinitely in the host at the initial site of infection; known as persistent parasites [122, 123]. These parasites play an important role in maintaining protective immunity in the event of reinfection by providing a constant source of *Leishmania* antigen for immune stimulation [121, 124]. Both mice and humans who recover from CL maintain chronic subclinical infection at the lesion site and have been shown to be highly resistant to second challenge through sandfly transmitted infections [125]. Though, the immune response is unable to clear the primary infection, the immune system can facilitate concomitant immunity by IFNγ secreting $CD4^{+}$ T_H1 cells [126]. However, reactivation of disease causing infection has been documented for leishmaniasis when the immune system is no longer able to control this low level chronic parasite infection [127, 128]. This is frequently observed when persistently infected individuals become immunosuppressed, such as during infection with the human immunodeficiency virus (HIV) [127, 129].

Currently, vaccine programs have been unsuccessful to emulate the protective responses mediated by concomitant immunity as observed during subclinical infections with persistent parasites (reviewed in [130]). Similar, a sterile cure whereby the parasites are completely eliminated has not been achieved without consequently the loss of long-term immunity [131].

In the past the leishmanization live vaccine practice was employed by inoculating virulent *Leishmania* parasites into individuals, however this has since fallen out of practice due to safety concerns regarding development of non-healing lesions [132]. Since then, vaccine-candidates have failed to provide protection against natural exposure even though they demonstrate protective cell-mediated immunity in rodent models. It is thought that this is due to differences in experimental delivery versus the natural route of infection via the bite of a sandfly. Other challenges are observed when using whole killed parasites or subunit protein vaccine candidates only short-term protection in rodent models has been observed [123, 131].

The difference in protective immunity induced following natural infection and inoculation of whole killed parasites is not fully understood but it has been hypothesized that there is a difference in the immunologic memory responses, which is influenced by the presence of live versus killed parasites. Moreover, the adjuvant dose-quantity tested to date may not be sufficient to generate a memory T cell population [123, 128]. It is possible that vaccines utilizing live-attenuated parasites will most closely mimic natural infection, potentially providing long-term protection against infection and disease [131].

Recently, vector-associated factors have been identified to have an important impact on challenge models in vaccine-mediated immunity [130]. Following needle versus infected sandfly challenge in mice showed that various protein/adjuvant-based vaccines provided intermediate protection against needle challenge whereas sandfly challenge failed to provide protection. Despite generating antigen-specific T_H1 immune responses prior to and following challenge, vaccines failed to protect against infected sandfly challenge [125, 133]. The sandfly vector challenge model clearly emphasizes important factors induced by the sandfly, such as the impact of recruited inflammatory cells and immune-mediated host cell activation by the vector.

5. Concluding remarks

The leishmaniases are one of the most important groups of neglected tropical diseases estimated to affect 1 million people annually in nearly 100 countries [1]. The fact that an effective vaccine has yet to be developed reflects the gap in our understanding of host responses to *Leishmania* species, disease pathogenesis and what actually constitutes a protective immune response. The different *Leishmania* parasites inducing different host immune responses, which are further impacted by host genetics, have made it difficult to achieve consensus among experimental studies regarding the role of the different immune components in *Leishmania* infection. Furthermore, research to date highlights the inadequacies of small animal models in understanding human host responses to *Leishmania*. The increase in *in vitro*/*ex vivo* characterization of *Leishmania*-specific immune responses using samples derived from human clinical studies has provided more information on human CL, however more efforts towards human clinical studies (cohort and case control-studies) including human *ex vivo* infection models should be emphasized to gain a better understanding of the human immune response to *Leishmania* parasites. An interesting recent focus has been the use of humanized mice to further examine the role of specific immune cells and responses in *Leishmania* infection; this could further inform the development of novel vaccine strategies [134].

Additionally, there are other important vector and parasite-derived components affecting host immune responses, which were outside the scope of this chapter but are important to consider in terms of host-parasite interactions. Recent experimental studies are providing new insights into host immune responses by employing a sandfly challenge model using the natural route of parasite inoculation via phlebotomine sandflies [46]. Vector-derived components have been shown to contribute to early immune responses in infection [14]. For example, tissue damage caused by the phlebotomine sandfly's proboscis and the delivery of sandfly saliva triggers the rapid recruitment of neutrophils which induce inflammation [41]. *Leishmania*-derived components have also been shown to play a role during inoculation and *Leishmania* exosomes have been shown to modulate immune cells and host responses through direct and indirect contact [135].

This chapter has highlighted the complexity associated with CL and how host immune cells can both be protective and pathogenic depending on the interaction with *Leishmania* species parasite and host genetic. Employing a human CL model that provides a better understanding and more accurately represents parasite-host interactions will be critical for the development of an effective vaccine capable of inducing long-lasting protective immunity.

Conflict of interest

The authors declare no conflict of interest.

Author details

Elina Panahi[1], Danielle I. Stanisic[1], Christopher S. Peacock[2,3] and Lara J. Herrero[1]*

1 Institute for Glycomics, Griffith University, Southport, Queensland, Australia

2 The Marshall Centre for Infectious Disease Research and Training, School of Biomedical Sciences, The University of Western Australia, Perth, Western Australia, Australia

3 Telethon Kids Institute, Perth Children's Hospital, Nedlands, Western Australia, Australia

*Address all correspondence to: l.herrero@griffith.edu.au

References

[1] Burza S, Croft SL, Boelaert M. Leishmaniasis. Lancet. 2018;**392**:951-970. DOI: 10.1016/S0140-6736(18)31204-2

[2] Dostálová A, Volf P. Leishmania development in sand flies: Parasite-vector interactions overview. Parasites & Vectors. 2012;**5**:276. DOI: 10.1186/1756-3305-5-276

[3] Martínez-López M, Soto M, Iborra S, Sancho D. Leishmania Hijacks myeloid cells for immune escape. Frontiers in Microbiology. 2018;**9**. DOI: 10.3389/fmicb.2018.00883

[4] Andrade-Narvaez FJ, Loría-Cervera EN, Sosa-Bibiano EI, Van Wynsberghe NR. Asymptomatic infection with American cutaneous leishmaniasis: Epidemiological and immunological studies. Memórias do Instituto Oswaldo Cruz. 2016;**111**:599-604. DOI: 10.1590/0074-02760160138

[5] van Henten S, Adriaensen W, Fikre H, Akuffo H, Diro E, Hailu A, et al. Cutaneous Leishmaniasis Due to Leishmania aethiopica. EClinicalMedicine 2018;**6**:69-81. DOI: 10.1016/j.eclinm.2018.12.009

[6] Fikre H, Mohammed R, Atinafu S, van Griensven J, Diro E. Clinical features and treatment response of cutaneous leishmaniasis in North-West Ethiopia. Tropical Medicine & International Health. 2017;**22**:1293-1301. DOI: 10.1111/tmi.12928

[7] Padovese V, Terranova M, Toma L, Barnabas GA, Morrone A. Cutaneous and mucocutaneous leishmaniasis in Tigray, northern Ethiopia: clinical aspects and therapeutic concerns. Transactions of the Royal Society of Tropical Medicine and Hygiene. 2009;**103**:707-711. DOI: 10.1016/j.trstmh.2009.02.023

[8] Masmoudi A, Hariz W, Marrekchi S, Amouri M, Turki H. Old World cutaneous leishmaniasis: diagnosis and treatment. Journal of Dermatological Case Reports. 2013;7:31-41. DOI:10.3315/jdcr.2013.1135

[9] Siriwardana Y, Deepachandi B, Gunasekara C, Warnasooriya W, Karunaweera ND. Leishmania donovani Induced Cutaneous Leishmaniasis: An Insight into Atypical Clinical Variants in Sri Lanka. Journal of Tropical Medicine. 2019;**2019**:1-11. DOI: 10.1155/2019/4538597

[10] Hashiguchi Y, Gomez EL, Kato H, Martini LR, Velez LN, Uezato H. Diffuse and disseminated cutaneous leishmaniasis: Clinical cases experienced in Ecuador and a brief review. Tropical Medicine and Health. 2016;**44**(1):2. Available from: http://tropmedhealth.biomedcentral.com/articles/10.1186/s41182-016-0002-0

[11] Ives A, Ronet C, Prevel F, Ruzzante G, Fuertes-Marraco S, Schutz F, et al. Leishmania RNA virus controls the severity of mucocutaneous leishmaniasis. Science. 2011;**331**:775-778. DOI: 10.1126/science.1199326

[12] Osero BO, Aruleba RT, Brombacher F, Hurdayal R. Unravelling the unsolved paradoxes of cytokine families in host resistance and susceptibility to Leishmania infection. Cytokine X. 2020;**2**:100043. DOI: 10.1016/j.cytox.2020.100043

[13] Loeuillet C, Bañuls A-L, Hide M. Study of Leishmania pathogenesis in mice: Experimental considerations. Parasites & Vectors. 2016;**9**:144. DOI: 10.1186/s13071-016-1413-9

[14] Dey R, Joshi AB, Oliveira F, Pereira L, Guimarães-Costa AB, Serafim TD, et al. Gut microbes egested during bites of infected sand flies augment severity of leishmaniasis via inflammasome-derived IL-1β. Cell Host & Microbe. 2018;**23**:134-143.e6. DOI: 10.1016/j.chom.2017.12.002

[15] Kimblin N, Peters N, Debrabant A, Secundino N, Egen J, Lawyer P, et al. Quantification of the infectious dose of Leishmania major transmitted to the skin by single sand flies. Proceedings of the National Academy of Sciences of the United States of America. 2008;**105**:10125-10130. DOI: 10.1073/pnas.0802331105

[16] Scott P, Novais FO. Cutaneous leishmaniasis: Immune responses in protection and pathogenesis. Nature Reviews. Immunology. 2016;**16**:581-592. DOI: 10.1038/nri.2016.72

[17] Gurung P, Kanneganti T-D. Innate immunity against Leishmania infections. Cellular Microbiology. 2015;**17**:1286-1294. DOI: 10.1111/cmi.12484

[18] Puentes SM, Da Silva RP, Sacks DL, Hammer CH, Joiner KA. Serum resistance of metacyclic stage Leishmania major promastigotes is due to release of C5b-9. Journal of Immunology. 1990;**145**:4311-4316

[19] Domínguez M, Moreno I, López-Trascasa M, Toraño A. Complement interaction with trypanosomatid promastigotes in normal human serum. The Journal of Experimental Medicine. 2002;**195**: 451-459. DOI: 10.1084/jem.20011319

[20] Yao C, Gaur Dixit U, Barker JH, Teesch LM, Love-Homan L, Donelson JE, et al. Attenuation of Leishmania infantum chagasi metacyclic promastigotes by sterol depletion. Infection and Immunity. 2013;**81**: 2507-2517. DOI: 10.1128/IAI.00214-13

[21] Joshi PB, Kelly BL, Kamhawi S, Sacks DL, McMaster WR. Targeted gene deletion in Leishmania major identifies leishmanolysin (GP63) as a virulence factor. Molecular and Biochemical Parasitology. 2002;**120**:33-40. DOI:10.1016/s0166-6851(01)00432-7

[22] Ricardo-Carter C, Favila M, Polando RE, Cotton RN, Bogard Horner K, Condon D, et al. Leishmania major inhibits IL-12 in macrophages by signalling through CR3 (CD11b/CD18) and down-regulation of ETS-mediated transcription. Parasite Immunology. 2013;**35**:409-420. DOI: 10.1111/pim.12049

[23] de Veer MJ, Curtis JM, Baldwin TM, DiDonato JA, Sexton A, McConville MJ, Handman E, Schofield L. MyD88 is essential for clearance of Leishmania major: possible role for lipophosphoglycan and Toll-like receptor 2 signaling. European Journal of Immunology. 2003;**33**:2822-2831. DOI: 10.1002/eji.200324128

[24] Vargas-Inchaustegui DA, Tai W, Xin L, Hogg AE, Corry DB, Soong L. Distinct roles for MyD88 and Toll-like receptor 2 during *Leishmania braziliensis* infection in mice. Infection and Immunity. 2009;**77**:2948-2956. DOI: 10.1128/IAI.00154-09

[25] Guerra CS, Macedo Silva RM, Carvalho LOP, Calabrese K d S, Bozza PT, Côrte-Real S. Histopathological analysis of initial cellular response in TLR-2 deficient mice experimentally infected by *Leishmania* (L.) *amazonensis*. International Journal of Experimental Pathology. 2010;**91**:451-459. DOI: 10.1111/j.1365-2613.2010.00717.x

[26] Franco LH, Beverley SM, Zamboni DS. Innate immune activation and subversion of mammalian functions by Leishmania lipophosphoglycan. Journal of Parasitology Research. 2012;**2012**:1-11. DOI: 10.1155/2012/165126

[27] Rogers ME. The role of Leishmania proteophosphoglycans in sand fly transmission and infection of the mammalian host. Frontiers in Microbiology. 2012;**3**. DOI: 10.3389/fmicb.2012.00223

[28] Filardy AA, Pires DR, Nunes MP, Takiya CM, Freire-de-Lima CG, Ribeiro-Gomes FL, et al. Proinflammatory clearance of apoptotic neutrophils induces

an IL-12 low IL-10 high regulatory phenotype in macrophages. Journal of Immunology. 2010;**185**:2044-2050. DOI: 10.4049/jimmunol.1000017

[29] Kopf M, Brombacher F, Köhler G, Kienzle G, Widmann KH, Lefrang K, et al. IL-4-deficient Balb/c mice resist infection with *Leishmania major*. The Journal of Experimental Medicine. 1996;**184**: 1127-1136. DOI: 10.1084/jem.184.3.1127

[30] Carneiro PP, Conceição J, Macedo M, Magalhães V, Carvalho EM, Bacellar O. The role of nitric oxide and reactive oxygen species in the killing of Leishmania braziliensis by monocytes from patients with cutaneous leishmaniasis. PLoS One. 2016;**11**:e0148084. DOI: 10.1371/journal.pone.0148084

[31] Polari LP, Carneiro PP, Macedo M, Machado PRL, Scott P, Carvalho EM, et al. Leishmania braziliensis infection enhances toll-like receptors 2 and 4 expression and triggers TNF-α and IL-10 production in human cutaneous leishmaniasis. Frontiers in Cellular and Infection Microbiology. 2019;**9**:120. DOI: 10.3389/fcimb.2019.00120

[32] Weinkopff T, Mariotto A, Simon G, La TYH, Auderset F, Schuster S, et al. Role of toll-like receptor 9 signaling in experimental leishmania braziliensis infection. Infection and Immunity. 2013;**81**:1575-1584. DOI: 10.1128/IAI.01401-12

[33] Vieira ÉLM, Keesen TSL, Machado PR, Guimarães LH, Carvalho EM, Dutra WO, et al. Immunoregulatory profile of monocytes from cutaneous leishmaniasis patients and association with lesion size. Parasite Immunology. 2013;**35**:65-72. DOI: 10.1111/ pim.12012

[34] Flandin J-F, Chano F, Descoteaux A. RNA interference reveals a role for TLR2 and TLR3 in the recognition of *Leishmania donovani* promastigotes by interferon-γ-primed macrophages. European Journal of Immunology. 2006;**36**:411-420. DOI: 10.1002/eji.200535079

[35] Regli IB, Passelli K, Martínez-Salazar B, Amore J, Hurrell BP, Müller AJ, et al. TLR7 sensing by neutrophils is critical for the control of cutaneous Leishmaniasis. Cell Reports. 2020;**31**:107746. DOI: 10.1016/j.celrep.2020.107746

[36] Charmoy M, Hurrell BP, Romano A, Lee SH, Ribeiro-Gomes F, Riteau N, et al. The Nlrp3 inflammasome, IL-1β, and neutrophil recruitment are required for susceptibility to a nonhealing strain of Leishmania major in C57BL/6 mice. European Journal of Immunology. 2016;**46**:897-911. DOI: 10.1002/eji.201546015

[37] Kautz-Neu K, Kostka SL, Dinges S, Iwakura Y, Udey MC, von Stebut E. IL-1 signalling is dispensable for protective immunity in Leishmania-resistant mice. Experimental Dermatology. 2011;**20**:76-78. DOI: 10.1111/j.1600-0625.2010.01172.x

[38] Satoskar AR, Okano M, Connaughton S, Raisanen-Sokolwski A, David JR, Labow M. Enhanced Th2-like responses in IL-1 type 1 receptor-deficient mice. European Journal of Immunology. 1998;**28**:2066-2074. DOI: 10.1002/(SICI)1521-4141(199807)28:07<2066::AID-IMMU2066>3.0.CO;2-X

[39] Lima-Junior DS, Costa DL, Carregaro V, Cunha LD, Silva ALN, Mineo TWP, et al. Inflammasome-derived IL-1β production induces nitric oxide–mediated resistance to Leishmania. Nature Medicine. 2013;**19**: 909-915. DOI: 10.1038/nm.3221

[40] Gurung P, Karki R, Vogel P, Watanabe M, Bix M, Lamkanfi M, et al. An NLRP3 inflammasome–triggered Th2-biased adaptive immune response promotes leishmaniasis. The Journal of

Clinical Investigation. 2015;**125**: 1329-1338. DOI: 10.1172/JCI79526

[41] Peters NC, Egen JG, Secundino N, Debrabant A, Kimblin N, Kamhawi S, et al. In vivo imaging reveals an essential role for neutrophils in Leishmaniasis transmitted by sand flies. Science (80-). 2008;**321**:970-974. DOI: 10.1126/science.1159194

[42] Passelli K, Billion O, Tacchini-Cottier F. The impact of neutrophil recruitment to the skin on the pathology induced by Leishmania infection. Frontiers in Immunology. 2021;**12**:649348. DOI: 10.3389/fimmu.2021. 649348

[43] Ribeiro-Gomes FL, Sacks D. The influence of early neutrophil-Leishmania interactions on the host immune response to infection. Frontiers in Cellular and Infection Microbiology. 2012;**2**:59. DOI: 10.3389/fcimb.2012.00059

[44] van Zandbergen G, Klinger M, Mueller A, Dannenberg S, Gebert A, Solbach W, et al. Cutting edge: Neutrophil granulocyte serves as a vector for leishmania entry into macrophages. Journal of Immunology. 2004;**173**:6521-6525. DOI: 10.4049/jimmunol.173.11.6521

[45] Charmoy M, Brunner-Agten S, Aebischer D, Auderset F, Launois P, Milon G, et al. Neutrophil-derived CCL3 is essential for the rapid recruitment of dendritic cells to the site of Leishmania major inoculation in resistant mice. PLoS Pathogens. 2010;**6**:e1000755. DOI: 10.1371/ journal.ppat.1000755

[46] Chaves MM, Lee SH, Kamenyeva O, Ghosh K, Peters NC, Sacks D. The role of dermis resident macrophages and their interaction with neutrophils in the early establishment of *Leishmania major* infection transmitted by sand fly bite. PLoS Pathogens. 2020;**16**:e1008674. DOI: 10.1371/journal.ppat.1008674

[47] Romano A, Carneiro MBH, Doria NA, Roma EH, Ribeiro-Gomes FL, Inbar E, et al. Divergent roles for Ly6C+CCR2+CX3CR1+ inflammatory monocytes during primary or secondary infection of the skin with the intra-phagosomal pathogen *Leishmania major*. PLoS Pathogens. 2017;**13**:e1006479

[48] Aga E, Katschinski DM, van Zandbergen G, Laufs H, Hansen B, Müller K, et al. Inhibition of the spontaneous apoptosis of neutrophil granulocytes by the intracellular parasite *Leishmania major*. Journal of Immunology. 2002;**169**:898-905. DOI: 10.4049/jimmunol.169.2.898

[49] Novais FO, Santiago RC, Báfica A, Khouri R, Afonso L, Borges VM, et al. Neutrophils and macrophages cooperate in host resistance against *Leishmania braziliensis* infection. Journal of Immunology. 2009;**183**:8088-8098. DOI: 10.4049/jimmunol.0803720

[50] Ribeiro-Gomes FL, Roma EH, Carneiro MBH, Doria NA, Sacks DL, Peters NC. Site-dependent recruitment of inflammatory cells determines the effective dose of *Leishmania major*. Infection and Immunity. 2014;**82**:2713-2727. DOI: 10.1128/IAI.01600-13

[51] Tacchini-Cottier F, Zweifel C, Belkaid Y, Mukankundiye C, Vasei M, Launois P, et al. An immunomodulatory function for neutrophils during the induction of a CD4 + Th2 response in BALB/c mice infected with *Leishmania major*. Journal of Immunology. 2000;**165**:2628-2636. DOI: 10.4049/jimmunol.165.5.2628

[52] Charmoy M, Megnekou R, Allenbach C, Zweifel C, Perez C, Monnat K, et al. Leishmania major induces distinct neutrophil phenotypes in mice that are resistant or susceptible to infection. Journal of Leukocyte Biology. 2007;**82**:288-299. DOI: 10.1189/jlb.0706440

[53] Sousa LMA, Carneiro MBH, Resende ME, Martins LS, dos Santos LM, Vaz LG, et al. Neutrophils have a protective role during early stages of *Leishmania amazonensis* infection in BALB/c mice. Parasite Immunology. 2014;**36**:13-31. DOI: 10.1111/pim.12078

[54] Conceição J, Davis R, Carneiro PP, Giudice A, Muniz AC, Wilson ME, et al. Characterization of neutrophil function in human cutaneous Leishmaniasis caused by *Leishmania braziliensis*. PLoS Neglected Tropical Diseases. 2016;**10**:e0004715. DOI: 10.1371/journal.pntd.0004715

[55] Tavares NM, Araújo-Santos T, Afonso L, Nogueira PM, Lopes UG, Soares RP, et al. Understanding the mechanisms controlling leishmania amazonensis infection in vitro: The role of LTB4 derived from human neutrophils. The Journal of Infectious Diseases. 2014;**210**:656-666. DOI: 10.1093/infdis/jiu158

[56] Tavares N, Afonso L, Suarez M, Ampuero M, Prates DB, Araújo-Santos T, et al. Degranulating neutrophils promote leukotriene B 4 production by infected macrophages to kill *Leishmania amazonensis* parasites. Journal of Immunology. 2016;**196**:1865-1873. DOI: 10.4049/jimmunol.1502224

[57] Goncalves R, Zhang X, Cohen H, Debrabant A, Mosser DM. Platelet activation attracts a subpopulation of effector monocytes to sites of *Leishmania major* infection. The Journal of Experimental Medicine. 2011;**208**:1253-1265. DOI: 10.1084/jem.20101751

[58] Olekhnovitch R, Ryffel B, Müller AJ, Bousso P. Collective nitric oxide production provides tissue-wide immunity during Leishmania infection. The Journal of Clinical Investigation. 2014;**124**:1711-1722. DOI: 10.1172/JCI72058

[59] Novais FO, Nguyen BT, Beiting DP, Carvalho LP, Glennie ND, Passos S, et al. Human classical monocytes control the intracellular stage of *Leishmania braziliensis* by reactive oxygen species. The Journal of Infectious Diseases. 2014;**209**:1288-1296. DOI: 10.1093/infdis/jiu013

[60] Scharton TM, Scott P. Natural killer cells are a source of interferon gamma that drives differentiation of CD4+ T cell subsets and induces early resistance to *Leishmania major* in mice. The Journal of Experimental Medicine. 1993;**178**:567-577. DOI: 10.1084/jem.178.2.567

[61] Wei X, Charles IG, Smith A, Ure J, Feng G, Huang F, et al. Altered immune responses in mice lacking inducible nitric oxide synthase. Nature. 1995;**375**:408-411. DOI: 10.1038/375408a0

[62] Roma EH, Macedo JP, Goes GR, Gonçalves JL, De CW, Cisalpino D, et al. Impact of reactive oxygen species (ROS) on the control of parasite loads and inflammation in *Leishmania amazonensis* infection. Parasites & Vectors. 2016;**9**:193. DOI: 10.1186/s13071-016-1472-y

[63] Gantt KR, Goldman TL, McCormick ML, Miller MA, Jeronimo SMB, Nascimento ET, et al. Oxidative responses of human and murine macrophages during phagocytosis of *Leishmania chagasi*. Journal of Immunology. 2001;**167**:893-901. DOI: 10.4049/jimmunol.167.2.893

[64] Tibúrcio R, Nunes S, Nunes I, Rosa Ampuero M, Silva IB, Lima R, et al. Molecular aspects of dendritic cell activation in Leishmaniasis: An immunobiological view. Frontiers in Immunology. 2019;**10**:227. DOI: 10.3389/fimmu.2019.00227

[65] Sato N, Ahuja SK, Quinones M, Kostecki V, Reddick RL, Melby PC, et al. Cc chemokine receptor (Ccr)2 is required for langerhans cell migration and localization of T Helper Cell Type 1 (Th1)-inducing dendritic cells. The

Journal of Experimental Medicine. 2000;**192**:205-218. DOI: 10.1084/jem.192.2.205

[66] Carvalho AM, Guimarães LH, Costa R, Saldanha MG, Prates I, Carvalho LP, et al. Impaired Th1 response is associated with therapeutic failure in patients with cutaneous Leishmaniasis caused by *Leishmania braziliensis*. The Journal of Infectious Diseases. 2021;**223**:527-535. DOI: 10.1093/infdis/jiaa374

[67] de Lima CMF, Magalhães AS, Costa R, Barreto CC, Machado PRL, Carvalho EM, et al. High anti-leishmania IgG antibody levels are associated with severity of mucosal Leishmaniasis. Frontiers in Cellular and Infection Microbiology. 2021;**11**:652956. DOI: 10.3389/fcimb.2021.652956

[68] Christensen SM, Belew AT, El-Sayed NM, Tafuri WL, Silveira FT, Mosser DM. Host and parasite responses in human diffuse cutaneous leishmaniasis caused by *L. amazonensis*. PLoS Neglected Tropical Diseases. 2019;**13**:e0007152. DOI: 10.1371/journal.pntd.0007152

[69] Kostka SL, Knop J, Konur A, Udey MC, von Stebut E. Distinct roles for IL-1 receptor type I signaling in early versus established *Leishmania major* infections. Journal of Investigative Dermatology. 2006;**126**(7):1582-1589. Available from: https://linkinghub.elsevier.com/retrieve/pii/S0022202X15329900

[70] Rutz S, Eidenschenk C, Ouyang W. IL-22, not simply a Th17 cytokine. Immunological Reviews. 2013;**252**:116-1132. DOI: 10.1111/imr.12027

[71] Araujo Flores GV, Sandoval Pacheco CM, Sosa Ochoa WH, Gomes CMC, Zúniga C, Corbett CP, et al. Th17 lymphocytes in atypical cutaneous leishmaniasis caused by *Leishmania* (L.) *infantum* chagasi in Central America. Parasite Immunology. 2020;**42**:e12772. DOI: 10.1111/pim.12772

[72] Alexander J, Brombacher F. T Helper1/T Helper2 cells and resistance/susceptibility to Leishmania infection: Is this paradigm still relevant? Frontiers in Immunology. 2012;**3**:80. DOI: 10.3389/fimmu.2012.00080

[73] Voronov E, Dotan S, Gayvoronsky L, White RM, Cohen I, Krelin Y, et al. IL-1-induced inflammation promotes development of leishmaniasis in susceptible BALB/c mice. International Immunology. 2010;**22**(4):245-257

[74] Malek TR. The main function of IL-2 is to promote the development of T regulatory cells. Journal of Leukocyte Biology. 2003;**74**:961-965. DOI: 10.1189/jlb.0603272

[75] Oliveira PRS, Dessein H, Romano A, Cabantous S, de Brito MEF, Santoro F, et al. IL2RA genetic variants reduce IL-2–dependent responses and aggravate human cutaneous Leishmaniasis. Journal of Immunology. 2015;**194**:2664-2672. DOI: 10.4049/jimmunol.1402047

[76] Biedermann T, Zimmermann S, Himmelrich H, Gumy A, Egeter O, Sakrauski AK, et al. IL-4 instructs TH1 responses and resistance to *Leishmania major* in susceptible BALB/c mice. Nature Immunology [Internet]. 2001;**2**(11):1054-1060. Available from: http://www.nature.com/articles/ni725

[77] Poudel B, Yorek MS, Mazgaeen L, Brown SA, Kanneganti T-D, Gurung P. Acute IL-4 governs pathogenic T cell responses during *Leishmania major* infection. ImmunoHorizons. 2020;**4**:546-560. DOI: 10.4049/immunohorizons.2000076

[78] Titus RG, Dekrey GK, Morris RV, Soares MBP. Interleukin-6 deficiency influences cytokine expression in susceptible BALB mice infected with

Leishmania major but does not alter the outcome of disease. Infection and Immunity. 2001;**69**:5189-5192. DOI: 10.1128/IAI.69.8.5189-5192.2001

[79] Laufs H, Müller K, Fleischer J, Reiling N, Jahnke N, Jensenius JC, et al. Intracellular survival of *Leishmania major* in neutrophil granulocytes after uptake in the absence of heat-labile serum factors. Infection and Immunity. 2002;**70**:826-835. DOI: 10.1128/IAI.70.2.826-835.2002

[80] Buxbaum LU, Scott P. Interleukin 10- and Fcγ receptor-deficient mice resolve *Leishmania mexicana* lesions. Infection and Immunity. 2005;**73**:2101-8. DOI: 10.1128/IAI.73.4.2101-2108.2005

[81] Park AY, Hondowicz BD, Scott P. IL-12 is required to maintain a Th1 response during *Leishmania major* infection. Journal of Immunology [Internet]. 2000;**165**(2):896-902. Available from: http://www.jimmunol.org/lookup/doi/10.4049/jimmunol.165.2.896

[82] Matthews DJ, Emson CL, McKenzie GJ, Jolin HE, Blackwell JM, McKenzie ANJ. IL-13 is a susceptibility factor for *Leishmania major* infection. Journal of Immunology [Internet]. 2000;**164**(3):1458-1462. Available from: http://www.jimmunol.org/lookup/doi/10.4049/jimmunol.164.3.1458

[83] Banerjee A, Bhattacharya P, Joshi AB, Ismail N, Dey R, Nakhasi HL. Role of pro-inflammatory cytokine IL-17 in Leishmania pathogenesis and in protective immunity by Leishmania vaccines. Cellular Immunology [Internet]. 2016;**309**:37-41. Available from: https://linkinghub.elsevier.com/retrieve/pii/S0008874916300533

[84] Lopez Kostka S, Dinges S, Griewank K, Iwakura Y, Udey MC, von Stebut E. IL-17 promotes progression of cutaneous leishmaniasis in susceptible mice. Journal of Immunology [Internet]. 2009;**182**(5):3039-3046. Available from: http://www.jimmunol.org/lookup/doi/10.4049/jimmunol.0713598

[85] Monteforte GM, Takeda K, Rodriguez-Sosa M, Akira S, David JR, Satoskar AR. Genetically resistant mice lacking IL-18 gene develop Th1 response and control cutaneous *Leishmania major* infection. Journal of Immunology [Internet]. 2000;**164**(11):5890-5893. Available from: http://www.jimmunol.org/lookup/doi/10.4049/jimmunol.164.11.5890

[86] Gimblet C, Loesche MA, Carvalho L, Carvalho EM, Grice EA, Artis D, et al. IL-22 protects against tissue damage during cutaneous leishmaniasis. PLoS One. 2015

[87] Anderson CF, Stumhofer JS, Hunter CA, Sacks D. IL-27 regulates IL-10 and IL-17 from CD4 + cells in nonhealing *Leishmania major* infection. Journal of Immunology[Internet]. 2009;**183**(7):4619-4627. Available from: http://www.jimmunol.org/lookup/doi/10.4049/jimmunol.0804024

[88] Farias Amorim CO, Novais F, Nguyen BT, Nascimento MT, Lago J, Lago AS, et al. Localized skin inflammation during cutaneous leishmaniasis drives a chronic, systemic IFN-γ signature. PLoS Neglected Tropical Diseases. 2021;**15**:e0009321 10.1371/journal.pntd.0009321

[89] Pinheiro RO, Rossi-Bergmann B. Interferon-gamma is required for the late but not early control of *Leishmania amazonensis* infection in C57Bl/6 mice. Memórias do Instituto Oswaldo Cruz [Internet]. 2007;**102**(1):79-82. Available from: http://www.scielo.br/scielo.php?script=sci_arttext&pid=S0074-02762007000100013&lng=en&tlng=en

[90] Fromm PD, Kling JC, Remke A, Bogdan C, Körner H. Fatal leishmaniasis in the absence of TNF despite a strong Th1 response. Frontiers in Microbiology.

2016;**6**:1520. DOI: 10.3389/fmicb.2015.01520

[91] Melby PC, Andrade-Narvaez FJ, Darnell BJ, Valencia-Pacheco G, Tryon VV, Palomo-Cetina A. Increased expression of proinflammatory cytokines in chronic lesions of human cutaneous leishmaniasis. Infection and Immunity. 1994;**62**:837-842. DOI: 10.1128/IAI.62.3.837-842.1994

[92] Heinzel FP, Schoenhaut DS, Rerko RM, Rosser LE, Gately MK. Recombinant interleukin 12 cures mice infected with *Leishmania major*. The Journal of Experimental Medicine. 1993;**177**:1505-1509. DOI: 10.1084/jem.177.5.1505

[93] Sypek JP, Chung CL, Mayor SEH, Subramanyam JM, Goldman SJ, Sieburth DS, et al. Resolution of cutaneous leishmaniasis: Interleukin 12 initiates a protective T helper type 1 immune response. The Journal of Experimental Medicine. 1993;**177**: 1797-1802. DOI: 10.1084/jem.177.6.1797

[94] Carneiro MB, Lopes ME, Hohman LS, Romano A, David BA, Kratofil R, et al. Th1-Th2 cross-regulation controls early leishmania infection in the skin by modulating the size of the permissive monocytic host cell reservoir. Cell Host & Microbe. 2020;**27**:752-768.e7. DOI: 10.1016/j.chom.2020.03.011

[95] Mendez S, Reckling SK, Piccirillo CA, Sacks D, Belkaid Y. Role for CD4+ CD25+ regulatory T cells in reactivation of persistent Leishmaniasis and control of concomitant immunity. The Journal of Experimental Medicine. 2004;**200**:201-210. DOI: 10.1084/jem.20040298

[96] Sadick MD, Heinzel FP, Holaday BJ, Pu RT, Dawkins RS, Locksley RM. Cure of murine leishmaniasis with anti-interleukin 4 monoclonal antibody. Evidence for a T cell-dependent, interferon gamma-independent mechanism. The Journal of Experimental Medicine. 1990;**171**:115-127. DOI: 10.1084/jem.171.1.115

[97] Kane MM, Mosser DM. The role of IL-10 in promoting disease progression in Leishmaniasis. Journal of Immunology. 2001;**166**:1141-1147. DOI: 10.4049/jimmunol.166.2.1141

[98] Belkaid Y, Piccirillo CA, Mendez S, Shevach EM, Sacks DL. CD4+CD25+ regulatory T cells control *Leishmania major* persistence and immunity. Nature. 2002;**420**:502-507. DOI: 10.1038/nature01152

[99] Nylén S, Sacks D. Interleukin-10 and the pathogenesis of human visceral leishmaniasis. Trends in Immunology. 2007;**28**:378-384. DOI: 10.1016/j.it.2007.07.004

[100] Carneiro MBH, Lopes MEDM, Vaz LG, Sousa LMA, Dos Santos LM, De Souza CC, et al. IFN-γ-dependent recruitment of CD4+ T cells and macrophages contributes to pathogenesis during leishmania amazonensis infection. Journal of Interferon & Cytokine Research. 2015;**35**:935-947. DOI: 10.1089/jir.2015.0043

[101] Novais FO, Scott P. CD8+ T cells in cutaneous leishmaniasis: The good, the bad, and the ugly. Seminars in Immunopathology. 2015;**37**:251-259. DOI: 10.1007/s00281-015-0475-7

[102] Belkaid Y, Von Stebut E, Mendez S, Lira R, Caler E, Bertholet S, et al. CD8 + T cells are required for primary immunity in C57BL/6 mice following low-dose, intradermal challenge with *Leishmania major*. Journal of Immunology. 2002;**168**:3992-4000. DOI: 10.4049/jimmunol.168.8.3992

[103] Novais FO, Carvalho LP, Graff JW, Beiting DP, Ruthel G, Roos DS, et al. Cytotoxic T cells mediate pathology and metastasis in cutaneous Leishmaniasis. PLoS Pathogens. 2013;**9**:e1003504. DOI: 10.1371/ journal.ppat.1003504

[104] Soong L, Chang CH, Sun J, Longley BJ, Ruddle NH, Flavell RA, et al. Role of CD4+ T cells in pathogenesis associated with *Leishmania amazonensis* infection. Journal of Immunology. 1997;158:5374-5383. PMID: 9164958

[105] Uzonna JE, Joyce KL, Scott P. Low dose *Leishmania major* promotes a transient T helper cell type 2 response that is down-regulated by interferon γ–producing CD8+ T cells. The Journal of Experimental Medicine. 2004;**199**:1559-1566. DOI: 10.1084/jem.20040172

[106] Novais FO, Nguyen BT, Scott P. Granzyme B inhibition by tofacitinib blocks the pathology induced by CD8 T cells in cutaneous Leishmaniasis. The Journal of Investigative Dermatology. 2021;**141**:575-585. DOI: 10.1016/j.jid.2020.07.011

[107] Bertholet S, Debrabant A, Afrin F, Caler E, Mendez S, Tabbara KS, et al. Antigen requirements for efficient priming of CD8+ T cells by *Leishmania major*-infected dendritic cells. Infection and Immunity. 2005;**73**:6620-6628. DOI: 10.1128/ IAI.73.10.6620-6628.2005

[108] Da-Cruz AM, Oliveira-Neto MP, Bertho ÁL, Mendes-Aguiar CO, Coutinho SG. T cells specific to Leishmania and other nonrelated microbial antigens can migrate to human Leishmaniasis skin lesions. The Journal of Investigative Dermatology. 2010;**130**: 1329-1336. DOI: 10.1038/jid.2009.428

[109] Cardoso TM, Machado Á, Costa DL, Carvalho LP, Queiroz A, Machado P, et al. Protective and pathological functions of CD8 + T Cells in *Leishmania braziliensis* infection. Infection and Immunity. 2015;**83**: 898-906. DOI: 10.1128/IAI.02404-14

[110] Santos CDS, Boaventura V, Ribeiro Cardoso C, Tavares N, Lordelo MJ, Noronha A, et al. CD8+ granzyme B+–mediated tissue injury vs. CD4+IFNγ+–mediated parasite killing in human cutaneous Leishmaniasis. The Journal of Investigative Dermatology. 2013;**133**:1533-1540. DOI: 10.1038/ jid.2013.4

[111] Novais FO, Carvalho AM, Clark ML, Carvalho LP, Beiting DP, Brodsky IE, et al. CD8+ T cell cytotoxicity mediates pathology in the skin by inflammasome activation and IL-1β production. PLoS Pathogens. 2017;**13**:e1006196. DOI: 10.1371/journal.ppat.1006196

[112] Faria DR, Souza PEA, Durães FV, Carvalho EM, Gollob KJ, Machado PR, et al. Recruitment of CD8(+) T cells expressing granzyme A is associated with lesion progression in human cutaneous leishmaniasis. Parasite Immunology. 2009;**31**:432-439. DOI: 10.1111/j.1365-3024.2009.01125.x

[113] Yurchenko E, Tritt M, Hay V, Shevach EM, Belkaid Y, Piccirillo CA. CCR5-dependent homing of naturally occurring CD4+ regulatory T cells to sites of *Leishmania major* infection favors pathogen persistence. The Journal of Experimental Medicine. 2006;**203**: 2451-2460. DOI: 10.1084/jem.20060956

[114] Suffia IJ, Reckling SK, Piccirillo CA, Goldszmid RS, Belkaid Y. Infected site-restricted Foxp3+ natural regulatory T cells are specific for microbial antigens. The Journal of Experimental Medicine. 2006;**203**:777-788. DOI: 10.1084/jem.20052056

[115] Okwor I, Liu D, Beverley SM, Uzonna JE. Inoculation of killed *Leishmania major* into immune mice rapidly disrupts immunity to a secondary challenge via IL-10-mediated process. Proceedings of the National Academy of Sciences. 2009;**106**:13951-13956. DOI: 10.1073/pnas.0905184106

[116] Ji J, Masterson J, Sun J, Soong L. CD4 + CD25 + regulatory T cells restrain pathogenic responses during *Leishmania amazonensis* infection. Journal of

Immunology. 2005;**174**:7147-7153. DOI: 10.4049/jimmunol.174.11.7147

[117] Woelbing F, Kostka SL, Moelle K, Belkaid Y, Sunderkoetter C, Verbeek S, et al. Uptake of Leishmania major by dendritic cells is mediated by Fcγ receptors and facilitates acquisition of protective immunity. The Journal of Experimental Medicine. 2006;**203**: 177-188. DOI: 10.1084/jem.20052288

[118] Miles SA, Conrad SM, Alves RG, Jeronimo SMB, Mosser DM. A role for IgG immune complexes during infection with the intracellular pathogen Leishmania. The Journal of Experimental Medicine. 2005;**201**: 747-754. DOI: 10.1084/jem.20041470

[119] Hurdayal R, Ndlovu HH, Revaz-Breton M, Parihar SP, Nono JK, Govender M, et al. IL-4–producing B cells regulate T helper cell dichotomy in type 1- and type 2-controlled diseases. Proceedings of the National Academy of Sciences of the United States of America. 2017;**114**:E8430-E8439. DOI: 10.1073/ pnas.1708125114

[120] Radwanska M, Cutler AJ, Hoving JC, Magez S, Holscher C, Bohms A, et al. Deletion of IL-4Rα on CD4 T cells renders BALB/c mice resistant to *Leishmania major* infection. PLoS Pathogens. 2007;**3**:e68. DOI: 10.1371/ journal.ppat.0030068

[121] Mandell MA, Beverley SM. Continual renewal and replication of persistent *Leishmania major* Parasites in concomitantly immune hosts. Proceedings of the National Academy of Sciences of the United States of America. 2017;**114**:E801-E810. DOI: 10.1073/ pnas.1619265114

[122] Mendonça MG, de Brito MEF, Rodrigues EHG, Bandeira V, Jardim ML, Abath FGC. Persistence of Leishmania parasites in scars after clinical cure of American cutaneous leishmaniasis: Is there a sterile cure? The Journal of Infectious Diseases. 2004;**189**: 1018-1023. DOI: 10.1086/382135

[123] Okwor I, Uzonna J. Persistent parasites and immunologic memory in cutaneous leishmaniasis: Implications for vaccine designs and vaccination strategies. Immunologic Research. 2008;**41**:123-136. DOI: 10.1007/ s12026-008-8016-2

[124] Pagán AJ, Peters NC, Debrabant A, Ribeiro-Gomes F, Pepper M, Karp CL, et al. Tracking antigen—specific CD4 + T cells throughout the course of chronic *Leishmania major* infection in resistant mice. European Journal of Immunology. 2013;**43**:427-438. DOI: 10.1002/ eji.201242715

[125] Peters NC, Kimblin N, Secundino N, Kamhawi S, Lawyer P, Sacks DL. Vector transmission of Leishmania abrogates vaccine-induced protective immunity. PLoS Pathogens. 2009;**5**:e1000484. DOI: 10.1371/ journal.ppat.1000484

[126] Peters NC, Pagán AJ, Lawyer PG, Hand TW, Henrique Roma E, Stamper LW, et al. Chronic parasitic infection maintains high frequencies of short-lived Ly6C+CD4+ effector T Cells that are required for protection against re-infection. PLoS Pathogens. 2014;**10**:e1004538. DOI: 10.1371/journal. ppat.1004538

[127] Alvar J, Aparicio P, Aseffa A, Den Boer M, Cañavate C, Dedet J-P, et al. The relationship between Leishmaniasis and AIDS: The second 10 years. Clinical Microbiology Reviews. 2008;**21**:334-359. DOI: 10.1128/CMR.00061-07

[128] Bogdan C. Mechanisms and consequences of persistence of intracellular pathogens: Leishmaniasis as an example. Cellular Microbiology. 2008;**10**:1221-1234. DOI: 10.1111/ j.1462-5822.2008.01146.x

[129] Parmentier L, Cusini A, Müller N, Zangger H, Hartley M-A, Desponds C,

et al. Severe cutaneous leishmaniasis in a human immunodeficiency virus patient coinfected with *Leishmania braziliensis* and its endosymbiotic virus. The American Journal of Tropical Medicine and Hygiene. 2016;**94**: 840-843. DOI: 10.4269/ajtmh.15-0803

[130] Hohman LS, Peters NC. CD4+ T cell-mediated immunity against the phagosomal pathogen Leishmania: Implications for vaccination. Trends in Parasitology. 2019;**35**:423-435. DOI: 10.1016/j.pt.2019.04.002

[131] Nylén S, Gautam S. Immunological perspectives of leishmaniasis. Journal of Global Infectious Diseases. 2010;**2**:135. DOI: 10.4103/0974-777X.62876

[132] Okwor I, Mou Z, Liu D, Uzonna J. Protective immunity and vaccination against cutaneous leishmaniasis. Frontiers in Immunology. 2012;**3**:128. DOI: 10.3389/fimmu.2012.00128

[133] Peters NC, Bertholet S, Lawyer PG, Charmoy M, Romano A, Ribeiro-Gomes FL, et al. Evaluation of recombinant leishmania polyprotein plus glucopyranosyl lipid A stable emulsion vaccines against sand fly-transmitted *Leishmania major* in C57BL/6 mice. Journal of Immunology. 2012;**189**:4832-4841 10.4049/jimmunol.1201676

[134] Fischer MR, Schermann AI, Twelkmeyer T, Lorenz B, Wegner J, Jonuleit H, et al. Humanized mice in cutaneous leishmaniasis—Suitability analysis of human PBMC transfer into immunodeficient mice. Experimental Dermatology. 2019;**28**:1087-1090. DOI: 10.1111/exd.13999

[135] Atayde VD, Aslan H, Townsend S, Hassani K, Kamhawi S, Olivier M. Exosome secretion by the parasitic protozoan Leishmania within the sand fly midgut. Cell Reports. 2015;**13**:957-967. DOI: 10.1016/j.celrep.2015.09.058

Chapter 3

Extracellular Vesicles Released by *Leishmania*: Impact on Disease Development and Immune System Cells

Rogéria Cristina Zauli, Andrey Sladkevicius Vidal, Talita Vieira Dupin, Aline Correia Costa de Morais, Wagner Luiz Batista and Patricia Xander

Abstract

Leishmania spp. release extracellular vesicles (EVs) containing parasite molecules, including several antigens and virulence factors. These EVs can interact with the host cells, such as immune cells, contributing to the parasite–host relationship. Studies have demonstrated that *Leishmania*-EVs can promote infection in experimental models and modulate the immune response. Although the immunomodulatory effect has been demonstrated, *Leishmania*-EVs can deliver parasite antigens and therefore have the potential for use as a new diagnostic tool and development of new therapeutic and vaccine approaches. This review aims to bring significant advances in the field of extracellular vesicles and *Leishmania*, focusing on their role in the cells of the immune system.

Keywords: extracellular vesicles, exosomes, microvesicles, *Leishmania*, immune response, leishmaniasis

1. Introduction

The host–parasite communication and the parasite's intercellular interactions are crucial in the life cycle of the *Leishmania* parasites [1, 2]. In addition, several bioactive molecules released by the parasites have shown an important role in the parasite's adaptation in the host [3]. In mammalian hosts, molecules released by *Leishmania* contribute to the parasite's infectivity and the physiopathology of the leishmaniasis, acting by several mechanisms, such as subverting the immune response and favoring the intracellular multiplication of the parasite [3].

Several works have demonstrated that *Leishmania* species can release proteins and other molecules in extracellular vesicles (EVs) [4–6]. EVs is a generic term used to describe particles spontaneously released by prokaryotic and eukaryotic cells [7]. Deoxyribonucleic acid (DNA), ribonucleic acid (RNA), proteins, lipids, and cellular metabolites are present in EVs that can deliver information from one cell to another [8]. Thus, EVs are now considered a new mechanism of intercellular communication [7].

Leishmania-EVs carry parasites molecules, such as small RNA, heat shock proteins (HSPs), and virulence factors (glycoprotein 63 - GP63 and lipofosfoglican - LPG) [4, 5, 9]. Functional studies showed immunomodulatory and signaling-inducing activities properties of the *Leishmania*-EVs [10]. They are present in the intestinal lumen of sandflies and are regurgitated along with promastigote forms during the blood meal [6]. In addition, these particles modulate the macrophage's activation and alter the course of the parasite infection [4–6, 11]. Although immunomodulatory properties have been demonstrated in experimental models, additional studies are necessary to better understand the role of EVs in the parasite–host relationship. Next, we describe an overview of the extracellular vesicles relevant to *Leishmania* infection and the main findings related to EVs released by *Leishmania* parasites.

2. Extracellular vesicles (EVs): an overview

EVs can be detected in body fluids, including urine, saliva, blood, plasma, amniotic fluid, breast milk, ascites, synovial fluid, and cerebrospinal fluid [7, 12]. Structurally, they present a spherical shape with a double layer composed of lipids and proteins and can be filled with biomolecules from the cell of origin [13]. EVs are classified based on their biogenesis, composition, and size, namely—exosomes, microvesicles (MVs), and apoptotic bodies (ABs) [8, 13]. Although MVs and exosomes show structural similarities, they are different in size, content, lipid composition, and biogenesis [7]. ABs are released by apoptotic cells and have specific characteristics [12] that will not be covered in this review.

Exosomes present sizes between 20 and 100 nm [14]. They are formed by the internal invagination of the endosomal membrane, originating the multivesicular bodies (MVBs) [8]. After maturation, exosomes are secreted by exocytosis via fusion of MBVs with the cell surface, or they may be digested by lysosomes [14, 15]. Exosomes are rich in lipids (mainly phosphatidylserine, cholesterol, and ceramides), nucleic acids, and proteins [8]. In addition, proteins such as endosomal sorting complexes required for transport (ESCRT), Alix, tumor susceptibility gene 101 (TSG101), heat shock cognate 70 (HSC70), HSP90β, HSP60 and HSP70, proteins from the annexin family, and tetraspanins (cluster of differentiation 63 - CD63, CD9, CD81, and CD82) participate in the process of formation of exosomes [8, 16]. These molecules are increased in exosomes, but they are not exclusive markers of these EVs types [7].

MVs are a group of EVs with a diameter between 100 and 1,000 nm [7]. They are originated from the protrusion of the cytoplasmic membrane, and they can carry molecules of cell surface such as membrane receptors, integrins, adhesins, and others [8]. Some studies have shown that structures such as actin and microtubules (cytoskeleton), kinesins and myosins, and soluble NSF attachment receptors (SNAREs) play a role in the formation of MVs [17]. However, the molecular pathway is not well understood [8, 13, 18], and specific markers of MVs have not yet been described. The releasing of MVs and exosomes occurs under physiological cell conditions, but the quantity and content can be altered after stimuli, such as low oxygen and nitrogen content, oxidative stress, among others [4, 5, 19].

Different vesicle isolation techniques have been performed; however, centrifugation/ultracentrifugation and size exclusion chromatography are the most commonly used [7]. Flow cytometry, Western blotting, nanoparticle tracking technique (NTA), mass spectrometry, and electron microscopy have been used to quantify and better characterize the isolated EVs (exosomes and/or MVs) [7]. The inclusion of new methodologies and the discovering of specific EVs markers will bring a new perspective to understand the role of these nanoparticles in the biology and the pathophysiology of several diseases. In addition, there is a great expectation of the applications of EVs in diagnostics, treatments, and vaccine development.

Currently, there is a consensus that EVs play an important role in cell–cell communication being a vehicle for transporting molecules between cells, even cross-kingdom [8, 18, 20]. The effects on the recipient cells depend on the cell type, the origin of EVs, their content, and EVs can act locally and/or systemically. The changes in the recipient cells include modulation of the intracellular signaling pathways, gene regulation, post-transcriptional regulation, activation, or inhibition of different cell types [21–23]. After target cell recognition, EVs can interact with surface receptors, followed by fusion with the plasma membrane for releasing their content, and signaling different intracellular events. However, EVs can also be endocytosed by target cells or collapse after their secretion, delivering their contents into the intracellular space [8, 15].

In parasitic diseases, EVs have brought an exciting field to investigate since they can act as mediators in parasite–host interaction, allowing the transfer of virulence factors and effector molecules from the parasites to the host [24–26]. Parasites EVs are related to the pathogen adhesion, the spread of the parasites, and play a role in regulating the host's immune system. In addition, immune cells infected and/or stimulated with parasite components can release EVs [23] containing messenger RNA (mRNA), small noncoding RNAs (microRNA), chromosomal and mitochondrial DNA, retrotransposons, parasites antigens, and major histocompatibility complex (MHC) I and II [23, 27]. The effects in immunity are diverse, including modulation of innate immune response and antigen presentation.

The production and releasing of EVs by parasites or parasitized cells have been described and characterized in several parasitic infections [25]. For example, in *Leishmania*, several biological markers and virulence factors have been described in EVs released by the parasites [10, 28]. Thus, EVs released by these pathogens can have a role in the disease progression and the host's immune response to the parasite, contributing to the strategy to bypass the immune system.

3. EVs released by *Leishmania spp*

Leishmania species can release proteins and other molecules in EVs. Although the mechanisms for exosome/MVs secretion in *Leishmania* are still unclear, proteomics analysis of EVs has shed light on the functions and properties of these particles. Initial work showed that *Leishmania donovani* could use EVs as a protein transport vehicle [29]. Additional studies confirmed that *L. donovani* releases EVs. *Leishmania major*, *Leishmania mexicana*, and *Leishmania amazonensis* also used EVs as an important mechanism for protein secretion [4, 5, 30]. The presence of EVs in the intestinal lumen of sandflies and their release together with the parasites during the blood meal reinforce the hypothesis that these EVs contribute to the process of infection and development of leishmaniasis [6].

The release of EVs by *Leishmania* is related to the temperature. Promastigotes of *L. mexicana* and *L. donovani* increased the release of EVs after parasite cultivation at 37°C (mammalian host temperature), compared to the EVs obtained from parasites incubated at 26°C (vector temperature) [30]. Furthermore, to *L. donovani*, differences in the content of the EVs obtained at 37°C and 26°C [4] were also observed, suggesting a possible parasite strategy for establishment in the host. However, *L. amazonensis* showed a different pattern in EVs releasing since a higher number of particles were detected after cultivation at 26°C, compared to the parasite incubated at 34°C or 37°C [5]. Altogether these observations suggest that *Leishmania* species can adapt differently to the release of EVs.

Proteomic studies showed the presence of the metalloprotease GP63 in EVs released by *Leishmania* cultivated *in vitro* and by the parasite infecting sandflies. GP63 is the main surface glycoprotein of *Leishmania* and is considered a virulence factor since it contributes to the parasite escape of immune response [31–34]. Evaluating the proteomic profile of EVs released by *Leishmania infantum* in three different phases (logarithmic, stationary, and metacyclic stages) showed that the metacyclic phase had a higher abundance of GP63. In contrast, EVs of parasites in the logarithmic phase had the lowest abundance [35]. In a similar approach, higher concentrations of GP63 were detected in EVs released by *L. infantum* in the stationary phase while parasites in the logarithmic phase showed enrichment of ribosomal proteins [36]. However, proteomic analysis of EVs from *Leishmania infantum chagasi* showed no significant biological differences in EVs released by parasites in logarithmic or stationary phases [37].

Besides GP63, other proteins have already been identified in *L. donovani*-EVs, such as elongation factor-1α (EF-1α), fructose-1,6-bisphosphate aldolase FBA, HSP70, and HSP90 [4]. A comparative study of *L. infantum*-EVs from drug-resistance parasites identified differences in their morphology, size, distribution, and protein content. Identifying proteins related to drug resistance in EVs from resistant parasites can bring new possibilities to predict prognostics and treatments in leishmaniasis [38].

The presence of small noncoding RNAs was identified in EVs released by *L. donovani* and *Leishmania braziliensis*, suggesting the regulatory role of these EVs in the host cells [39]. Additional studies to address the EVs content from different *Leishmania* species may clarify the role of these particles in visceral and cutaneous leishmaniasis. Furthermore, these studies may provide the use of *Leishmania*-EVs in diagnostics, the development of a vaccine, and promising therapeutic alternatives.

4. *Leishmania*-EVs and immune response

Some evidence have pointed that *Leishmania*-EVs present immunomodulatory effects, altering the immune response and contributing to the disease progression. The treatment of human monocytes with *L. donovani*-EVs induced the production of interleukin 10 (IL-10) and inhibited the tumor necrosis factor-alpha (TNF-α) production, even after challenging with interferon-gamma (IFN-γ) [11]. Similar effects were observed in dendritic cells (DC) treated with these EVs since the production of cytokines IL-12p70, TNF-α and IL-10 were inhibited and there was impaired in the ability of these cells to stimulate the differentiation naive CD4 T lymphocytes into T helper 1 (Th1) profile [11]. On the other hand, EVs released by *L. amazonensis* increased the expression of IL-10 and IL-6 in bone marrow-derived macrophages (BMDM) [5]. In fact, EVs released by different *Leishmania* species seem to induce different responses in human macrophages [40]. EVs from *L. infantum* and *L. braziliensis* failed to induce an inflammatory response in human macrophages. However, *L. amazonensis*-EVs stimulated human macrophages to produce nitric oxide (NO), TNF-α, IL-6, and IL-10 via Toll-like receptor 4 (TLR4) and TLR2 (**Figure 1A**) [40].

Few studies have proposed mechanisms of intracellular signaling pathways activated by *Leishmania*-EVs into phagocytes cells. EVs released by *L. amazonensis* amastigotes containing DNA fragments were capable of inducing the CD200 expression in macrophages [41]. The high expression of this molecule leads to the inhibition of NO production, contributing to the parasite survival [41]. In addition, evidence suggests that the composition of EVs can influence the outcome of cell

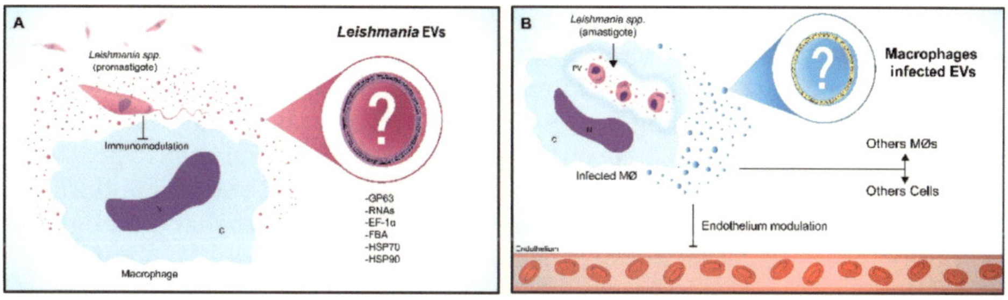

Figure 1.
Leishmania EVs and their influence on the modulation of immune and endothelial cells. (A) Macrophage modulation by EVs released by Leishmania spp. promastigotes. (B) Macrophages infected with Leishmania spp. release EVs with modulating activities. C - cytoplasm; N - nucleus; PV - parasitophorous vacuole; Mϕ(s) – Macrophages.

signaling. *Leishmania* EVs-containing *Leishmania* RNA virus (LRV1) released by *Leishmania guyanensis* trigger TLR3/TRIF (TIR domain-containing adaptor inducing interferon-β signaling), inducing inflammatory cytokines (pro-IL-1b, TNF-a, and IL-12), and the autophagy by impairing NLRP3 (NOD-, LRR and pyrin domain-containing protein 3) inflammasome network [42, 43] (**Figure 1B**). Thus, these initial studies demonstrated a refined and complex intracellular signaling pathway induced by EVs, which depends on the species and evolutionary form that is releasing the EVs and the presence or absence of *Leishmania* virus.

Besides macrophages and DCs, *Leishmania*-EVs can modulate other immune cells. EVs released by *L. infantum* inhibited the expansion of peripheral iNKT (Invariant Natural Killer T) cells and the production of IL-4 and IFN-γ by this cell type [44]. Experiments using CD1d specific ligands (glycolipid α-GalactosylCeramide (α-GalCer) suggest that lipids present in *L. infantum*-EVs and other exocomponents released by the parasites may compete for the CD1 binding site, inhibiting iNKT activation [44]. In addition, our group showed that murine B-1 cells (a subtype of B lymphocytes) stimulated with EVs released by *L. amazonensis* produced higher levels of NO, compared to non-stimulated B-1 cells [45]. The increase in the expression of TLR-9, TNF-α, and transcriptional factors related to the differentiation of B-1 cells to phagocytes are important changes observed in B-1 cells treated with *L. amazonensis*-EVs [45]. These data suggest that *Leishmania*-EVs participate in the modulation of different cells and different levels of the immune response. Interestingly, some mechanisms seem conserved between species, but some specifies are related to *Leishmania* species making comparative studies necessary.

In a mammalian host, *Leishmania* is an intracellular parasite. Thus, studying changes in infected cells can provide important information about the parasite's biology. Silverman et al. [4] showed *Leishmania* exosomes and exosomal proteins in the cytosolic compartment of infected macrophages. In addition, EVs released by macrophages infected with *L. mexicana* containing GP63, and this finding instigated the investigation to uncover the role of these EVs in immunity [46]. Naïve macrophages exposed to EVs from *L. mexicana*-macrophages infected cells induced the activation of mitogen-activated protein (MAP) kinases (except c-Jun N-terminal kinase - JNK) and the nuclear translocation of nuclear factor-κB (NF-κB) and activator protein 1 (AP-1) [46]. BMDM infected with *L. amazonensis* released EVs which were able to activate naive macrophages to produce proinflammatory cytokines IL-12, IL-1β, and TNF-α, contributing both to modulate the immune system in favor of a Th1 immune response and to the elimination of the *Leishmania*, leading, therefore, to the control the infection [47] (**Figure 1B**).

Thus, infected macrophages are able to release EVs that deliver information to activate naïve macrophages, contributing to activate an innate immune response.

Evidence suggests that EVs released by *Leishmania*-infected cells can stimulate different cells, promoting a response against the parasite. EVs released by macrophages infected with *L. donovani* stimulated endothelial cells to produce granulocyte colony-stimulating factor (G-CSF)/CSF-3, and vascular endothelial growth factor A (VEGF-A), promoted an increase in epithelial cell migration and induced endothelial cell tube formation [48] (**Figure 1B**). A study with EVs released by B-1 cells infected with *L. amazonensis* showed the impact of these EVs on naive macrophages activation and the protective effect on the experimental infection with the parasite [49]. Macrophages treated with EVs from infected peritoneal B-1 cells alter the expression of inducible nitric oxide synthase (iNOS), IL-6, IL-10, and TNF-α [49]. Overall, these studies demonstrated that *Leishmania* infection changes the content of EVs from infected cells and suggest that these EVs participate in the activation of immune and nonimmune cells, actively participating in the pathophysiology of the *Leishmania* infection.

5. EVs and leishmaniasis progression

Experimental models have contributed to better understanding the role of EVs in the leishmaniasis progression. The treatment of mice with *L. donovani*-EVs before the parasite infection exacerbated the infection and induced IL-10 production in the spleen [11]. Furthermore, mice treated with *L. major*-EVs before challenge with the parasite showed an increased frequency of IL-4-producing CD4+ T cells in both the spleen and lymph nodes, leading to disease exacerbation [11]. These findings suggest that *Leishmania* EVs are predominantly immunosuppressive and favor the parasite. In fact, our group demonstrated that *L. amazonensis* EVs co-injected with the parasite led to disease exacerbation with a predominance of Th2 response in BALB/c mice [5]. Similar results were observed for *L. major*, but the co-injection of the parasite and related EVs induced an increase in the expression of IL-17 and IL-4 [6].

Changes in the content of EVs may impact the immune response and disease progression [9, 11]. Studies performed with genetically modified parasites showed that in a mouse model of air pouch formation (murine air pouch injection) EVs derived from *L. major* GP63 knockout (KO) (*L. major* GP63$^{-/-}$) induced greater recruitment of inflammatory cells, compared to EVs derived from wild parasites [9]. Furthermore, EVs derived from *L. donovani* exhibited an immunosuppressive effect and exacerbated the disease in animals challenged with the parasite, but EVs derived from *L. donovani* HSP100 KO (*L. donovani* HSP100$^{-/-}$) were able to induce a pro-inflammatory response and did not exacerbate the disease [11]. Thus, the hypothesis that EVs derived from parasites with different virulence profiles (virulent and attenuated) present relevant alterations in their protein content and can induce distinct immune responses in an experimental immunization model cannot be discarded.

The relevance of EVs in *Leishmania* infection's biology was shown by the demonstration that *Leishmania* promastigotes release EVs in the sandflies [6]. The experimental infection with *L. major* in the presence of EVs released by the parasite in the vector led to higher lesion size and parasite load, associated with impaired effector immune response [6]. Taken together, the *in vivo* studies suggest that EVs released by *Leishmania* participate in the infection, favoring the establishment of the parasite and the progression of the disease.

6. Conclusions

The knowledge acquired studying EVs has allowed understanding that these particles are related to intercellular communication and cross-kingdom relationship. The release of these EVs by *Leishmania* is related to initial infection, modulation of the immune system, and disease progression in the host (**Table 1**). However, several aspects of the biology and physiology of these molecules still need to be better investigated. Would releasing these EVs into the vector be related to the parasite's adaptation to that environment? Can EVs contribute to parasite multiplication in the vector? Is there population regulation and/or transfer of resistance factors and immune response escape by EVs between different *Leishmania* species? Do these transfers occur in the vector and/or in the mammalian host? Can vesicles released by *Leishmania* be used for the development of vaccines and new diagnostic approaches? Thus, the field of EVs released by *Leishmania* and other pathogens is fascinating and, there will be significant advances and contributions to the area in the future with the discovery of new therapeutic targets and new players in the host–parasite relationship.

Leishmania species	Biological function	Reference
L. donovani	• Increased IL-10 and inhibited TNF-α production by human monocytes; • Inhibited IL-12p70, TNF-α, and IL-10 production by DC; • Impaired the ability of DC to drive T cells differentiation into Th1; • In experimental infection: exacerbated the infection; promoted IL-10 production in the spleen.	[11]
L. amazonensis	• Increased the expression of IL-10 and IL-6 in BMDM; • In experimental infection: led to disease exacerbation with a predominance of Th2 response in BALB/c mice;	[5]
	• Increased the production of NO, TNF-α, IL-6, and IL-10 via TLR4 and TLR2 by human monocytes;	[40]
	• In B-1 cells: increased NO production; increased expression of TLR-9 and TNF-α; induced the expression of factors related to myeloid commitment;	[45]
	• Increased the CD200 expression and inhibited the NO production (EVs released by amastigotes)	[41]
L. guyanensis infected with *Leishmania* RNA Virus (LRV1)	• Triggered TLR3/TRIF signaling; • Impaired NLRP3 inflammasome network	[42]
L. infantum	• Inhibited iNKT activation and production of IL-4 and IFN-γ by these cells;	[44]
L. major	• In experimental infection: • Increased the disease progression; • Increased the expression of IL-17 and IL-4	[10]

Table 1.
Biological effects of the EVs released by different Leishmania species.

Acknowledgements

This work was supported by Fundação de Amparo à Pesquisa do Estado de São Paulo (grant number 2019/21614-3). Scholarships were provided by the Fundação de Amparo à Pesquisa do Estado de São Paulo (2021/01556-9), Conselho Nacional de Desenvolvimento Científico e Tecnológico (CNPq), and Coordenação de Aperfeiçoamento de Pessoal de Nível Superior (CAPES).

Conflict of interest

The authors declare no conflict of interest.

Author details

Rogéria Cristina Zauli[1,2]†, Andrey Sladkevicius Vidal[2]†, Talita Vieira Dupin[2], Aline Correia Costa de Morais[2], Wagner Luiz Batista[2] and Patricia Xander[2*]

1 Technical Support Center for Teaching, Research and Extension (NATEPE), Federal University of São Paulo, Campus Diadema, Diadema, Brazil

2 Laboratory of Cellular Immunology and Biochemistry of Fungi and Protozoa, Department of Pharmaceutical Sciences, Federal University of São Paulo, Campus Diadema, Diadema, Brazil

*Address all correspondence to: patricia.xander@unifesp.br

† These authors have contributed equally to this work.

References

[1] Burza S, Croft SL, Boelaert M, Leishmaniasis. Lancet. 2018;**392**: 951-970. DOI: 10.1016/S0140-6736(18)31204-2

[2] Scott P, Novais FO, Cutaneous leishmaniasis: Immune responses in protection and pathogenesis. Nature Reviews Immunology. 2016;**16(9)**: 581-592. DOI: 10.1038/NRI.2016.72

[3] de Morais CG, Castro Lima AK, Terra R, dos Santos RF, Da-Silva SA, Dutra PM. The Dialogue of the Host-Parasite Relationship: *Leishmania* spp. and *Trypanosoma cruzi* Infection. BioMed Research International. 2015;**2015**:324915. DOI: 10.1155/2015/324915

[4] Silverman JM, Clos J, de'Oliveira CC, Shirvani O, Fang Y, Wang C, et al. An exosome-based secretion pathway is responsible for protein export from *Leishmania* and communication with macrophages. Journal of Cell Science. 2010;**123**:842-852. DOI: 10.1242/jcs.056465

[5] Barbosa FMC, Dupin TV, Toledo MDS, Reis NFDC, Ribeiro K, Cronemberger-Andrade A, et al. Extracellular vesicles released by *Leishmania (Leishmania) amazonensis* promote disease progression and induce the production of different cytokines in macrophages and B-1 cells. Frontiers in Microbiology. 2018;**9**:3056. DOI: 10.3389/fmicb.2018.03056

[6] Atayde VD, Aslan H, Townsend S, Hassani K, Kamhawi S, Olivier M. Exosome secretion by the parasitic protozoan *Leishmania* within the sand fly midgut. Cell Reports. 2015;**13**(5):957-967. DOI: 10.1016/j.celrep.2015.09.058

[7] Théry C, Witwer KW, Aikawa E, Alcaraz MJ, Anderson JD, Andriantsitohaina R, et al. Minimal information for studies of extracellular vesicles 2018 (MISEV2018): A position statement of the International Society for Extracellular Vesicles and update of the MISEV2014 guidelines. Journal of Extracellular Vesicles. 2018;**7**(1): 1535750. DOI: 10.1080/20013078.2018.1535750

[8] van Niel G, D'Angelo G, Raposo G. Shedding light on the cell biology of extracellular vesicles. Nature Reviews Molecular Cell Biology. 2018;**19**(4): 213-228. DOI: 10.1038/nrm.2017.125

[9] Hassani K, Shio MT, Martel C, Faubert D, Olivier M. Absence of metalloprotease GP63 alters the protein content of *Leishmania* exosomes. PLoS ONE. 2014;**9**(4):e95007. DOI: 10.1371/journal.pone.0095007

[10] Atayde VD, Hassani K, da Silva Lira Filho A, Borges AR, Adhikari A, Martel C, et al. *Leishmania* exosomes and other virulence factors: Impact on innate immune response and macrophage functions. Cellular Immunology. 2016;**309**:7-18. DOI: 10.1016/j.cellimm.2016.07.013

[11] Silverman JM, Clos J, Horakova E, Wang AY, Wiesgigl M, Kelly I, et al. *Leishmania* exosomes modulate innate and adaptive immune responses through effects on monocytes and dendritic cells. Journal of Immunology. 2010; **185**(9):5011-5022. DOI: 10.4049/jimmunol.1000541

[12] Battistelli M, Falcieri E. Apoptotic bodies: Particular extracellular vesicles involved in intercellular communication. Biology (Basel). 2020;**9**(1):21. DOI: 10.3390/biology9010021

[13] Raposo G, Stoorvogel W. Extracellular vesicles: Exosomes, microvesicles, and friends. The Journal of Cell Biology. 2013;**200**:373-383. DOI: 10.1083/jcb.201211138

[14] Tkach M, Théry C. Communication by extracellular vesicles: Where we are

and where we need to go. Cell 2016; **164**(6):1226-1232. DOI: 10.1016/j.cell.2016.01.043

[15] Meldolesi J. Exosomes and ectosomes in intercellular communication. Current Biology. 2018;**28**(8):R435-RR44. DOI: 10.1016/j.cub.2018.01.059

[16] Kowal J, Arras G, Colombo M, Jouve M, Morath JP, Primdal-Bengtson B, et al. Proteomic comparison defines novel markers to characterize heterogeneous populations of extracellular vesicle subtypes. Proceedings of the National Academy of Sciences of the United States of America. 2016;**113**(8):E968-E977. DOI: 10.1073/pnas.1521230113

[17] Cai H, Reinisch K, Ferro-Novick S. Coats, tethers, Rabs, and SNAREs work together to mediate the intracellular destination of a transport vesicle. Developmental Cell. 2007;**12**(5):671-682. DOI: 10.1016/j.devcel.2007.04.005

[18] Yáñez-Mó M, Siljander PR, Andreu Z, Zavec AB, Borràs FE, Buzas EI, et al. Biological properties of extracellular vesicles and their physiological functions. Journal of Extracellular Vesicles. 2015;**4**:27066. DOI: 10.3402/jev.v4.27066

[19] Gavinho B, Sabatke B, Feijoli V, Rossi IV, da Silva JM, Evans-Osses I, et al. Peptidylarginine deiminase inhibition abolishes the production of large extracellular vesicles from *Giardia intestinalis*, Affecting host-pathogen interactions by hindering adhesion to host cells, Frontiers in Cellular Infection Microbiology. 2020;**10**:417. DOI: 10.3389/fcimb.2020.00417

[20] Schorey JS, Cheng Y, Singh PP, Smith VL. Exosomes and other extracellular vesicles in host-pathogen interactions. EMBO Reports. 2015;**16**(1):24-43. DOI: 10.15252/embr.201439363

[21] Campos JH, Soares RP, Ribeiro K, Andrade AC, Batista WL, Torrecilhas AC. Extracellular vesicles: Role in inflammatory responses and potential uses in vaccination in cancer and infectious diseases. Journal of Immunology Research. 2015;**2015**:832057. DOI: 10.1155/2015/832057

[22] Dong G, Filho AL, Olivier M. Modulation of host-pathogen communication by extracellular vesicles (EVs) of the protozoan parasite. Frontiers in Cellular and Infection Microbiology. 2019;**9**:100. DOI: 10.3389/fcimb.2019.00100

[23] Khosravi M, Mirsamadi ES, Mirjalali H, Zali MR. Isolation and functions of extracellular vesicles derived from parasites: The promise of a new era in immunotherapy, vaccination, and diagnosis. International Journal of Nanomedicine. 2020;**15**:2957-2969. DOI: 10.2147/IJN.S250993

[24] Montaner S, Galiano A, Trelis M, Martin-Jaular L, Del Portillo HA, Bernal D, et al. The role of extracellular vesicles in modulating the host immune response during parasitic infections. Frontiers in Immunology. 2014;**5**:433. DOI: 10.3389/fimmu.2014.00433

[25] Marcilla A, Martin-Jaular L, Trelis M, de Menezes-Neto A, Osuna A, Bernal D, et al. Extracellular vesicles in parasitic diseases. Journal of Extracelluar Vesicles. 2014;**3**:25040. DOI: 10.3402/jev.v3.25040

[26] Soares R, Xander P, Costa A, Marcilla A, Menezes-Neto A, Del Portillo H, et al. Highlights of the São Paulo ISEV workshop on extracellular vesicles in cross-kingdom communication. Journal of Extracellular Vesicles. 2017;**6**(1):1407213. DOI: 10.1080/20013078.2017.1407213

[27] Jeppesen DK, Fenix AM, Franklin JL, Higginbotham JN, Zhang Q, Zimmerman LJ, et al.

Reassessment of exosome composition. Cell. 2019;**177**(2):428-445. DOI: 10.1016/j.cell.2019.02.029

[28] Lambertz U, Silverman JM, Nandan D, McMaster WR, Clos J, Foster LJ, et al. Secreted virulence factors and immune evasion in visceral leishmaniasis. Journal of Leukocyte Biology. 2012;**91**(6):887-899. DOI: 10.1189/jlb.0611326

[29] Silverman JM, Chan SK, Robinson DP, Dwyer DM, Nandan D, Foster LJ, et al. Proteomic analysis of the secretome of *Leishmania donovani*. Genome Biology. 2008;**9**(2):R35. DOI: 10.1186/gb-2008-9-2-r35

[30] Hassani K, Antoniak E, Jardim A, Olivier M. Temperature-induced protein secretion by *Leishmania mexicana* modulates macrophage signalling and function. PLoS ONE. 2011;**6**(5):e18724. DOI: 10.1371/journal.pone.0018724

[31] Gomez MA, Contreras I, Hallé M, Tremblay ML, McMaster RW, Olivier M. *Leishmania* GP63 alters host signaling through cleavage-activated protein tyrosine phosphatases. Sci Signal. 2009;**2**(90):ra58. DOI: 10.1126/scisignal.2000213

[32] Hallé M, Gomez MA, Stuible M, Shimizu H, McMaster WR, Olivier M, et al. The *Leishmania* surface protease GP63 cleaves multiple intracellular proteins and actively participates in p38 mitogen-activated protein kinase inactivation. The Journal of Biological Chemistry. 2009;**284**(11):6893-6908. DOI: 10.1074/jbc.M805861200

[33] Isnard A, Shio MT, Olivier M. Impact of *Leishmania* metalloprotease GP63 on macrophage signaling. Frontiers in Cellular and Infection Microbiology. 2012;**2**:72. DOI: 10.3389/fcimb.2012.00072

[34] Olivier M, Atayde VD, Isnard A, Hassani K, Shio MT. *Leishmania* virulence factors: Focus on the metalloprotease GP63. Microbes and Infection. 2012;**14**(15):1377-1389. DOI: 10.1016/j.micinf.2012.05.014

[35] Marshall S, Kelly PH, Singh BK, Pope RM, Kim P, Zhanbolat B, et al. Extracellular release of virulence factor major surface protease via exosomes in *Leishmania infantum* promastigotes. Parasites & Vectors. 2018;**11**(1):355. DOI: 10.1186/s13071-018-2937-y

[36] Santarém N, Racine G, Silvestre R, Cordeiro-da-Silva A, Ouellette M. Exoproteome dynamics in *Leishmania infantum*. Journal of Proteomics. 2013;**84**:106-118. DOI: 10.1016/j.jprot.2013.03.012

[37] Forrest DM, Batista M, Marchini FK, Tempone AJ, Traub-Csekö YM. Proteomic analysis of exosomes derived from procyclic and metacyclic-like cultured *Leishmania infantum chagasi*. Journal of Proteomics. 2020; **227**:103902. DOI: 10.1016/j.jprot.2020.103902

[38] Douanne N, Dong G, Douanne M, Olivier M, Fernandez-Prada C. Unravelling the proteomic signature of extracellular vesicles released by drug-resistant *Leishmania infantum* parasites. PLoS Neglected Tropical Diseases. 2020;**14**(7):e0008439. DOI: 10.1371/journal.pntd.0008439

[39] Lambertz U, Oviedo Ovando ME, Vasconcelos EJ, Unrau PJ, Myler PJ, Reiner NE. Small RNAs derived from tRNAs and rRNAs are highly enriched in exosomes from both old and new world *Leishmania* providing evidence for conserved exosomal RNA Packaging. BMC Genomics. 2015;**16**:151. DOI: 10.1186/s12864-015-1260-7

[40] Nogueira PM, de Menezes-Neto A, Borges VM, Descoteaux A, Torrecilhas AC, Xander P, et al. Immunomodulatory Properties of *leishmania* extracellular vesicles during

host-parasite interaction: Differential activation of TLRs and NF-κB translocation by dermotropic and viscerotropic species. Frontiers in Cellular and Infection Microbiology. 2020;**10**:380. DOI: 10.3389/fcimb.2020.00380

[41] Sauter IP, Madrid KG, de Assis JB, Sá-Nunes A, Torrecilhas AC, Staquicini DI, et al. TLR9/MyD88/TRIF signaling activates host immune inhibitory CD200 in *Leishmania* infection. JCI Insight. 2019;**4**(10). DOI: 10.1172/jci.insight.126207

[42] de Carvalho RVH, Lima-Junior DS, da Silva MVG, Dilucca M, Rodrigues TS, Horta CV, et al. *Leishmania* RNA virus exacerbates Leishmaniasis by subverting innate immunity via TLR3-mediated NLRP3 inflammasome inhibition. Nature Communications. 2019;**10**(1):5273. DOI: 10.1038/s41467-019-13356-2

[43] Olivier M, Zamboni DS. *Leishmania Viannia guyanensis*, LRV1 virus and extracellular vesicles: A dangerous trio influencing the faith of immune response during muco-cutaneous leishmaniasis. Current Opinion in Immunology. 2020;**66**:108-113. DOI: 10.1016/j.coi.2020.08.004

[44] Belo R, Santarém N, Pereira C, Pérez-Cabezas B, Macedo F, Leite-de-Moraes M, et al. Exoproducts Inhibit Human Invariant NKT Cell Expansion and Activation. Frontiers in Immunology. 2017;**8**:710. DOI: 10.3389/fimmu.2017.00710

[45] Reis NFC, Dupin TV, Costa CR, Toledo MDS, de Oliveira VC, Popi AF, et al. Promastigotes or extracellular vesicles modulate B-1 cell activation and differentiation. Frontiers in Cellular and Infection Microbiology. 2020;**10**:573813. DOI: 10.3389/fcimb.2020.573813

[46] Hassani K, Olivier M. Immunomodulatory impact of *leishmania*-induced macrophage exosomes: A comparative proteomic and functional analysis. PLoS Neglected Tropical Diseases. 2013;**7**(5):e2185. DOI: 10.1371/journal.pntd.0002185

[47] Cronemberger-Andrade A, Aragão-França L, de Araujo CF, Rocha VJ, Borges-Silva MaC, Figueira CP, et al. Extracellular vesicles from *Leishmania*-infected macrophages confer an anti-infection cytokine-production profile to naïve macrophages. PLoS Neglected Tropical Diseases. 2014;**8**(9):e3161. DOI: 10.1371/journal.pntd.0003161

[48] Gioseffi A, Hamerly T, Van K, Zhang N, Dinglasan RR, Yates PA, et al. Leishmania-infected macrophages release extracellular vesicles that can promote lesion development. Life Science Alliance. 2020;**3**(12):e202000742. DOI: 10.26508/lsa.202000742

[49] Toledo MDS, Cronemberger-Andrade A, Barbosa FMC, Reis NFC, Dupin TV, Soares RP, et al. Effects of extracellular vesicles released by peritoneal B-1 cells on experimental *Leishmania (Leishmania) amazonensis* infection. Journal of Leukocyte Biology. 2020;**108**(6):1803-1814. DOI: 10.1002/JLB.3MA0220-464RR

Section 2

Medicine

Chapter 4

Treatment of Leishmaniasis

R. Sivayogana, Aishwarya Krishnakumar, S. Kumaravel, Rajesh Rajagopal and P. Ravikanth

Abstract

Treatment of Leishmaniasis is always not satisfactory despite advancement all these years. This chapter will discuss the standard treatment options like Amphotericin, oral miltefosine, topical paromycin, add more details about newer emerging drugs and alternative therapies, surgical treatment modalities for resistant cases. Will discuss few information regarding vaccines. Special precautions to be taken while travelling to endemic areas will be discussed. Management protocol for mucocutaneous and visceral type will be highlighted. Side-effects of drugs used in the treatment of Leishmaniasis will be discussed in short and measures to monitor these side effects will be discussed. Long term monitoring of relapse will also be discussed.

Keywords: leishmaniasis, treatment, amphotericin B, miltefosine, pentavalent antimonials

1. Introduction

The main goal of treatment is parasite eradication and clinical healing. Generally, parasite eradication is seen long before clinical re-epithelialization. Treatment for each case varies so it needs to be individualised depending upon various factors affecting the treatment outcome [1] (**Table 1**). The clinical manifestation of leishmaniasis can be broadly classified as cutaneous and visceral types. In this chapter, treatment for various clinical manifestations will be discussed in detail.

Host	Agent	Environment
Age of patient	Various species of parasite	Geographic region (endemicity)
Immune status	Drug resistance	Cost and availability of treatment
Nutritional status	Tissue tropism	
Genetic background		
Presence of intercurrent disease (e.g.; HIV infection)		
Site and severity of infection		
Toxicity of therapeutic options		

Table 1.
Factors affecting the treatment outcome.

IntechOpen

2. Treatment of leishmaniasis

Choice of treatment depends on the clinical presentation. Treatment options vary from a mere observation in spontaneously healing lesions, topical/local therapy and parenteral treatment.

Old world leishmaniasis caused by *Leishmania major* resolves spontaneously in 2–4 months whereas *Leishmania tropica* resolves by 6–15 months. New World leishmaniasis caused by resolves spontaneously in 3–4 months in 75% of cases [2]. Single lesions can be managed with local treatment options like heat therapy, cryotherapy and topical preparations. For cutaneous and mucocutaneous lesions, the drugs of choice are pentavalent antimony and miltefosine. Amphotericin B is considered the drug of choice for visceral leishmaniasis (**Table 2**).

Cutaneous leishmaniasis	
Drugs of choice	• Sodium stibogluconate • Miltefosine
Alternatives	**Systemic** • Liposomal amphotericin • Amphotericin B • Pentamidine • Fluconazole **Topicals -** • Paromomycin 15% and MBCL 12% ointment • Paromomycin 15% and gentamicin 0.5% cream • Heat therapy • Cryotherapy with liquid nitrogen **Intralesional Alternatives** • sodium stibogluconate (Pentostam) • meglumine antimoniate (Glucantime)
Mucocutaneous leishmaniasis	
Drugs of choice	Sodium stibogluconate Liposomal amphotericin Amphotericin B Miltefosine
Alternative	Pentamidine
Visceral leishmaniasis	
Drugs of choice	liposomal amphotericin B
Alternatives	Miltefosine Paromomycin Pentavalent antimonials Amphotericin B

Table 2.
Treatment recommendations for leishmaniasis.

3. Indications of systemic treatment

1. Lesions over face, genitalia, over joints

2. Mucosal lesions

3. Immunocompromised host

4. Single lesion >5 cm in size

5. > 4 lesions (~1 cm in size)

6. Persistent, progressive, deep, sporotrichoid, and secondarily infected lesions

7. Markedly enlarged lymph nodes

8. New World leishmaniasis caused by *Leishmania braziliensis* complex

Drugs used in systemic treatment

4. Pentavalent antimonials

The pentavalent antimonials [3] are the drug of choice for the treatment of cutaneous leishmaniasis (both old world and new world). Given as a single daily dose via the intravenous or intramuscular route. It is used only in areas (East Africa, Central Asia and South America) where the species causing the disease are still sensitive to this drug.

4.1 Drugs and dose

Sodium stibogluconate (Pentostam) IM/IV 20 mg/kg/day for 15 to 20 days.
Meglumine antimoniate (Glucantime) IM/IV 20 mg/kg/day for 20 days.

4.2 Mechanism of action

Leishmania amastigote converts the pentavalent form of SSG to a toxic trivalent form by a specific reductase enzyme. This in turn promotes the efflux of glutathione and reduced thiols within the parasite and increases oxidative damage. Other action includes inhibition of glycolysis and oxidation of fatty acids of the parasite. Accumulation of SSG within macrophages is responsible for its prolonged inhibitory action against the parasite.

4.3 Adverse events

The most serious side effects are cardiotoxicity and nephrotoxicity. Most patients on antimony will develop pancreatitis (either subclinical or severe abdominal pain). The dose-dependent side effects include pain at the injection site, myalgia, hepatitis, bone marrow suppression, QT prolongation, headache, fatigue, rash, and nausea, vomiting, metallic taste. These problems resolve with a reduction in the dose of antimonial. Other side-effects include sterile abscess, stiffness in the injected muscle, mental symptoms.

Relative contraindication: >60% resistance is seen in species in India and Nepal, hence not used as a first-line drug.

5. Oral miltefosine

This drug [4] is a derivative of alkyl phosphocholine with potent activity against leishmaniasis. It is the FDA-approved drug for the treatment of mucosal and visceral leishmaniasis due to *L. braziliensis, Leishmania guyanensis, and Leishmania panamensis.*

Dose (Table 3).

Available as 10 and 50 mg capsules.

Dose-1.5 to 2.5 mg/kg/day for 28 days orally up to 150 mg/day.

Weight	Dose
Adult >50 kgs	150 mg/day
Adult >12 years weighing >25 kgs	50 mg BID
Adult >12 years weighing <25 kgs	50 mg OD
Children (2–11 years)	2.5 mg/kg/day (as 10 mg capsules)

Table 3.
Dose of miltefosine according to age and bodyweight.

5.1 Mechanism of action

As a phosphocholine analogue, it is thought to interfere with cell-signalling pathways, and it may interfere with parasite lipid biosynthetic enzyme synthesis. Mutation limiting the transport of drug into cell membrane can cause resistance to its action. This can be overcome by combination treatment with liposomal Amp B or paromomycin.

5.2 Adverse events

Diarrhoea, anorexia, nausea, vomiting, reproductive toxicity in animals. These are common reactions during the first week of treatment so the drug should be taken in divided doses with meals to diminish nausea, vomiting, diarrhoea. Miltefosine is known to cause reversible nephrotoxicity and hepatotoxicity, hence monitoring (once a week) of renal and liver function tests is recommended during the treatment period.

5.3 Contraindications

Pregnancy (teratogenic) and lactation. The female patient should avoid pregnancy during and till 3 months after stopping treatment.

6. Amphotericin B (AMB)

Amphotericin B [5] is the first-line drug for visceral leishmaniasis and the second choice of drug for mucocutaneous leishmaniasis. Can be used in leishmaniasis associated with HIV disease, pregnancy and breastfeeding patients.

6.1 Dose and formulations

This drug is available in two forms- a less expensive formulation with deoxycholate (AMB-DOC) and a highly expensive form incorporated with liposomes (L-AMB). Since the toxicity is less with L-AMB it is most commonly used for treatment and research purposes.

6.2 Dose of L-AMB

Indian subcontinent: 10 mg/kg or 3 mg/kg/day for 5 consecutive days (total 15 mg/kg).

Mediterranean region: Two infusions of 10 mg/kg for children was found to be successful.

Other regions: Total dose of 18-21 mg/kg.

6.3 Mechanism of action

Binding to sterols present in parasite's membrane causing a change in permeability. This drug highly concentrates in the reticuloendothelial cells in the spleen and liver, hence best suited for visceral leishmaniasis.

6.4 Adverse events

Infusion reaction like fever, chills, pain all over the body, dyspnoea occurs due to raised cytokines levels of Interleukin and TNF- alpha. Other side effects of amphotericin include nephrotoxicity, hypokalaemia and anaemia. Liposomal amphotericin is less toxic than amphotericin.

7. Paromomycin

It is an [6] aminoglycoside antibiotic that has been tried in the treatment of visceral leishmaniasis in India and Africa. It shows a promising cure in areas with species resistant to SSG. Moreover, it is less expensive, easy to administer than AMB.

Dose: 11 mg/kg/day given as intramuscular injection for 21 days.

Adverse drug effect: ototoxicity, injection site pain, the reversible elevation of serum transaminase, renal toxicity (rare).

Adverse effects and laboratory monitoring of the above mentioned drugs has been discussed in (**Table 4**).

Drug	Adverse events	Laboratory Monitoring for toxicity
Amphotericin B	Infusion related reactions, hypokalaemia, hypomagnesemia, nephrotoxicity and anaemia	CBC, RFT, LFT, serum electrolytes. ECG and urinalysis –baseline and twice weekly.
Liposomal amphotericin B	Same as above but better tolerated than amphotericin B. Infusion related reactions to liposomal amphotericin B also can be caused by pseudollergy due to liposome induced complement activation	Same as above
Pentavalent antimonials: 1. sodium stibogluconate 2. meglumine antimoniate	1. Myalgia, large joint arthralgia, headache, malaise, fatigue, anorexia, nausea commonly noted as treatment progresses. 2. Laboratory abnormalities are usually reversible includes elevated Aminotransferases, lipase/amylase values. 3. ECG abnormalities (e.g. Non-specific ST-T wave changes, QTc prolongation) 4. Pancytopenia	Baseline and weekly monitoring of serum chemistry values (Aminotransferases, lipase/amylase, potassium, creatinine, BUN, glucose), CBC and ECG
Miltefosine	GI symptoms, dizziness/motion sickness, scrotal pain, decreased or absent ejaculate, nephrotoxicity, hepatotoxicity	Renal function, hepatic function and CBC –baseline and weekly monitoring

Table 4.
Adverse effects and laboratory monitoring of major anti-leishmanial drugs.

8. Combination therapy

A combination of two drugs [7] in the treatment of leishmaniasis has been tried to overcome the drug resistance, to achieve higher efficacy and cure rate, for better compliance and to reduce the overall dose, cost and side effect of each drug.

The following 3 combinations have been tested in various studies:

1. L-AMB (5 mg/kg daily as single i.v dose) + oral miltefosine daily for 7 days

2. L-AMB (5 mg/kg daily as single i.v dose) + Paromomycin (i.m) daily for 10 days

3. Oral miltefosine daily for 7 days + Paromomycin (i.m) daily for 10 days

9. Other miscellaneous drugs used in the treatment of leishmaniasis

Antimony resistance can be overcome by combining antimonials with paromomycin, pentoxifylline, allopurinol, IFN-γ, granulocyte-macrophage colony-stimulating factor, azithromycin and topical imiquimod.

Pentamidine

It causes the inhibition [8] of the active transport system and the mitochondrial topoisomerase II which in turn leads to parasitic death.
Dose: 2 to 4 mg/kg/day IM or IV on alternate days for 4 to 7 days.

Adverse events

Hypotension and hypoglycaemia are serious side effects of this drug. Hence it is recommended in antimony-resistant/ contraindicated or when serious hepatic or cardiac side-effects occur during antimonial therapy.

Oral azoles

Mechanism of action- Azoles block ergosterol synthesis and cause the accumulation of 14-methyl sterols leading to inhibition of leishmaniasis growth.

DOSE: Fluconazole 200 mg daily for 6 weeks.
Ketoconazole 600 mg daily for 28 days (not used now).

Allopurinol

A combination of a low dose of meglumine antimoniate (30 mg/kg/day) with allopurinol (20 mg/kg/day) was found to be effective in the treatment of cutaneous leishmaniasis. The addition of allopurinol increases the antimonial effect of meglumine antimonials [9].

Doxycycline

Doxycycline, [10] though it's not the first choice of medication, still is considered equally efficacious to pentavalent antimony. It is known to have good intracellular penetration and acts directly on the body of leishmania. Due to its anti-inflammatory effect, there will be immediate relief in signs of local inflammation. Oral route of administration, low cost, easy availability and ack of major adverse effects, make doxycycline a good alternative option in the treatment of leishmaniasis. It is given in the dose of 200 mg/day.

Azithromycin

The efficacy of [11] azithromycin is questionable. It has been used in children, pregnant females and elderly patients when other classical drugs are contraindicated. Dose of 500 mg daily for 10 days, repeated every 1 to 2 months. Total of 3–4 cycles given.

Zinc sulphate

It acts by Boosting of Th1 reaction as well as phagocytosis of parasites.
Dose-2.5 to 10 mg/kg/day orally for 30 to 40 days.

Others: Rifampicin, dapsone, terbinafine, metronidazole, cotrimoxazole, nifurtimox, quinolones, pyrimethamine, anti-IL10 has been reported in the treatment of leishmaniasis [12].

10. Drugs used in topical therapy

1. Paromomycin 15% and MBCL (methyl benzethonium chloride)12% ointment

It is applied topically twice a day for 10 days and the cycle is repeated after 10 days of the waiting period. Methlybenzethonium itself has some antileishmanial activity and it helps in the penetration of paromomycin. Topical preparation may cause local inflammation [13].

2. Paromomycin 15% and gentamicin 0.5% cream

Applied topically once a day for 20 days [14].

11. Heat therapy

This treatment [15] is done in a single session. Under aseptic precautions, the lesion is anaesthetized with 2% lidocaine. With the ThermoSurgery instrument (fork-like applicator), heat is applied at 50° C for 30 seconds. This will cover an area of 3x 4 mm. Then the applicator is moved to an adjacent area and the same heat is applied, this process is continued until the lesion is fully covered. The entire session takes about 4-5 min. The lesion should then be covered with a gauze bandage. This is FDA approved for the treatment of cutaneous leishmaniasis.

12. Cryotherapy with liquid nitrogen

Freeze (15–20 secs) thaw (20-60secs) freeze (15-20 sec) cycle is followed until 1-2 mm of normal circumferential skin is frozen. A total of 3 applications will be given once in 3 weeks.

13. Intralesional antimonial therapy

Sodium stibogluconate (100 mg antimony/ml) or meglumine antimoniate is injected into all sides of the lesion until it blanches on alternate days. A total of 10 injections is given. This treatment is combined with cryotherapy for better results [16]

Other local therapy options: Surgical excision, curettage, laser ablation, photodynamic therapy, sodium chloride (moist wound therapy), topical azoles, topical glyceryl trinitrate, topical amphotericin B, intralesional interferon-gamma and intralesional metronidazole [17].

14. Assessing response to treatment

Clinical symptoms will take time to improve in cutaneous leishmaniasis. Time taken vary from patient to patient. After effective treatment, it takes around 4 to 6 weeks for the ulcer to show signs of healing, which includes re-epithelialization, reduction in the size of the ulcer, reduction of signs of local inflammation. Healing continues till 12 weeks' time, at which decisions about continued observation versus retreatment should be made. Because of the chances of relapse in cutaneous leishmaniasis, complete responses are not measured until 6 to 12 months after successful therapy.

15. Treatment of leishmaniasis in returned traveller

Intravenous or intralesional treatment with sodium stibogluconate and other less frequently used agents resulted in resolution for most of these patients. Avoiding blood donation for 1 year is recommended in travellers from endemic areas with a history or suspicion of leishmaniasis [18].

16. Prevention of leishmaniasis

The first step in prevention is promotion and use of personal protective measures like use of protective clothing (wear long-sleeved shirts, long pants, and socks), usage of permethrin-treated bed nets, insect repellents containing 30–35% N, N-diethyl-3-methylbenzamide (DEET); avoid visits to endemic areas; staying indoors in the evening as during this time the sandflies are most active.

17. Vaccines

Preventive [19] vaccines are the best and most cost-effective protective measure against pathogens and are saving millions of lives every year around the world. The development of the *Leishmania* vaccine has proven to be a difficult and challenging task, because of the inadequate knowledge of parasite pathogenesis and the complex immune responses needed for protection. Killed/live attenuated / plasmid DNA based vaccines with or without bacilli Calmette-Guerin seems to be useful in endemic areas. But none of the vaccines is FDA approved for safe prophylactic use in humans. A vaccine for dogs is available and approved.

Author details

R. Sivayogana*, Aishwarya Krishnakumar, S. Kumaravel, Rajesh Rajagopal and P. Ravikanth
Meenakshi Medical College Hospital and Research Institute, Kanchipuram, Tamilnadu, India

*Address all correspondence to: drsivayogananew1@gmail.com

References

[1] Von Stebut E. Leishmaniasis and other protozoan infections. In: Kang S, Amagai M, Bruckner AL, Enk AH, Margolis DJ, McMichael AJ, et al., editors. Fitzpatrick's Dermatology. 9th ed. New York: McGraw-Hill Publishing; 2019. pp. 3228-3231

[2] Downing C, Tyring S. Parasitic disease. In: Burns T, Breathnach S, Neil C, Griffiths C, editors. Rook's Textbook of Dermatology. 9th ed. West Susex: Blackwell Publishing Ltd; 2012. pp. 1061-1064

[3] Arevalo J, Ramirez L, Adaui V, Zimic M, Tulliano G, Miranda-Verástegui C, et al. Influence of Leishmania (Viannia) species on the response to antimonial treatment in patients with American tegumentary leishmaniasis. Journal of Infectious Diseases. 2007;**195**(12):1846-1851. DOI: 10.1086/518041

[4] Soto J, Arana BA, Toledo J, et al. Miltefosine for new world cutaneous leishmaniasis. Clinical Infectious Disease. 2004;**38**:1266-1272

[5] Tripathi KD. Essentials of Medical Pharmacology. 8th ed. New Delhi, India: Jaypee Brothers Medical; 2018

[6] Wiwanitkit V. Interest in paromomycin for the treatment of visceral leishmaniasis (kala-azar). Therapeutics and Clinical Risk Management. 2012;**8**:323-328

[7] Van Griensven J, Balasegaram M, Meheus F, Alvar J, Lynen L, Boelaert M. Combination therapy for visceral leishmaniasis. The Lancet Infectious Diseases. 2010 Mar;**10**(3):184-194

[8] Yang G, Choi G, No JH. Antileishmanial mechanism of diamidines involves targeting kinetoplasts. Antimicrobial Agents and Chemotherapy. 21 Oct 2016;**60**(11):6828-6836

[9] Momeni AZ, Reiszadae MR, Aminjavaheri M. Treatment of cutaneous leishmaniasis with a combination of allopurinol and low dose meglumine antimoniate. International Journal of Dermatology. 2002;**41**:441-443

[10] Masmoudi A, Dammak A, Chaaben H, Maalej N, Akrout F, Turki H. Doxycycline for the treatment of cutaneous leishmaniasis. Dermatology Online Journal. 2008;**14**:22

[11] Prata A, Silva-Vergara ML, Costa L, Rocha A, Krolewiecki A, Silva JC, et al. Efficacy of azithromycin in the treatment of cutaneous leishmaniasis. Revista da Sociedade Brasileira de Medicina Tropical. Jan-Feb 2003;**36**(1): 65-69

[12] Aronson N, Herwaldt BL, Libman M, Pearson R, Lopez-Velez R, Weina P, et al. Diagnosis and treatment of Leishmaniasis: Clinical practice guidelines by the Infectious Diseases Society of America (IDSA) and the American Society of Tropical Medicine and Hygiene (ASTMH). The American Journal of Tropical Medicine and Hygiene. 11 Jan 2017;**96**(1):24-45

[13] Arana B, Mendoza C, Rizzo N, et al. Randomized, controlled, double-blind trial of topical treatment of cutaneous leishmaniasis with paromomycin plus methylbenzethonium chloride ointment in Guatemala. The American Journal of Tropical Medicine and Hygiene. 2001;**65**:466-470

[14] Sosa N, Pascale JM, Jiménez AI, et al. Topical paromomycin for new world cutaneous leishmaniasis. PLoS Neglected Tropical Diseases. 2019;**13**(5): e0007253

[15] Reithinger R, Mohsen M, Wahid M, et al. Efficacy of thermotherapy to treat cutaneous leishmaniasis caused by Leishmania tropica in Kabul Afghanistan:

A randomized, controlled trial. Clinical Infectious Diseases. 2005;**40**:1148-1155

[16] Mehmet G, Tatli N, Hatice O, Erel O, Seyrek A, Abdurrahim K, et al. Efficacy of cryotherapy and intralesional pentostam in treatment of cutaneous leishmaniasis. Journal of the Egyptian Society of Parasitology. 2000;**30**:169-176

[17] Berman JD. Human leishmaniasis: Clinical, diagnostic and chemotherapeutic developments in the last 10 years. Clinical Infectious Diseases. 1997;**24**:684-703

[18] Magill AJ. Cutaneous leishmaniasis in the returning traveler. Infectious Disease Clinics of North America. 2005;**19**:241-266

[19] Moafi M, Rezvan H, Sherkat R, Taleban R. Leishmania vaccines entered in clinical trials: A review of literature. International Journal of Preventive Medicine. 07 Jun 2019;**10**:95

Chapter 5

Visceral Leishmaniasis: Asymptomatic Facts

Medhavi Sudarshan and Sumit Sharan

Abstract

Visceral Leishmaniasis (VL) caused by protozoan parasite *Leishmania* is a vector borne disease and infection is limited not to human but also to animals worldwide. For infection identification and prevalence in both *Leishmania* endemic and nonendemic regions, several serological and genetic techniques are used. Although diagnostic techniques and clinical symptoms can establish illness status, it is extremely difficult to diagnose infection in the absence of symptoms. Asymptomatic are healthy people who have an infection but are unaware of it. The epidemiology of asymptomatic Leishmaniasis is critical for its eradication. Only a small percentage of infected people are clinically suspected of having VL, as the majority of them may not show any symptoms and remain asymptomatic. Some asymptomatic infections may go away after a while, or they may linger for years, or they may develop to illness with clinical signs. Asymptomatic infection varies per endemic location, but almost all of them point to this hidden category of parasite infection. It is now critical to understand many factors such as diagnostic markers, genetic markers, and immunological markers along with different risk factors. All of these criteria, as well as some innovative techniques to diagnosing and controlling asymptomatic leishmaniasis, will be covered in this chapter. The main focus will be on asymptomatic condition of Indian Visceral Leishmaniasis, which is caused by *Leishmania donovani* and spreads via female sand fly *P. argentipes* biting. The numerous criteria that play a role in asymptomatic to symptomatic conversion in a specific time period will also be discussed in this chapter.

Keywords: *Leishmania*, infection, asymptomatic, markers

1. Introduction

Leishmaniasis is a serious public health problem in many countries throughout the world. The illness is caused by numerous intracellular protozoan parasites of the genus *Leishmania*. The most frequent vectors of this neglected infectious illness are phlebotomine sandflies, *Phlebotomus* and *Lutzomyia*, which is most widespread in the tropics and subtropics of Africa, Asia, America, and southern Europe. This illness is the world's second most lethal parasitic killer (after malaria). It's multi-faceted. It can be a deadly murderer in certain forms, or a merciless mutilator who disfigures its victims for life in others. There are now an estimated 12 million cases of leishmaniasis in 98 countries, with 1.5–2 million new cases emerging annually, 1–1.5 million instances of cutaneous leishmaniasis, and 5,00,000 cases of visceral leishmaniasis (VL). VL can create large-scale epidemics with a high case fatality rate. VL (kala-azar) is a latent danger to more than 147 million people residing in the disease-endemic South East Asia region of the Indian subcontinent, which is caused by *Leishmania donovani*. Out of the five VL-affected nations in the area (India, Bangladesh, Nepal, Thailand, and Bhutan), India accounts for more than 80% of recorded cases, while Bhutan and Thailand have sporadic reports. Bihar is the most VL-endemic state in India, accounting for 90 percent of all VL cases in the country [1]. *L. infantum, L. chagasi,* or *Leishmania donovani* are the parasites that cause Visceral Leishmaniasis (VL) in North Africa and Southern Europe as well as Latin America and East Africa respectively [2]. The transmission of *L. donovani* is usually thought to be anthroponomic. Its prevalence is gradually growing around the world, creating a public health issue in the VL endemic zone. The classic WHO definition of Visceral Leishmaniasis is "a person with clinical symptoms (primarily persistent irregular fever, splenomegaly and weight loss) and serological and/or parasitological evidence." Leishmaniasis Post Kala Azar (PKDL) has been related to Visceral Leishmaniasis (VL). According to WHO, probable PKDL affects individuals from VL endemic areas who have numerous hypopigmented maculae, papules, plaques, or nodules but no corresponding loss of sensitivity. However, these are the circumstances in which *Leishmania* infection manifests as symptoms. Many people in endemic locations are infected with the parasite yet show no symptoms of the sickness, according to previous research. These are classified as asymptomatic stages of *Leishmania* infection. *L. donovani* infection can range from asymptomatic carrier to full-blown symptomatic illness with persistent fever, splenomegaly, pancytopenia, and hypergammaglobulinemia. Visceral leishmaniasis has an asymptomatic incubation period of variable duration [3]. A large majority of those who have been exposed to the parasite are asymptomatic, with just a tiny number of people exhibiting clinical manifestations [4, 5]. A disease is considered asymptomatic if it lacks the visible symptoms that are normally associated with it. Asymptomatic conditions may not be detected unless medical tests are performed. Importantly, doctors lack the tools necessary to tell apart asymptomatic patients from those who are suffering from something more subtle [6]. In a Mexican cutaneous leishmaniasis region in 1953, the term asymptomatic in *Leishmania* infection was first used [7]. Asymptomatic *Leishmania* infection was used initially in 1974 by Pampiglione but the description has remained ambiguous five decades later. At this time, there is no way of knowing who of the asymptomatically infected persons would acquire VL illness and when. Asymptomatic people are those who live in an endemic region and have an immune response to *Leishmania* (either antibodies or a particular cellular response), or who have parasites—or parasite DNA—in their blood, but are otherwise healthy [8]. Escalating asymptomatic leishmaniasis due to distinct *Leishmania* species like *L. donovani* and *L. infantum* is critical for determining trends in the disease's prevalence. This first interaction between parasite and host is known as infection. The parasite can be killed by inherent or acquired immunity in the host, or it might persist by using an effective mechanism that bypasses the host's defenses. If the parasite persists, it may lead to a fascinating dynamic interaction between the host and parasite, where the host becomes an asymptomatic carrier when everything is in balance. Due to co-evolution, it is quite frequent in several parasite illnesses for the number of patients to be less when compared to the vast number of persons with asymptomatic infection (in general, an infected person who is asymptomatic is not necessarily a patient). Because of this, asymptomatic instances of VL are common in regions with the disease [9, 10].

2. Epidemiology

It is essential to understand the global prevalence of asymptomatic leishmaniasis. In addition, it's critical to look at the variables that contribute to asymptomatic infection. The variation arises because of changes in parasite virulence and host demographic characteristics, as well as from research designs and the tests employed to determine asymptomatic infection. Worldwide epidemiological statistics show that asymptomatic VL can come from both endemic and non-endemic areas. Those who are infected may unintentionally transfer the disease to others. They may go away on their own, or they may develop symptoms at a later time. As per some findings Asymptomatic infections are those who remain seropositive for many (up to 10–12) years without developing into active disease [11, 12], and are more prevalent in VL endemic regions [13]. In the New World, asymptomatic leishmaniasis was considerably more frequent than in the Old World. The higher prevalence might be explained by the greater diversity of leishmaniasis in the New World as a result of the vector's adoption of new hosts and climate change [14]. Asymptomatic leishmaniasis was less common in children than in the general population. This difference, however, was insignificant on a statistical basis. It was hypothesized that the rise in infection prevalence with age was owing to young children's reduced exposure to infectious sandfly bites [15]. Some indicators indicate that in VL endemic locations, the ratio of asymptomatic vs. active VL patients varies: 2.4:1 in Sudan, 4:1 in Kenya, 5.6:1 in Ethiopia, between 4:1 and 17:1 in the Indian subcontinent, and 50:1 in Spain [16]. Reports from the other endemic regions also confirm the existence of parasitic DNA in all VL causing species in asymptomatic individuals.

According to a meta-analysis of original articles reporting asymptomatic leishmaniasis, the prevalence of asymptomatic leishmaniasis was 11.3%, 95% confidence interval (CI) 8.6%–14.4%] in general population, 36.7% [95% CI 27.6%–46.8%] in inhabitants living in the same or neighboring household to the symptomatic patients, and 11.8% [95% CI 7.1–19%] in HIV infected patient. Meta-regression analysis also showed no significant change in the prevalence of asymptomatic leishmaniasis during the last 40 years [17]. From 1982 to 2015, the trend of total leishmaniasis' asymptomatic proportion did not change considerably, according to the meta-regression study [coefficient = 0.0350 (95% CI, −0.0213 to 0.0913), P = 0.2233] [17]. But, while the disease's geographical range is broad, it is not continuous. The study also suggest, for *L. donovani*, the pattern of asymptomatic infection has not altered over time [coefficient = 0.0015 (95 CI, −0.0531 to 0.0561), P = 0.9564]. In contrast, the frequency of asymptomatic *L. infantum* infection has grown with time, although this shift is statistically insignificant [coefficient = 0.0824 (95 percent CI, −0.0126 to 0.1774), P = 0.0892]. According to research on *L. infantum* in the New World, the prevalence has considerably grown over time [coefficient = 0.0908 (95% CI, 0.0321 to 0.1496), P = 0.002]. The frequency of asymptomatic leishmaniasis in children is also rising over time [coefficient = 0.0599 (95% CI, 0.0066 to 0.1133), P = 0.028]. Drought, hunger, and high population density all contribute to the spread of the illness. The infection-to-disease ratio varies from village to village and also changes over time within the same community [18]. Asymptomatic incident *L. donovani* infection is nine times more common than incident VL illness in VL high-endemic foci in India and Nepal [19]. Within the next 18 months, around 1 in 50 of new yet latent infections developed into VL. There is one important asymptomatic category comprises those individuals of endemic regions who turn seronegative in due course of time [19]. These people most likely acquire the required level of immune response following parasite exposure, which protects them from future illness development by efficiently removing living parasites. They are most likely not carrying live parasites and can be called real resistant instances. The spontaneous change of seropositive to seronegative status ranges from 33–86% [19–22]. However, a research conducted in Bangladesh found that this conversion rate drops to as low as 6.3% after a year among those with high antibody titers [23]. These people give more tangible proof that a threshold immune response level is required to protect the host against parasites. Despite the fact that the majority of seropositive asymptomatic people go on to become seronegative, these individuals are known to contribute to the spread of disease outside of endemic areas [24, 25].

3. Diagnosis

Diagnosis of VL is done by serological tests and molecular test along with direct parasite identification technique. Direct techniques are *Leishmania* parasite isolation from spleen, bone marrow, or blood for microscopy or culture. Different serological tests are ELISA, direct agglutination test (DAT), immunofluorescence antibody test (IFAT), indirect immunofluorescence (IIF), western blot (WB), rK39 immuno-chromatographic strip test while molecular tests include polymerase chain reaction (PCR), qRT-PCR and k-DNA southern blot whereas immunological test include Montenegro Skin Test (MST)/Leishmania skin test (LST) or Interferon Gamma Release Assay (IGRA). The lack of a good biomarker makes defining *Leishmania* asymptomatic infections extremely difficult. It's also unclear how to distinguish parasite persistence in an asymptomatically infected person from new infections that develop after the first episode, i.e. old parasites eliminated by the immune response followed by new infectious parasite populations that would follow the same destiny. Asymptomatic infections cannot be diagnosed with a single, widely approved test. It cannot be diagnosed using any standard or commercially available methods. Patients who are infected with *Leishmania* do not show any symptoms, but tests such as the polymerase chain reaction (PCR) or leishmania skin test (LST)/Montenegro skin test (MST) are positive regardless of whether they show any symptoms [22]. Population-based demographic and immunological surveys showed high but variable prevalence of leishmanial antibodies in the population of Bihar [26]. Serological test DAT/ELISA can perform in epidemiological studies as is noninvasive. But is indirect methodology and tells antibody response due to *Leishmania* infection. Because of the varying durations between infection and seroconversion (ranging from 3 months to 7 years), serology may not be a useful predictor of infection when employed in cross-sectional research [19]. The most often used techniques include an intradermal skin test that indicates the cellular immune response associated with prior exposure to *Leishmania* and the identification of anti-Leishmania antibodies, a less specific indication of infection or continuing illness [27]. Conventional PCR is direct tool as show presence of *Leishmania* specific DNA in interest of samples (blood, buccal swab, urine). Sensitivity and specificity vary for selection of primers. These above mentioned techniques are in use worldwide in epidemiological study to know prevalence of *Leishmania* infection in healthy individuals. But when data compare is compare with active *Leishmania* cases tough to distinguish healthy infection, i.e. asymptomatic. Using DAT seroconversion as a measure of infection, studies found that asymptomatic infection was nine times more common than acute VL illness in high-endemic foci in Bihar [19]. However, in any longitudinal epidemiological investigation, seroconversion should be the primary criteria for detecting asymptomatic infection. The variation in the ratio of VL cases versus asymptomatic cases in different *L. donovani* and *L. infantum* endemic areas from 2.4:1 in Sudan to 50:1 in Spain [28] reflects variations in parasite virulence and host features, However, this may also be due to variations in research design and the methodologies used to diagnose asymptomatic infection. Cell immunity generally lasts for several years, and in some cases, for the rest of a person's life [29, 30]. Serological indicators, on the other hand, can go from positive to negative in as little as four months after the initial sample is examined [22]. In endemic locations where mean parasitemia levels are low or intermittent, serology is generally unreliable for identifying silent Leishmania infection [6]. Cytokine release assays are useful for detecting asymptomatic individuals among immunocompetent subjects in VL-endemic areas; they can also detect the same among immunosuppressed subjects following solid organ transplantation [31]. When compared with the reference test SLA-lymphoproliferative assay, IL-2 appears as a new, 100% sensitive and specific marker for asymptomatic individuals with a positive cellular response (compared with 100% and 84.78%, respectively, for IFN-γ) [32]. Some laboratory tests, including SLA-stimulated PBMC assay, may be difficult to perform under certain conditions. In contrast, the WBA holds much promise as a test at the point-of-care level [33]. The WHO recently recommended screening healthy populations for leishmaniasis infection using SLA-stimulated blood. There are ways to diagnose those who have asymptomatic *Leishmania* infection by whole blood stimulation with the soluble *Leishmania* antigen (SLA), followed by plasma cytokine and chemokine measurements. Combining these diagnostic tests with molecular studies might assist in estimating the real scope of the *Leishmania* outbreak in the endemic region. CXCL10 and CXCL9 DPS were shown to be reliable indicators for identifying asymptomatic individuals in *L. infantum* and *L. donovani* endemic regions. In distant areas, it makes samples more accessible and reduces the cost of epidemiological and epidemic investigations [34].

The immunological determinants such as Adenosine deaminase (ADA), Interferon gamma (IFN-γ), Tumor Necrosis Factor alpha (TNF-α) and Interleukin 10 (IL-10) were examined to predict probable biomarkers for conversion to symptomatic VL. Asymptomatic cases were also earlier reported to harbor the parasite in their blood [35, 36]. Many immunological methods such as direct agglutination test (DAT) and lateral flow immune-chromatographic tests, such as rK39 and rkE-16 have been introduced to screen large number of individuals in endemic areas [37–39]. *Leishmania infantum/chagasi* infection is endemic in Sicily. Approximately 47% of residents live in areas at risk of infection. The prevalence of asymptomatic carriers is unknown. In asymptomatic subjects, IFAT showed sensitivity (30.1%) higher than rK39-ELISA (26.3%) for the detection of cryptic infection, even though a lower specificity was reported (63.4 vs. 76.3%).

Molecular methods are the most suited due to the lack of a gold standard and the limitations of conventional diagnostic procedures, where parasitology is ethically impractical for persons without symptoms and serological tests do not discriminate between past and present illness. Recent molecular methods, such as conventional polymerase chain reaction (PCR) and quantitative real time PCR assay (qPCR), have made considerable advances in screening, diagnosis, and post-therapy follow-up, allowing for better sensitivity than prior serological assays. Quantitative PCR (qPCR) is now a days promising tool for detection and quantification of Leishmania and able to describe threshold as well as reference value for asymptomatic infection.

There are several types of molecular methodologies, and the choice of use should be based on what results are expected to be achieved. While in the conventional Polymerase Chain Reaction (cPCR) the results are only qualitative, quantitative products can be obtained in the Real-Time technique (qPCR), such as the levels of parasitic DNA circulating in the blood [40]. The sensitivity of the assays may vary according to the types of targets and samples used. The most used amplification targets are: kinetoplast DNA (kDNA) [41, 42], internal non-coding spacer region (ITS-1) [43] and the smaller ribosomal subunits (SSU - rRNA) [44–46]. Sudarshan et al. [35] when performing a qPCR, analyzed the level of circulating parasites to differentiate a possible disease progression. They obtained a minimum level of detection of 0.001 parasitic genomes/mL of blood and 34.79% of positive samples by the technique, using the kDNA and hydrolysis probes of the TaqMan type, as a target and method of visualizing the products. Likewise, Kaushal et al. [6, 47] (S. Das et al., 2014; Kaushalet al., 2017, [6, 47] (S. Das et al., 2014; Kaushal et al., 2017) (Das et al. 2014, Kaushal et al. 2017, ([6, 47], when carrying out a study to detect asymptomatic individuals, obtained an amount < 5 parasites/mL of blood and a positive sample rate of 21.54%, using kDNA as a target and SYBR Green I as a result detection system. Sudarshan et al. [48], affirm that Leishmania DNA may be used as a marker of infection since it is detected before the seroconversion of antibodies. Individuals can be diagnosed as seronegative when they are tested before the development of immunity or when it is in a very low quantity, not being identified by serological methods. Similar data were also suggested by Costa et al. [27] and Bhattarai et al. [49], wherein asymptomatic infections detected by molecular methods have been observed in seronegative people. This demonstrates that possibly due to the limitations of serological methods, molecular tests are more suitable for the identification of asymptomatic cases. Although parasitic DNA is considered the first infection marker before immunological conversion [35], there are controversies regarding its use. The limitation of the use of DNA as a target is found in a possible detection of the genetic material of the parasite when it is already dead, although this is discussed, the half-life of the nucleic acid in the body is around 24 hours, which can cause flaws in distinguishing viable parasites from detecting fragments of lifeless parasites. Lack of standardization of a methodology still becomes a gap that can lead mainly to problems and delays in detection of the cases. Moreover, the use of nanoparticle techniques represents a trend for diagnosis, immunotherapy, and programs to eliminate VL. These methodologies bring a new approach with new forms of diagnosis and drugs, where improvements in efficacy and less toxicity can be observed. There will be continuous and significant improvements to all their current roles in diagnostics and will also provide multiple roles in terms of recognizing other DNA or materials, using fluorophores or other active molecules. it is reasonable to have a lower value of serum hemoglobin, hematocrit, and albumin among symptomatic patients. So, they would be considered as a marker of symptomatic diseases rather than a risk or protective factor. Studies are going on to define asymptomatic as yet there is no or very less agreement between different markers. Although Gold standard for Leishmaniasis detection is parasitological confirmation by microscopy which need splenic aspirate. But for asymptomatics it is not possible as ethical issues are very high because of invasive nature of samples. As the use of spleen or bone marrow aspirate is not ethical in asymptomatic subjects, the negative predictive value (NPV) cannot be exactly evaluated.

4. Immunology

Asymptomatic cases differ considerably from VL patients, and it is assumed that a mixed profile is crucial not only for the management of parasite replication but also for the preservation of these people' immune state. The increased number of cells expressing different cytokines demonstrates this. However, in VL-endemic areas, the clinical form is frequently asymptomatic, followed by protective immunity with a predominant type 1 T-cell response [50]. Asymptomatic seemed to have mixed profile having an increase of IFN-γ + neutrophils/eosinophils and NK cells, of IL-12+ eosinophils/monocytes, along with increase of IL-4+ neutrophils and NK cells and IL-10+ eosinophils/monocytes [51]. Despite earlier findings of a constant type 1 T-lymphocyte immune response during asymptomatic VL it was recently shown that asymptomatic patients' PBMC generated significant amounts of IL-10 when stimulated with *L. infantum* recombinant antigens [52].

Different findings point to the idea that IL-10 is a key immunomodulator in asymptomatic people, dampening host defense mechanisms and favoring immune response regulation following parasite elimination. Furthermore, CD4+ T cells from asymptomatic patients infected with *L. infantum* have been shown to generate significant amounts of IL-5 [53]. In immunocompetent people, leishmania infection is typically asymptomatic, although the percentage of HIV+ people infected with the parasite who stay asymptomatic is unknown. HIV+ individuals might still have a Th1-type cellular response to Leishmania despite their weakened immune system. These people may be identified using cytokine release tests, which identify IFN-γ in the supernatants of SLA-stimulated PBMC and IFN-γ and IL-2 in SLA-stimulated whole blood. These biomarkers appear to be 100% reliable for detecting asymptomatic immune responders to Leishmania among HIV+ patients [33]. Analyses of cytokine responses in symptomatic and asymptomatic VL patients' peripheral blood mononuclear cells (PBMCs) indicated that the production of Th17 cytokines was highly linked with the asymptomatic status [54, 55]. It was discovered by Carvalho et al. that peripheral blood mononuclear cells (PBMCs) from people with subclinical or asymptomatic infection (positive serology and skin test for Leishmania antigen) react to stimulation with Leishmania antigen by producing IL-2, IFN- and IL-12 [50]. An Indian study found that active disease elicited a mixed IFN-/IL-10 response, but asymptomatic infections (IFN- release assay [IGRA]–positive endemic healthy controls) did not trigger an antigen-driven whole-blood IL-10 response [56]. Surprisingly, the frequency of CD4+ T cells is higher in people with asymptomatic infections who have positive LST [57], Furthermore high levels of IFN- are produced by CD8+ T cells isolated from asymptomatic patients, which implies that CD8+ cells play a role in human resistance to Leishmania infection. Furthermore, researchers discovered that in asymptomatic people, a distinct subpopulation of CD4+ cells that produced both IFN- and IL-5 was important for infection management [22, 53]. A longitudinal study conducted in Sudan recently suggested that Th17 cells may play a protective role in human VL, and it was found that *L. donovani* stimulates the production of IL-17 and IL-22 by exposed PBMCs from healthy and resistant subjects who did not develop VL before or after cytokine response testing. In addition, elevated levels of IFN-γ, C reactive protein, nitric oxide, and IL-12 in the blood have also been reported to offer resistance in asymptomatic patients [58]. Disease resistant endemic individuals have an immune response that shields them against pathogenesis in response to an insect bite which are quite similar to those of VL immunology, and as a result, they cannot be utilized to provide a clear picture of protective immune parameters in asymptomatic patients. Besides the protective immune response, it appears that these people either possess a large number of long-lived memory B cells that continuously secrete antibodies or they are continually exposed to *Leishmania* but do not acquire VL as a result of the protective immunological response [59]. The quantity of antibodies in blood has been connected to the incidence of asymptomatic to symptomatic VL conversion. Although it will be difficult to track these instances, they may aid in the discovery of host immunological mechanisms that influence disease susceptibility and resistance. Strong cell mediated immunity, a broad repertoire of memory T and B cells, and short-lived plasma cells may be linked with the immune biology of resistant asymptomatic infections (they do not show seropositivity for a longer period). Focused research on these people might disclose the characteristics of protective immunity that are needed to build a preventive vaccination candidate. In asymptomatic patients, the levels of ADA, IL-10, and IFN-γ were continuously high, with ADA and IL-10, but not IFN-γ, remaining higher as clinical symptoms progressed into active VL. ADA and IL-10 might be used as a biomarker in the transition from asymptomatic to symptomatic VL [60]. Due to their high innate cellular immunity, many asymptomatic individuals become seronegative without acquiring

VL. IFN- γ became high in asymptomatic infection but dropped after conversion, but TNF-α levels did not alter much at either stage of illness. The cytokine profile might be utilized to better treat VL patients with autoimmune diseases, as well as to identify and protect individuals with asymptomatic infection who are at risk of developing illness. Assays for cytokine release are already being utilized to detect asymptomatic individuals [31, 61]. Cytokines, which operate on macrophages, are receiving a lot of attention these days because of their ability to alter the immune response. Studies on the function of cytokines in asymptomatic infections and/or subclinical VL cases are scarce in the literature, and these investigations generally assess cytokine levels just once, before any clinical symptoms arise. Research into immune responses shows that patients with low levels of IL-10 production have additional flaws. In VL, IL-10 mRNA expression is highly expressed, and this cytokine's involvement in reducing T cell responses in these individuals has been well established. According to the finding, the balance between the production of IFN-γ and IL-10 may be a significant factor in determining whether or not patients develop illness after contracting *L. chagasi* infection even while they are asymptomatic [62].

5. Genetics

For many years, there has been speculation that, in VL, the Leishmania genotypic differences involve in asymptomatic or symptomatic forms of the disease. There was findings that the Leishmania Internal Transcribed Spacer 1 (ITS1) from symptomatic VL and asymptomatic cases has significant genetic differences in southern Iran [63]. Several investigations have shown that the genotypic characteristics of symptomatic and asymptomatic VL patients might differ [64, 65]. Researchers identified significant genetic diversity between *Leishmania* species isolated from asymptomatic and symptomatic patients, particularly those with HIV/VL coinfection, in a study done in southern France. The study also discovered that asymptomatic isolates had a modest polymorphism in their parasite genome [64]. In Southern France, MLMT showed parasite genotype appear to differs in *Leishmania* patients compared with asymptomatic related carriers [66].

Aside from the parasite genotype, the host's genetic background may have a role in determining whether VL is asymptomatic or symptomatic [67]. Study also linked symptomatic VL to a gene that codes for a receptor for transforming growth factor beta (TGF-β) whereas the asymptomatic is connected to gene encoding II-a receptor for the Fc fragment of IgG [67]. However, the association between SNP/HLA genotyping and progression from asymptomatic or seroconversion to VL overt disease has been insignificant [68]. Polymorphism at SLC11A1 has been shown to be linked [69, 70] and associated in regulating susceptibility with human VL in Sudan. However, no evidence of such an association was found in an Indian population [71]. Few studies indicate that host genetic association and development of clinical symptoms is linked to NRAMP1, TNF-α, IL-4 and IFN-γ receptor (IFNGR1)], TGF β, IL-8, C-X-C chemokine receptor 1 (CXCR1) and C-X-C chemokine receptor 2 (CXCR2), IL-2R, Delta-like1 (DLL1), and mannan binding lectin genes [48, 69, 72, 73]. In one of the recent most studies on asymptomatic VL, were able to link several HLA-DRβ allele groups with the progression of VL [68].

6. Other risk factors

Besides, serological methodologies performed on individuals without symptoms may have low sensitivity due to a weak humoral response [74]. Risk factors have been analyzed by some studies, taking into account that contact with the parasite is necessary, but it is not sufficient for the development of the active disease. These characteristics can play an important role in the cycle of asymptomatic individuals [6]. The male gender is one of the individual factors that demonstrate a positive association with asymptomatic infection [75]. Although other hosts and parasite variables may be additional causes, the conversion of asymptomatic infections to symptomatic VL also indicates the survival of parasites in these people [76]. The extrinsic variables such as age and nutritional state, as well as a weakened host immunological system, are thought to be significant in the progression from asymptomatic to symptomatic infection. Poor dietary status has been linked to an increased chance of developing clinical VL in addition to hereditary risk. The relationship between malnutrition and the course of VL at the cellular level is poorly understood. A better understanding of these mechanisms might open new opportunities for prevention or therapeutic dietary intervention [16].

There were evidences that suspected individuals living in households with family history, were at particularly high risk of infection. Although the cohort studied did not contain population-specific genetic markers, the addition of such factors might help predict outcomes when molecular diagnostics and serodiagnostic testing are combined. Even if they have a competent immune response, persons who have come into touch with the parasite do not inevitably acquire the symptomatic version of the condition [16]. Age, genetic, immunological, and dietary features, the existence of other diseases, and vector density are all potential risk factors for the disease's development [75], and type of "asymptomatic" definition applied to the study [28]. Despite being practical and easy, methodologies handling have some limitations: (i) do not differentiate past disease from recent [75, 77] (ii) there is the possibility of cross-reactivity with other related parasites [78]. Asymptomatic infection is usually observed in family members or in direct contact to clinical VL cases, suggesting that family members are at risk of infection. In a research from India, it is discovered that family members of VL patients had 1.8 times the risk of becoming infected as compared to those who did not have VL in the house. Kala-azar patients were younger ($P < 0.001$) and reported lower red meat consumption ($P < 0.01$) than asymptomatic seropositive individuals. Retinol and zinc levels were lower in current kala-azar patients and those who later developed kala-azar compared with uninfected and asymptomatically infected subjects. The characteristics that help determine whether an infection leads to overt disease appear to include age and dietary factors such as intake of iron- and zinc-rich red meat [79, 80]. Kala-azar patients were younger ($P < 0.001$) and reported lower red meat consumption ($P < 0.01$) than asymptomatic seropositive individuals. In comparison to uninfected and asymptomatically infected people, active kala-azar patients and those who later acquired kala-azar had decreased retinol and zinc levels. In contrast with different groups, kala-azar patients had greater CRP values. A population at increased risk of symptomatic illness may have a low red meat intake and low zinc and retinol levels.

7. Conclusion

Control efforts for leishmaniasis (especially asymptomatic VL), particularly in endemic regions, need a detailed understanding of *Leishmania* ecology and epidemiology. Those infected with viscerotropic *Leishmania* species, on the other hand, may remain asymptomatic, which is the most typical result of infection in endemic regions. However, it is impossible to offer reliable estimates of the number of infected vs. those at risk. The number of persons infected but asymptomatic is far greater than the number of people infected and presenting with clinical disease.

As a result, it is critical to understand how many infected people will acquire illness and how they may be identified before clinical symptoms appear. Different studied found that utilizing anti-rK39 ELISA to screen family members and contacts might be a very reliable technique for early diagnosis and planning preventive treatment of latently infected asymptomatic carriers in order to eradicate kala-azar. Although there have been isolated instances of parasite circulation in the peripheral blood of asymptomatic individuals with *L. donovani* and *Leishmania tropica* infection. Various study findings explain the immune response as tracked prospectively and its diagnostic value in predicting the fate of latent infection in a relatively large number of patients. Serologically positive state a relatively transient increase in serum antibodies caused by recent infection that lasts for months, whereas LST positive thought to indicate long-term cell-mediated immunity after asymptomatic infection or clinical cure of kala-azar. A favorable LST result may take months to years to manifest after effective kalaazar therapy, but it lasts for decades after exposure. There are few data on risk factors for asymptomatic leishmaniasis, and its epidemiology is unknown. Such knowledge is critical for efforts to prevent and control visceral leishmaniasis, such as the eradication programs. In a Brazilian research, sand flies fed on kala-azar patients were sick in 25% of cases, while none of the sand flies fed on asymptomatically afflicted individuals became infected. Seroepidemiologic data from disease-endemic areas of India are scarce and based on small sample sizes. Serologic status is not a good predictor for conversion to clinical VL. Studies confirmed that 33% persons were serologically positive, only 3.48% seropositive persons showed disease conversion. However, 2.57%seronegative persons at baseline showed disease conversion also [11]. Human instances of transfusion-transmitted visceral leishmaniasis (VL) have been reported in both endemic and non-endemic locations, with clinical characteristics and outcomes comparable to those of natural infection [81].

When innate immune cells from asymptomatic carriers were stimulated with antigens in vitro, they exhibited a regulated rise in cytokine production that differed from that seen in non-infected subjects. This implies that using more than one diagnostic approach makes it easier to identify a substantial proportion of asymptomatic carriers. One often mentioned flaw in these research is the difficulty in identifying those who are briefly and quietly infected with the parasite. A recent study of asymptomatic people' innate and adaptive immunity revealed that a mixed cytokine profile is crucial not just for parasite replication control, but also for the preservation of these individuals' immune state [51]. Only 20% of those infected with *L. chagasi* in endemic regions of VL develop classical VL, according to research. Even before extremely sensitive molecular diagnostic technologies became available, it was established that the majority of infected people living in an endemic region have asymptomatic self-cured illnesses [82]. Nonetheless, despite the PCR assays' excellent sensitivity and specificity in identifying *Leishmania* DNA in clinically sick patients' peripheral blood, a proportion of asymptomatic persons with positive serological tests had no detectable circulating *Leishmania* DNA. As a result, the co-positivity between the PCR assay and different serological assays was astonishingly low. It's conceivable that these apparent differences might be explained by how an illness develops in people. The parasite can be identified in the peripheral blood at a certain point (providing a positive PCR assay), followed by adaptive-mediated immunity with the generation of antibodies and a T lymphocytes-mediated immune response. Because these biological moments are never-ending, it's possible to analyze certain people when they are in a state of transition. Other non-invasive and extremely sensitive techniques, such as PCR in peripheral blood, have recently been available. This has made it possible to identify asymptomatic carriers of *Leishmnia* who otherwise would not have been detected using just serological methods [83]. Research findings suggest that the method used to diagnose an infection may have an impact on infection-related variables including risk factors and treatment results [61]. At the moment, it is impossible to determine who among the asymptomatically infected persons will acquire VL illness and when. A research from Bangladesh further indicates that about 80% of asymptomatic individuals contribute to disease transmission, compared to 8–10% of VL and PKDL patients [13].

The question of why just a few exposed asymptomatic people acquire full-blown illness symptoms but not all remains unsolved. The major immunological variables that promote the conversion of asymptomatic patients to symptomatic stage of visceral leishmaniasis have been attempted to explicate in several research. It is crucial to note that the use of five diagnostic techniques as a regular strategy would be impractical in endemic situations. Before a particular recommendation can be made, more research is needed to confirm the optimal diagnostic method [61]. The important checkpoints for determining disease resistance or susceptibility are cytokines that control cellular immunity [84, 85]. Despite substantial understanding of host–parasite interactions and immunobiology, reliable protective immunity criteria have yet to be discovered. Asymptomatic instances of human VL can be diagnosed using qPCR using RNA targets. There are also questions about whether or not using RNA as a gene target can help discover asymptomatic instances of VL. By combining this methodology with epidemiological data analysis, it will be possible to improve the detection and treatment of asymptomatic cases. Priority should be given to stepping up efforts to better characterize asymptomatic illness in endemic areas and to develop a uniform case definition for leishmanial infection. Self-clearing infections vs. illness development must have all of their factors examined thoroughly. The problems in parasite and sand fly management methods, as well as changes in the epidemiology of VL in disease-endemic countries, are important threats to its eradication. In addition, the movement of infected but asymptomatic people from endemic areas has resulted in additional infections in non-endemic areas [86]. The xenodiagnosis approach validates whether asymptomatic infected people can be infectious to sand flies and might be a crucial step in determining whether or not to modify the existing VL management strategy. One study used xenodiagnosis to identify VL infection in HIV-positive people and found even asymptomatic patients in the early stages of the infection were able to infect others [87]. Although Xenodiagnosis findings from an Indian investigation indicate that neither asymptomatic nor treated patients were infected by vector sandflies [88]. Asymptomatic infected persons are not now the focus of drug research efforts. This is because the asymptomatic state is not clearly defined, but largely because an intervention is less of a priority as long as the role of asymptomatically infected people in transmission is not clarified. There have been significant gains in reducing infection rates thanks to the eradication programs, but there are still some obstacles to overcome along the way. Considering that humans are the sole reservoir for *Leishmania donovani*, the effectiveness of a control programme hinges heavily on treating both symptomatic and potentially asymptomatic persons, if such individuals are found to also function as a reservoir. The lack of techniques to identify live parasites in silent infections and their relationship to disease transmission, sterile cure characteristics, and PKDL development remains a serious danger to the disease's eradication. There has been tremendous progress in the control or elimination of tropical illnesses, with a large drop in the incidence of these diseases. Although it is critical to comprehend these underlying causes for each illness, asymptomatic carriers are a common component that can contribute to resurgence; their effect in terms of population percentage and function in transmission must be established. More study is needed to completely understand the determinants.

Conflict of interest

None.

Author details

Medhavi Sudarshan[1*] and Sumit Sharan[2]

1 Jagat Narain Lal College, Khagaul, Patliputra University, Patna, Bihar, India

2 Nidan Health Care and Diagnostic Centre, Patna, Bihar, India

*Address all correspondence to: medhavisudarshan@gmail.com

References

[1] Poché DM, Grant WE, Wang HH. Visceral Leishmaniasis on the Indian Subcontinent: Modelling the Dynamic Relationship between Vector Control Schemes and Vector Life Cycles. PLoS Negl Trop Dis. 2016;10(8):e0004868.

[2] Sundar S. Visceral leishmaniasis. Trop Parasitol. 2015;5(2):83-85.

[3] Rodrigues V, Cordeiro-da-Silva A, Laforge M, Silvestre R, Estaquier J. Regulation of immunity during visceral Leishmania infection. Parasit Vectors. 2016;9:118.

[4] Singh S, Kumari V, Singh N. Predicting kala-azar disease manifestations in asymptomatic patients with latent Leishmania donovani infection by detection of antibody against recombinant K39 antigen. Clin Diagn Lab Immunol. 2002;9(3):568-572.

[5] Bimal S, Singh SK, Das VN, Sinha PK, Gupta AK, Bhattacharya SK, et al. Leishmania donovani: effect of therapy on expression of CD2 antigen and secretion of macrophage migration inhibition factor by T-cells in patients with visceral leishmaniasis. Exp Parasitol. 2005;111(2):130-132.

[6] Das S, Matlashewski G, Bhunia GS, Kesari S, Das P. Asymptomatic Leishmania infections in northern India: a threat for the elimination programme? Trans R Soc Trop Med Hyg. 2014; 108(11):679-684.

[7] BIAGI F. [Intradermal reactions with leishmanine in Escarcega, Campeche, Mexico]. Medicina (Mex). 1953;33(677): 255-60.

[8] Alvar J, Alves F, Bucheton B, Burrows L, Büscher P, Carrillo E, et al. Implications of asymptomatic infection for the natural history of selected parasitic tropical diseases. Semin Immunopathol. 2020;42(3):231-246.

[9] Schaefer KU, Kurtzhals JA, Gachihi GS, Muller AS, Kager PA. A prospective sero-epidemiological study of visceral leishmaniasis in Baringo District, Rift Valley Province, Kenya. Trans R Soc Trop Med Hyg. 1995; 89(5):471-475.

[10] Sinha PK, Bimal S, Pandey K, Singh SK, Ranjan A, Kumar N, et al. A community-based, comparative evaluation of direct agglutination and rK39 strip tests in the early detection of subclinical Leishmania donovani infection. Ann Trop Med Parasitol. 2008;102(2):119-125.

[11] Gidwani K, Kumar R, Rai M, Sundar S. Longitudinal seroepidemiologic study of visceral leishmaniasis in hyperendemic regions of Bihar, India. Am J Trop Med Hyg. 2009;80(3):345-346.

[12] Gidwani K, Picado A, Ostyn B, Singh SP, Kumar R, Khanal B, et al. Persistence of Leishmania donovani antibodies in past visceral leishmaniasis cases in India. Clin Vaccine Immunol. 2011;18(2):346-348.

[13] Hirve S, Boelaert M, Matlashewski G, Mondal D, Arana B, Kroeger A, et al. Transmission Dynamics of Visceral Leishmaniasis in the Indian Subcontinent - A Systematic Literature Review. PLoS Negl Trop Dis. 2016;10(8):e0004896.

[14] Steverding D. The history of leishmaniasis. Parasit Vectors. 2017;10(1):82.

[15] Staff PNTD. Correction: Age trends in asymptomatic and symptomatic Leishmania donovani infection in the Indian subcontinent: A review and analysis of data from diagnostic and epidemiological studies. PLoS Negl Trop Dis. 2019;13(2):e0007150.

[16] Singh OP, Hasker E, Sacks D, Boelaert M, Sundar S. Asymptomatic

Leishmania infection: a new challenge for Leishmania control. Clin Infect Dis. 2014;58(10):1424-1429.

[17] Mannan SB, Elhadad H, Loc TTH, Sadik M, Mohamed MYF, Nam NH, et al. Prevalence and associated factors of asymptomatic leishmaniasis: a systematic review and meta-analysis. Parasitol Int. 2021;81:102229.

[18] Khalil EA, Zijlstra EE, Kager PA, El Hassan AM. Epidemiology and clinical manifestations of Leishmania donovani infection in two villages in an endemic area in eastern Sudan. Trop Med Int Health. 2002;7(1):35-44.

[19] Ostyn B, Gidwani K, Khanal B, Picado A, Chappuis F, Singh SP, et al. Incidence of symptomatic and asymptomatic Leishmania donovani infections in high-endemic foci in India and Nepal: a prospective study. PLoS Negl Trop Dis. 2011;5(10):e1284.

[20] Das VN, Siddiqui NA, Verma RB, Topno RK, Singh D, Das S, et al. Asymptomatic infection of visceral leishmaniasis in hyperendemic areas of Vaishali district, Bihar, India: a challenge to kala-azar elimination programmes. Trans R Soc Trop Med Hyg. 2011;105(11):661-666.

[21] Bimal S, Das VN, Sinha PK, Gupta AK, Verma N, Ranjan A, et al. Usefulness of the direct agglutination test in the early detection of subclinical Leishmania donovani infection: a community-based study. Ann Trop Med Parasitol. 2005;99(8):743-749.

[22] Hasker E, Kansal S, Malaviya P, Gidwani K, Picado A, Singh RP, et al. Latent infection with Leishmania donovani in highly endemic villages in Bihar, India. PLoS Negl Trop Dis. 2013;7(2):e2053.

[23] Bern C, Haque R, Chowdhury R, Ali M, Kurkjian KM, Vaz L, et al. The epidemiology of visceral leishmaniasis and asymptomatic leishmanial infection in a highly endemic Bangladeshi village. Am J Trop Med Hyg. 2007;76(5): 909-914.

[24] Saha S, Mondal S, Ravindran R, Bhowmick S, Modak D, Mallick S, et al. IL-10- and TGF-beta-mediated susceptibility in kala-azar and post-kala-azar dermal leishmaniasis: the significance of amphotericin B in the control of Leishmania donovani infection in India. J Immunol. 2007; 179(8):5592-5603.

[25] Stauch A, Sarkar RR, Picado A, Ostyn B, Sundar S, Rijal S, et al. Visceral leishmaniasis in the Indian subcontinent: modelling epidemiology and control. PLoS Negl Trop Dis. 2011;5(11):e1405.

[26] Singh SP, Picado A, Boelaert M, Gidwani K, Andersen EW, Ostyn B, et al. The epidemiology of Leishmania donovani infection in high transmission foci in India. Trop Med Int Health. 2010;15 Suppl 2:12-20.

[27] Costa CH, Stewart JM, Gomes RB, Garcez LM, Ramos PK, Bozza M, et al. Asymptomatic human carriers of Leishmania chagasi. Am J Trop Med Hyg. 2002;66(4):334-337.

[28] Chappuis F, Sundar S, Hailu A, Ghalib H, Rijal S, Peeling RW, et al. Visceral leishmaniasis: what are the needs for diagnosis, treatment and control? Nat Rev Microbiol. 2007;5(11): 873-882.

[29] Kar K. Serodiagnosis of leishmaniasis. Crit Rev Microbiol. 1995;21(2):123-152.

[30] Werneck GL, Rodrigues L, Santos MV, Araújo IB, Moura LS, Lima SS, et al. The burden of Leishmania chagasi infection during an urban outbreak of visceral leishmaniasis in Brazil. Acta Trop. 2002;83(1): 13-18.

[31] Carrillo E, Carrasco-Antón N, López-Medrano F, Salto E, Fernández L, San Martín JV, et al. Cytokine Release Assays as Tests for Exposure to Leishmania, and for Confirming Cure from Leishmaniasis, in Solid Organ Transplant Recipients. PLoS Negl Trop Dis. 2015;9(10):e0004179.

[32] Ibarra-Meneses AV, Carrillo E, Sánchez C, García-Martínez J, López Lacomba D, San Martin JV, et al. Interleukin-2 as a marker for detecting asymptomatic individuals in areas where Leishmania infantum is endemic. Clin Microbiol Infect. 2016;22(8): 739.e1-4.

[33] Botana L, Ibarra-Meneses AV, Sánchez C, Castro A, San Martin JV, Molina L, et al. Asymptomatic immune responders to Leishmania among HIV positive patients. PLoS Negl Trop Dis. 2019;13(6):e0007461.

[34] Ibarra-Meneses AV, Mondal D, Alvar J, Moreno J, Carrillo E. Cytokines and chemokines measured in dried SLA-stimulated whole blood spots for asymptomatic Leishmania infantum and Leishmania donovani infection. Sci Rep. 2017;7(1):17266.

[35] Sudarshan M, Singh T, Singh AK, Chourasia A, Singh B, Wilson ME, et al. Quantitative PCR in epidemiology for early detection of visceral leishmaniasis cases in India. PLoS Negl Trop Dis. 2014;8(12):e3366.

[36] Sudarshan M, Sundar S. Parasite load estimation by qPCR differentiates between asymptomatic and symptomatic infection in Indian visceral leishmaniasis. Diagn Microbiol Infect Dis. 2014;80(1):40-42.

[37] Harith AE, Kolk AH, Kager PA, Leeuwenburg J, Muigai R, Kiugu S, et al. A simple and economical direct agglutination test for serodiagnosis and sero-epidemiological studies of visceral leishmaniasis. Trans R Soc Trop Med Hyg. 1986;80(4):583-536.

[38] Boelaert M, El-Safi S, Hailu A, Mukhtar M, Rijal S, Sundar S, et al. Diagnostic tests for kala-azar: a multi-centre study of the freeze-dried DAT, rK39 strip test and KAtex in East Africa and the Indian subcontinent. Trans R Soc Trop Med Hyg. 2008;102(1):32-40.

[39] Sundar S, Singh RK, Bimal SK, Gidwani K, Mishra A, Maurya R, et al. Comparative evaluation of parasitology and serological tests in the diagnosis of visceral leishmaniasis in India: a phase III diagnostic accuracy study. Trop Med Int Health. 2007;12(2):284-289.

[40] Sundar S, Singh OP. Molecular Diagnosis of Visceral Leishmaniasis. Mol Diagn Ther. 2018;22(4):443-457.

[41] Abbasi I, Aramin S, Hailu A, Shiferaw W, Kassahun A, Belay S, et al. Evaluation of PCR procedures for detecting and quantifying Leishmania donovani DNA in large numbers of dried human blood samples from a visceral leishmaniasis focus in Northern Ethiopia. BMC Infect Dis. 2013;13:153.

[42] Gualda KP, Marcussi LM, Neitzke-Abreu HC, Aristides SM, Lonardoni MV, Cardoso RF, et al. NEW PRIMERS FOR DETECTION OF Leishmania infantum USING POLYMERASE CHAIN REACTION. Rev Inst Med Trop Sao Paulo. 2015;57(5):377-383.

[43] Schönian G, Nasereddin A, Dinse N, Schweynoch C, Schallig HD, Presber W, et al. PCR diagnosis and characterization of Leishmania in local and imported clinical samples. Diagn Microbiol Infect Dis. 2003;47(1): 349-358.

[44] van den Bogaart E, Schoone GJ, Adams ER, Schallig HD. Duplex quantitative Reverse-Transcriptase PCR for simultaneous assessment of drug

activity against Leishmania intracellular amastigotes and their host cells. Int J Parasitol Drugs Drug Resist. 2014;4(1): 14-19.

[45] Gedda MR, Madhukar P, Shukla A, Mudavath SL, Srivastava ON, Singh OP, et al. Nanodiagnostics in leishmaniasis: A new frontiers for early elimination. Wiley Interdiscip Rev Nanomed Nanobiotechnol. 2021;13(2):e1675.

[46] Singh OP, Gedda MR, Mudavath SL, Srivastava ON, Sundar S. Envisioning the innovations in nanomedicine to combat visceral leishmaniasis: for future theranostic application. Nanomedicine (Lond). 2019;14(14):1911-1927.

[47] Kaushal H, Bhattacharya SK, Verma S, Salotra P. Serological and Molecular Analysis of. Am J Trop Med Hyg. 2017;96(6):1448-1455.

[48] Mehrotra S, Fakiola M, Mishra A, Sudarshan M, Tiwary P, Rani DS, et al. Genetic and functional evaluation of the role of DLL1 in susceptibility to visceral leishmaniasis in India. Infect Genet Evol. 2012;12(6):1195-1201.

[49] Bhattarai NR, Van der Auwera G, Khanal B, De Doncker S, Rijal S, Das ML, et al. PCR and direct agglutination as Leishmania infection markers among healthy Nepalese subjects living in areas endemic for Kala-Azar. Trop Med Int Health. 2009;14(4):404-411.

[50] Carvalho EM, Barral A, Pedral-Sampaio D, Barral-Netto M, Badaró R, Rocha H, et al. Immunologic markers of clinical evolution in children recently infected with Leishmania donovani chagasi. J Infect Dis. 1992; 165(3):535-540.

[51] Peruhype-Magalhães V, Martins-Filho OA, Prata A, Silva LeA, Rabello A, Teixeira-Carvalho A, et al. Immune response in human visceral leishmaniasis: analysis of the correlation between innate immunity cytokine profile and disease outcome. Scand J Immunol. 2005;62(5):487-495.

[52] de Carvalho LP, Soto M, Jerônimo S, Dondji B, Bacellar O, Luz V, et al. Characterization of the immune response to Leishmania infantum recombinant antigens. Microbes Infect. 2003;5(1):7-12.

[53] Mary C, Auriault V, Faugère B, Dessein AJ. Control of Leishmania infantum infection is associated with CD8(+) and gamma interferon- and interleukin-5-producing CD4(+) antigen-specific T cells. Infect Immun. 1999;67(11):5559-5566.

[54] Pitta MG, Romano A, Cabantous S, Henri S, Hammad A, Kouriba B, et al. IL-17 and IL-22 are associated with protection against human kala azar caused by Leishmania donovani. J Clin Invest. 2009;119(8):2379-2387.

[55] Ghosh K, Sharma G, Saha A, Kar S, Das PK, Ukil A. Successful therapy of visceral leishmaniasis with curdlan involves T-helper 17 cytokines. J Infect Dis. 2013;207(6):1016-1025.

[56] Singh OP, Gidwani K, Kumar R, Nylén S, Jones SL, Boelaert M, et al. Reassessment of immune correlates in human visceral leishmaniasis as defined by cytokine release in whole blood. Clin Vaccine Immunol. 2012;19(6):961-966.

[57] Hailu A, van Baarle D, Knol GJ, Berhe N, Miedema F, Kager PA. T cell subset and cytokine profiles in human visceral leishmaniasis during active and asymptomatic or sub-clinical infection with Leishmania donovani. Clin Immunol. 2005;117(2):182-191.

[58] Stanley AC, Engwerda CR. Balancing immunity and pathology in visceral leishmaniasis. Immunol Cell Biol. 2007;85(2):138-147.

[59] Pape KA, Taylor JJ, Maul RW, Gearhart PJ, Jenkins MK. Different B

cell populations mediate early and late memory during an endogenous immune response. Science. 2011;331(6021): 1203-1207.

[60] Das VNR, Bimal S, Siddiqui NA, Kumar A, Pandey K, Sinha SK, et al. Conversion of asymptomatic infection to symptomatic visceral leishmaniasis: A study of possible immunological markers. PLoS Negl Trop Dis. 2020; 14(6):e0008272.

[61] de Gouvêa Viana L, de Assis TS, Orsini M, da Silva AR, de Souza GF, Caligiorne R, et al. Combined diagnostic methods identify a remarkable proportion of asymptomatic Leishmania (Leishmania) chagasi carriers who present modulated cytokine profiles. Trans R Soc Trop Med Hyg. 2008; 102(6):548-555.

[62] Ghalib HW, Piuvezam MR, Skeiky YA, Siddig M, Hashim FA, el-Hassan AM, et al. Interleukin 10 production correlates with pathology in human Leishmania donovani infections. J Clin Invest. 1993;92(1):324-329.

[63] Rezaei Z, Azarang E, Shahabi S, Omidian M, Pourabbas B, Sarkari B. ITS1 Is Genetically Divergent in Asymptomatic and Symptomatic Visceral Leishmaniasis: Results of a Study in Southern Iran. J Trop Med. 2020;2020:5351098.

[64] Hide M, Marion E, Pomares C, Fisa R, Marty P, Bañuls AL. Parasitic genotypes appear to differ in leishmaniasis patients compared with asymptomatic related carriers. Int J Parasitol. 2013;43(5):389-397.

[65] Montoya L, Gállego M, Gavignet B, Piarroux R, Rioux JA, Portús M, et al. Application of microsatellite genotyping to the study of a restricted Leishmania infantum focus: different genotype compositions in isolates from dogs and sand flies. Am J Trop Med Hyg. 2007;76(5):888-895.

[66] Hide M, Marion E, Pomares C, Fisa R, Marty P, Banuls AL. Parasitic genotypes appear to differ in leishmaniasis patients compared with asymptomatic related carriers. Int J Parasitol. 2013;43(5):389-397.

[67] Weirather JL, Duggal P, Nascimento EL, Monteiro GR, Martins DR, Lacerda HG, et al. Comprehensive candidate gene analysis for symptomatic or asymptomatic outcomes of Leishmania infantum infection in Brazil. Ann Hum Genet. 2017;81(1):41-48.

[68] Chakravarty J, Hasker E, Kansal S, Singh OP, Malaviya P, Singh AK, et al. Determinants for progression from asymptomatic infection to symptomatic visceral leishmaniasis: A cohort study. PLoS Negl Trop Dis. 2019;13(3): e0007216.

[69] Bucheton B, Abel L, Kheir MM, Mirgani A, El-Safi SH, Chevillard C, et al. Genetic control of visceral leishmaniasis in a Sudanese population: candidate gene testing indicates a linkage to the NRAMP1 region. Genes Immun. 2003;4(2):104-109.

[70] Mohamed HS, Ibrahim ME, Miller EN, White JK, Cordell HJ, Howson JM, et al. SLC11A1 (formerly NRAMP1) and susceptibility to visceral leishmaniasis in The Sudan. Eur J Hum Genet. 2004;12(1):66-74.

[71] Mehrotra S, Oommen J, Mishra A, Sudharshan M, Tiwary P, Jamieson SE, et al. No evidence for association between SLC11A1 and visceral leishmaniasis in India. BMC Med Genet. 2011;12:71.

[72] Karplus TM, Jeronimo SM, Chang H, Helms BK, Burns TL, Murray JC, et al. Association between the tumor necrosis factor locus and the clinical outcome of Leishmania chagasi infection. Infect Immun. 2002;70(12): 6919-6925.

[73] Mehrotra S, Fakiola M, Oommen J, Jamieson SE, Mishra A, Sudarshan M, et al. Genetic and functional evaluation of the role of CXCR1 and CXCR2 in susceptibility to visceral leishmaniasis in north-east India. BMC Med Genet. 2011;12:162.

[74] Alborzi A, Pourabbas B, Shahian F, Mardaneh J, Pouladfar GR, Ziyaeyan M. Detection of Leishmania infantum kinetoplast DNA in the whole blood of asymptomatic individuals by PCR-ELISA and comparison with other infection markers in endemic areas, southern Iran. Am J Trop Med Hyg. 2008;79(6):839-842.

[75] Custodio E, Gadisa E, Sordo L, Cruz I, Moreno J, Nieto J, et al. Factors associated with Leishmania asymptomatic infection: results from a cross-sectional survey in highland northern Ethiopia. PLoS Negl Trop Dis. 2012;6(9):e1813.

[76] McCall LI, Zhang WW, Matlashewski G. Determinants for the development of visceral leishmaniasis disease. PLoS Pathog. 2013;9(1): e1003053.

[77] Gadisa E, Custodio E, Cañavate C, Sordo L, Abebe Z, Nieto J, et al. Usefulness of the rK39-immuno chromatographic test, direct agglutination test, and leishmanin skin test for detecting asymptomatic Leishmania infection in children in a new visceral leishmaniasis focus in Amhara State, Ethiopia. Am J Trop Med Hyg. 2012;86(5):792-798.

[78] Srivastava P, Dayama A, Mehrotra S, Sundar S. Diagnosis of visceral leishmaniasis. Trans R Soc Trop Med Hyg. 2011;105(1):1-6.

[79] Dye C, Williams BG. Malnutrition, age and the risk of parasitic disease: visceral leishmaniasis revisited. Proc Biol Sci. 1993;254(1339):33-39.

[80] Harrison LH, Naidu TG, Drew JS, de Alencar JE, Pearson RD. Reciprocal relationships between undernutrition and the parasitic disease visceral leishmaniasis. Rev Infect Dis. 1986; 8(3):447-453.

[81] Dey A, Singh S. Transfusion transmitted leishmaniasis: a case report and review of literature. Indian J Med Microbiol. 2006;24(3):165-170.

[82] Badaro R, Jones TC, Carvalho EM, Sampaio D, Reed SG, Barral A, et al. New perspectives on a subclinical form of visceral leishmaniasis. J Infect Dis. 1986;154(6):1003-1011.

[83] Fissore C, Delaunay P, Ferrua B, Rosenthal E, Del Giudice P, Aufeuvre JP, et al. Convenience of serum for visceral leishmaniasis diagnosis by PCR. J Clin Microbiol. 2004;42(11):5332-5333.

[84] Costa-Pereira C, Moreira ML, Soares RP, Marteleto BH, Ribeiro VM, França-Dias MH, et al. One-year timeline kinetics of cytokine-mediated cellular immunity in dogs vaccinated against visceral leishmaniasis. BMC Vet Res. 2015;11:92.

[85] Murray HW, Flanders KC, Donaldson DD, Sypek JP, Gotwals PJ, Liu J, et al. Antagonizing deactivating cytokines to enhance host defense and chemotherapy in experimental visceral leishmaniasis. Infect Immun. 2005; 73(7):3903-3911.

[86] Alvar J, Aparicio P, Aseffa A, Den Boer M, Cañavate C, Dedet JP, et al. The relationship between leishmaniasis and AIDS: the second 10 years. Clin Microbiol Rev. 2008;21(2):334-59, table of contents.

[87] Molina R, Jiménez M, García-Martínez J, San Martín JV, Carrillo E, Sánchez C, et al. Role of asymptomatic and symptomatic humans as reservoirs of visceral leishmaniasis in a

Mediterranean context. PLoS Negl Trop Dis. 2020;14(4):e0008253.

[88] Singh OP, Tiwary P, Kushwaha AK, Singh SK, Singh DK, Lawyer P, et al. Xenodiagnosis to evaluate the infectiousness of humans to sandflies in an area endemic for visceral leishmaniasis in Bihar, India: a transmission-dynamics study. Lancet Microbe. 2021;2(1):e23-e31.

Chapter 6

Geographical Distribution of Cutaneous Leishmaniasis and Pathogenesis

Mohammed Hassan Flaih

Abstract

Leishmaniasis is still considered to be a global health problem, which spreads in most countries in the world. *Leishmania* is an intracellular obligate protistan parasite that causes different clinical symptoms in infected humans and other animals. There are clinically different types of the disease including: visceral, cutaneous or muco-cutaneous leishmaniasis. Approximately, two million new infections occurring annually; 0.7 to 1.2 million cases are recorded with cutaneous leishmaniasis and 200,000–400,000 cases return for visceral leishmaniasis. However, Cutaneous leishmaniasis considers one of uncontrolled wobbling endemic diseases, especially in Iraq, which occurs at the skin to cause a dermal lesion. Usually, the lesion is spontaneously healed to leave a colorless depressed scar and permanent immunity.

Keywords: pathogenicity, dermal lesion, papule, Lipophosphoglycan, leishmanolysin

1. Introduction

Leishmaniasis considers one of the neglected tropical diseases with a wide global distribution (**Figure 1**) [2]. WHO mentioned that leishmaniasis is from the important tropical diseases and represents a serious health problem. It includes a broad

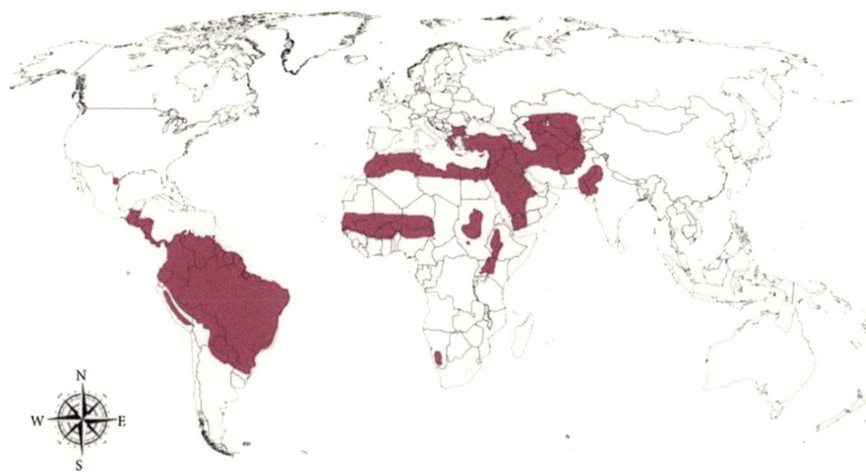

Figure 1.
Worldwide distribution of cutaneous leishmaniasis [1].

spectrum of clinical symptoms which may led to the fatal [3]. Leishmaniasis is endemic in 98 countries with over 350 million people at risk. There are more than 12 million infections with leishmaniasis and nearly 2 million new infections occurring annually; 0.7 to 1.2 million cases of cutaneous leishmaniasis and 200,000–400,000 cases of visceral leishmaniasis [4, 5]. Overall, two million new cases of cutaneous leishmaniasis are discovered annually in Afghanistan, Iran, Saudi Arabia, Syria, Iraq, Algeria, Brazil and Peru [6].

There are approximately 20 species confirmed for *Leishmania* are pathogenic to humans [7], that may cause different clinical symptoms (Cutaneous Leishmaniasis (CL), Muco-cutaneous Leishmaniasis (MCL) and Visceral Leishmaniasis (VL)) [8]. However, *Leishmania* parasites infect phagocytic cells. Virulence factors cause an inhibition or modification of host cell signaling pathways (interleukin and chemokine) which effect on other immune cells [9].

1.1 Prevalence of CL and geographical distribution

Although CL is considered as a global health problem, it remains as a neglected disease [10]. Leishmaniasis infections spread in geographically different regions. However, more infections occur in sub- or/and tropics of Africa, the Middle East, Southern and Central America and South Europe and Asia [11]. It is prevailing at a broad global level and there is an increase worldwide in recorded cases number, also is most neglectful diseases. There is a geographical expansion and a global increase in infection of visceral and cutaneous leishmaniasis, which is still associated with vector population expansion [12]. Environment conditions may overlap many biological processes that effect directly on geographically sandfly distribution, reproductive rates and abundance [13]. Further, *Leishmania* showed as an opportunistic pathogen with HIV-infected adults and even children [14]. Depending to recent reports, leishmaniasis considers an endemic disease in 98 countries and about 1.3 million new cases annually [15]. However, CL is an endemic disease in several countries in the Middle East and North Africa. Foci of *L. major* (zoonotic cutaneous leishmaniasis) are mainly in Sudan, Egypt, Libya, Tunisia, Jordan and Palestine while in Syria, Saudi Arabia, Iraq and Iran are endemic for both *L. tropica* (ACL) and *L. major* (ZCL) [16]. Nearly, there are 500,000 cases of ZCL occur annually, while ACL appear in 400,000 cases. Ninety percent of cutaneous leishmaniasis occur in Afghanistan, Ethiopia, Algeria, Syria, Saudi Arabia, Sudan, Iran, Iraq, Brazil and Peru [17]. In Sri Lanka, leishmaniasis has recorded 8487 cases from 2009 to 2016 [18]. In Pakistan, nearly 21,000–35,000 cases of CL are reported annually [19]. Moroccan Health Ministry mentioned that were 16,852 cases of ACL and 24,804 cases of ZCL in 2004–2013 [13]. Abdellatif *et al.* [20] observed 140 cases with cutaneous leishmaniasis in one provinces of Libya. Khosravi *et al.* [21] recorded 869 (4.7%) cases of CL after were examined 18,308 in Kerman province, Iran. In Syria, 22.882 cases via the period 2004–2008 [14], while 53,000 cases in 2012, only in the first half of 2013, were reported 41,000 cases [22]. In Iraq, Alsamarai and Alobaidi [23] are indicated to 107 cases with CL in Alhaweja General Hospital, Kirkuk. Al-Mayali [24] mentioned that infection rate in urban regions population high from rural regions, where most cases was in Diwania center. Al-Obaidi *et al.* [25] have conducted a survey based on Iraqi CDC database (2008–2015), 17,001 cases recorded in all parts Iraq. Flaih *et al.,* [26] recorded 247 cases of CL in Thi-Qar.

1.2 Pathogenesis

Leishmaniasis is caused by flagellated *Leishmania* parasites, obligate intracellular protozoa and infect humans and other mammals [27]. The infection is transmitted by infected females sandfly bite and the disease highly spreads in poor populations of tropical and subtropical countries [28]. The putative vectors of the disease are species belonging to the genus *Phlebotomus* and *Lutzomyia* [3].

Cutaneous leishmaniasis lesion continues in size and depth, about 4–6 weeks after the sandfly bite, to forms an ulcer that considers primary characteristic of late CL [29]. The clinical appearance of CL is determined by a genetic variation, complex, host immune status and response mechanism, site of the sandfly bite, size and duration of lesion and secondary infections. A combination of these factors is more likely to overlap [19]. Lesions of CL mostly appears on exposed body parts or that are mainly open to the environment as arm, legs, face and neck, but it a little occurs on body parts which are usually covered such as the back and abdomen [30, 31]. In addition, multiple lesions may be as result to the sandflies feeding behaviors which tend to occur multiple bites, prevalence of high numbers of infected insects or rubbing of the lesion to transmit for other areas [6].

CL is often leave a disfiguring scar, especially on visible body sites, causing also social, psychological, and economic problems [30]. Metacyclic promastigotes deposited into the mammalian host skin are engulfed, target host cells are macrophages. Promastigotes differentiate into amastigotes within it. Generally, amastigote replication leads to rupture of the macrophage. The free amastigotes invade other macrophages [7, 32]. Metacyclic promastigotes are highly motile, able to migrate via a collagen matrix, therefore phagocytosis of *Leishmania* may occur at far locations from the bite site [33]. When metacyclic promastigotes enter the host body, within minutes, the metacyclic promastigotes are engulfed by phagocytic cells, including: macrophages and neutrophils. Neutrophil has very short life span, so macrophages are the main host cells. Metacyclic differentiate into non-motile, small amastigote forms which reproduce by binary fission even rupturing the macrophages to infect other macrophages [32, 34]. However, neutrophils and dendritic cells are act as Trojan horses, which let the parasites to enter macrophages, *Leishmania* spp. does not activate parasite killing mechanisms (silent entry) [35]. *Leishmania* parasite can delay neutrophil apoptosis, which allows to the parasite replicates within these cells [36]. Although macrophages are host cells. Neutrophils, dendritic cells, and fibroblasts may be implicated in various stages of the infection [37]. Other cell types, as mast cells, natural killer cells (NK) and Langerhans cells are also involved in leishmaniasis establishment [38]. Both parasitic forms (amastigotes and promastigotes) have different ways, alter the structure of the parasitophorous vacuole and the environment of macrophage, to prevent series of cellular signaling events which lead to the parasite killing within the phagolysosome vacuole that provides an environment for parasite [35].

Leishmania must evade from the innate and adaptive immune responses. It is engulfed by macrophage but resist proteolysis and degradation in the phagolysosome [39, 40]. Macrophages engulf *Leishmania* directly via interactions with multiple cellular receptors as fibronectin receptor, mannose receptor, Toll-like receptors and CR1 and CR3 complement receptors, also engulf apoptotic neutrophils that contain Leishmanial parasites [7, 41]. Inside host cells, *Leishmania* parasites to be able to establish and survive. They resist and circumvent anti-parasitic immune response pathways. In some cases, *Leishmania* spp. smartly invest immune responses or induce cellular signaling pathways to facilitate entry and establishment of parasite [7]. An infection of any type of *Leishmania* depends on complex, virulence factors and host immunologic response [42].

The first sign of the infection appears as a small erythema around the site of the sandfly bite, amastigotes start to multiply inside dermal macrophages and after a variable incubation period. The erythema gradually converts to an inflammatory papule, usually few millimeters in diameter. It increases in a size and progresses to a nodule that often ulcerates to cause a non-painful ulcer, which appears discoloration of surrounding skin. The lesion may be multiple and/or small lesions surrounding the larger lesion. The development is slow range weeks to moths. The healing occurs after an adaptive cellular immune response that possible to fight the infection [43]. Ulcers become painful if accompanied secondary bacterial or fungal infection [44].

1.3 Essential virulence factors

A virulence is one of the important concepts which researches being on them. Also identification and determination of the virulence factors is a target for researchers in order to provide the road map of a vaccine design, identify of interactions with host defense mechanisms and a role of virulence factors in disease pathogenicity [45]. There are virulence factors have been identified of various *Leishmania* spp. that are possible at pathogenesis in the host. Some factors help in an engulfment and attachment of the parasite within host cells while other factors act as intracellular survival. Pathogen stops signaling pathways inside the host cell that activate immune response, thereby development of the disease [7].

The outcome of leishmaniasis infections depend both host status and pathogen virulence factors. *Leishmania* produces various virulence factors to facilitate transmission of parasite and infect mammalian host [46]. All of *Leishmania* surface coats with a glycocalyx that has a diversity in the composition. Notable, all of the surface-bound molecules share a common structural feature. They all contain a highly conserved glycosylphosphatidylinositol (GPI)-anchor. This type of GPI-lipid anchor is structurally different from those found in mammalian cells. The glycocalyx in the *Leishmania* promastigote is dominated by GPI-anchored phosphoglycosylated glycans. However, during the life cycle of the parasite, occur changes in composition of the *Leishmania* surface glycocalyx [47]. Metacyclic promastigote has a thick glycocalyx. The glycocalyx is made of glycoproteins and other glycosylated species anchored into the surface membrane via a glycosylphosphatidylinositol (GPI) linkage [39]. For survival inside macrophages containing microbicidal factors, *Leishmania* spp. modulate or/and inhibit cell signaling pathways cascades involved in their synthesis [9].

A number of important molecules that had identified as factors in parasite virulence as lipophosphoglycan (LPG), the surface protease (gp63), cysteine proteinases (CPs), proteophosphoglycan (PPG), glicoinositol-phospholipids (GIPLs) and the 11 kDa kinetoplastid membrane protein (KMP-11) [43, 48]. Glycoproteins, LPGs, PPGs, and GIPLs are GPI-anchored molecules in dense surface glycocalyx, Leishmanial parasites also secrete various glycoconjugates especially PPGs. Secreted and surface glycoconjugates for promastigote has importance in an infection, survival, or virulence but are not necessary in order to *Leishmania* viability inside culture [49].

2. Lipophosphoglycan (LPG)

LPG is most abundant glycolipid that densely coats surface of *Leishmania* promastigotes. It is composed of a glycan core which is joined a long polymer consist from repeating units of phosphoglycan (PGs) which is terminated with oligosaccharide capping structure. LPG connects to promastigote membrane by a phosphatidylinositol lipid (PI) anchor. The number of repeating units and the cap may differ between *Leishmania* spp. Also, the amount and structure of LPG varies during parasite life cycle [50, 51]. In all *Leishmania* species, LPG expresses high amounts on surface of procyclic and metacyclic promastigotes, in contrast with amastigotes [52]. LPG on metacyclic promastigote surface is much longer from procyclic and almost completely absent in amastigotes [39]. Indeed, this molecule has an important role not only in invertebrate and vertebrate host, but too during early steps for establishment of the infection [50]. *L. major* mutants which lack lpg1 and lpg2 genes are sensitive to host complement system. This leads to unable survival in both intermediate or definitive host [53]. LPG1 is one of the key enzymes in the LPG biosynthesis, that involved in the synthesis of the LPG glycan core [54]. As well as, *Leishmania* lack lpg1 gene expresses imperfect LPG, not contains PG domain [55]. *L. major* and *Labrus donovani* need LPG1 for infection establishment inside macrophages, phagocytosis eliminates LPG1- null mutants, then restoration of LPG expression given capacity to replication of parasite within macrophage [52, 54].

LPG acts as a ligand to attach promastigotes to midgut epithelium of sandfly and also protects promastigotes from destruction by proteolytic enzymes that are destined for blood meal digestion [56]. In mammalian host, leishmanial LPG plays an essential role to avoid the parasite lysis by the host complement system, either by prevent of complement molecules attachment or inactivate the assembly of complement complex on promastigote surface [47]. It has ability to modulation and creating an appropriateness environment in order to parasite survival but the mechanisms of underlying modulation remain completely unknown and not goodly understood [57]. LPGs delay lysosomes formation and allow *Leishmania* to covert to intracellular amastigote forms [58]. It has been shown to protection of the lysis by complement system, adhesion and entry in macrophages, inhibition of protein kinase C (PKC), inhibition of phagosomal maturation, modulation of nitric oxide (NO) production [59].

LPG interferes with the pro-inflammatory responses for host cell through binding with Toll-like receptor (TLR) 2 and 4 on macrophages and NK cells [57]. LPG-TLR interactions induce ERK phosphorylation, while suppressing of p38 MAP kinase phosphorylation (ERK and p38 MAP kinase are from components of MAP kinases), modulate production of reactive oxygen species (ROS) and nitric oxide and inhibit secretion of pro-inflammatory cytokine [47]. For example, if p38 MAP kinase activate will produced IL-12 and IL-10, that inhibit activation of ERK [57]. LPG binds with complement receptor (CR3) and anchored molecules on macrophage surface to facilitate parasite engulfment [7, 60]. Furthermore, Leishmanial LPG can to impair the nuclear translocation of NF-κB in monocytes which lead to decrease in IL-12 production, and this effects early immune response of the host [43].

3. Major surface protease: (MSP) GP63

GP63 is known leishmanolysin or called major surface protease (MSP) or promastigote surface protease (PSP), also called a zinc- dependent metalloprotease [50, 61, 62]. It is found at *Leishmania* surface connected through a glycophosphatidylinositol (GPI) anchor, or is direct secreted to an extracellular surrounding [50]. Fracture of GPI anchor by phospholipase C leads up to scattering gp63 in extracellular space, also is secreted directly by the flagellar pocket, as well as the presence of GP63 in intracellular pools [63].

GP63s are encoded by multiple genes that appear vary in their sequence (especially in untranslated regions), array in the *Leishmania* genome [63, 64]. Differences in the untranslated regions may lead to different gene expression [50]. These genes generate abundant proteins which lead to vary among species and forms of *Leishmania* that cause a different biological effect [65]. Genes of gp63 are expressed in promastigotes and amastigotes [61]. It is expressed in metacyclic more abundantly than procyclic promastigotes [62]. Also, gp63 has been observed at lower levels through its expression in amastigotes [50].

GP63 is a multifunction enzyme that related to an inhibition of complement components. The recent findings refer to a critical role played by gp63 as an important virulence factor that wide influence cellular signaling mechanisms and related pathways [65]. GP63 is responsible about migration of parasite through extracellular matrix, avoid lysis by the complement system, evasion from macrophagic intracellular hydrolysis [61] and facilitation of promastigotes phagocytosis by macrophage, matrix extracellular degradation, contribute to intracellular migration, NK inhibition and persistence and progression of infection [64, 66]. Also, inhibit nitric oxide production (Leishmanicidal) or macrophages pro-inflammatory cytokines [67].

This protease serves to cleaves complement protein C3b and converts to C3bi (inactivated form of C3b) and protects promastigote from complement-mediated lysis. Further, generation of C3bi leads to uptake promastigote by complement receptors such as CR3 which located at the surface of macrophage. The evidence suggests, promastigote ligates CR3 directly and via opsonized C3bi [7, 62]. C3bi acts as a bridge between complement receptor at surface of macrophage and gp63- bearing promastigote [68]. C3bi generation by enzymatic activity of gp63 bonded to promastigote surface, mediate phagocytosis process by complement receptors (CR1 andCR3) that leading to silent entry of parasite into macrophage [7, 62].

GP63 has been described to is not only to degradation and damage of transcription factors and various kinases, but also it modulates negative regulatory mechanisms of signaling pathways for example protein tyrosine phosphatases (PTP). Activation of PTP together with other signaling molecules leading to inhibition of leishmanicidal and inflammatory functions [63, 65]. GP63 is activate protein tyrosine phosphatases that result alteration of MAP, JAK, STAT1 and IRAK-1kinase pathways. In the nucleus, it is responsible for the inactivation of important transcription factors which activate specific chemokines, such as NF-κB [9, 65].

4. Cysteine proteinases (CPs)

Cysteine proteases (CPs) are degrading enzymes which cleave various proteins. They are act as essential virulence factors in leishmanial infection, as well play an important role in many pathogenic protozoa and other microorganisms [69]. At least from 6 classes proteases classified in the proteolysis: serine, cysteine, glutamate, metallo, threonine and aspartate proteases. Cysteine proteases (CPs) are classified into 72 families, so not all are expressed in parasitic protozoa [70]. In *Leishmania* genome, there are 154 peptidases include cysteine, aspartic, serine and metalloproteases. *Leishmania* protease are necessary for continuation and establishment of infection [71]. In several pathogenic organisms, including parasitic protozoa as *Entamoeba histolytica*, *Leishmania* and *Trypanosoma*, found CPs which are enzymes [72, 73]. *Leishmania* has three types from CPs: CPA, CPB, and CPC [72, 74]. CPs are expressed in higher levels in the mammalian amastigote [70]. Gene expression of CPA is maximal level in amastigote stage, while lower expression is in promastigote [73]. Also, CPB is expressed at high levels in the amastigote, is expressed at a very few level in procyclic-promastigotes [75]. CPB1 and CPB2 are expressed in higher levels of metacyclic promastigote, while CPC in procyclic-promastigote [70].

Although roles of CPs in pathogenesis of *Leishmania* are unclear, it has been showed that Leishmaniasis cannot continue in macrophages with the presence of

CP inhibitors [76]. Cysteine proteases play key roles in *Leishmania* biology and their inhibition is appearing as an important strategy to the elimination of the disease. They are necessary to metabolism, intracellular survival and reproduction of parasite [74], participate in exsheathing, excystment, also tissue invasion and some parasite immune-evasion [69]. CPs appears an essential role in pathogenicity and leads multi-processes such as modulation or evasion of the host immune response, cell/tissue degradation and damage, catalyze hydrolysis of various host proteins that are responsible of important cellular biological activities in pathways, differentiation of promastigote to amastigote and autophagy [70, 71]. Generally, CPA lead an essential key in the interactions of parasite with host cell [43, 77], while CPB modulates Th1 immune responses, and IFN-γ production via damage of transcription factor (NF- κB) and inhibition ofIL-12 production. Also CPB is modulate levels of parasite proteins as gp63 [70].

The inhibition of CPA and CPB or deletion their genes not only alters autophagy pathway but too prevents transformation into amastigotes, thus support hypothesis of autophagy is required for the differentiation [43, 78]. Parasites evidenced low growth, pathogenicity and efficacy after their treated with CP inhibitors [79]. There are efforts towards make it as vaccine candidates because their potential and their importance. For now, no effective drug or vaccine for leishmaniasis [69, 71, 74].

5. Proteophosphoglycan (PPG)

Leishmania expresses several types from proteophosphoglycans (PPGs). Some of PPGs are secreted and others found on surface of amastigotes and promastigotes [80]. PPGs are a large group from widely glycosylated proteins, have some unique features [81]. It is produce by both two parasite stages, is found on the parasite surface, Golgi, lysosome and flagellar pocket [53]. There are number of PPGs types, include filamentous proteophospho-glycan (fPPG) and GPI-anchored membranous proteophosphoglycan (mPPG), all of that are originally in stages of promastigotes within sandfly vector, there is also non-filamentous proteophosphoglycan (aPPG) which is a major product of amastigotes in mammalian host [82–84]. The ppg1 gene encodes membrane-bound PPG, and secreted non-filamentous PPG is encoded by ppg2 [85], while ppg3 gene is encode filamentous proteophosphoglycan [86]. Compositional analysis observed PPG contains 67% glycan, 28% protein and 5% phosphate. PPG is composed from repeating units of PGs that attach to protein backbone [81]. PG molecules are either connected to cell surface via GPI-lipid anchor, or secreted as protein-containing phosphoglycans [51]. PPG is proved to bind to macrophage receptors in order to facilitates parasite invasion, this may be explaining that PPG play an early role in infection and prevalence [53, 87, 88] are suggest possibilities of PPG in drug resistant mechanisms and PPG abundance of *L. donovani* is as evidence for resistant clinical isolates. PPG- null mutant *L. major* are more sensitive and less virulent to complement-lysis. In infected mice, not develop lesions in PPG- null mutant parasites [82]. Metacyclic promastigotes in sandfly midgut secrete fPPG which condenses to promastigote secretory gel (PSG), to formation a biological plug that block the anterior midgut, this is oblige sandfly to disgorge parasites though blood-feeding [89]. PSG is largest molecule that secretes by promastigotes within sandfly gut. Also, it is support both macrophage assemblage and infection [90]. Inside infected macrophages, amastigotes secrete aPPG which can reach to very high concentrations [90]. The membrane-bound PPG may play a direct important role in host–parasite interactions [90]. It is found on the surface of amastigotes and promastigotes [91]. Within macrophage, believed that aPPG is contribute in formation of parasitophorous vacuole, this protects infection in the mammalian cells, also PPG may contribute binding of *Leishmania* to host-cells and may be modulate biology of infected macrophage in the early infection [83].

6. Conclusion

CL has a global prevalence and there is an increase worldwide in recorded cases, and also considers from neglectful diseases. The dermal lesion is occurred by an obligate intracellular *Leishmania* parasite, which transmits via the bite of the female sandfly. The clinical appearances depend on *Leishmania* species, virulence factors and host immunologic response. Virulence factors have an important role in pathogenicity, so inhibition or absence one of them lead to effecting on parasite.

Author details

Mohammed Hassan Flaih
Department of Nursing Techniques, Al-Nasiriyah Technical Institute, Southern Technical University, Al-Nasiriyah, Iraq

*Address all correspondence to: moh.alqurayshi@stu.edu.iq

References

[1] Gabriel A et al. Cutaneous Leishmaniasis: The complexity of host's effective immune response against a polymorphic parasitic disease. Journal of Immunology Research. 2019;**2019**:1-16

[2] Abdoli A, Maspi N, Ghaffarifar F, Nasiri V. Viscerotropic leishmaniasis: A systematic review of the case reports to highlight spectrum of the infection in endemic countries. Parasitology Open. 2019;**4**:1-14

[3] Torres-guerrero E, Quintanilla-cedillo MR, Ruiz-esmenjaud J, Arenas R. Leishmaniasis: A review [Version 1; Referees: 2 Approved] referee status. F1000Res. 2017;**6**(750):1-15

[4] Akhoundi M et al. Leishmania infections: Molecular targets and diagnosis. Molecular Aspects of Medicine. 2017;**57**:1-29

[5] Izadi S et al. Molecular epidemiological survey of cutaneous Leishmaniasis in two highly endemic Metropolises of Iran, application of FTA cards for DNA extraction from Giemsa-stained slides. Jundishapur Journal of Microbiology. 2016;**9**(2):1-7

[6] Al-Khayat ZAY, Agha NFS, Alharmni KIF, Khudhur YJ. A clinico-epidemiological study on cutaneous leishmaniasis in Erbil, Iraq (2015-2017). International Journal of Research in Dermatology. 2018;**4**(1):1-7

[7] Oghumu S, Natarajan G, Satoskar AR. Pathogenesis of Leishmaniasis in humans. Human Emerging and Re-emerging Infections. 2015;**I**:337-348

[8] Kariyawasam UL et al. Genetic diversity of Leishmania donovani that causes cutaneous leishmaniasis in Sri Lanka : A cross sectional study with regional comparisons. BMC Infectious Diseases. 2017;**17**(791):1-11

[9] Gupta G, Oghumu S, Satoskar AR. Mechanisms of immune evasion in Leishmaniasis Gaurav. Advances in Applied Microbiology. 2013;**82**:155-184

[10] Ghatee MA et al. Population structure of Leishmania Tropica causing anthroponotic cutaneous Leishmaniasis in Southern Iran by PCR-RFLP of Kinetoplastid DNA. BioMed Research International. 2018;**2018**:1-11. DOI: 10.1155/2018/6049198

[11] Bessat M, El Shanat S. Leishmaniasis: Epidemiology, control and future perspectives with special emphasis on Egypt. Journal of Tropical Diseases. 2015;**3**(1):1-10

[12] Cunze S et al. Leishmaniasis in Eurasia and Africa: Geographical distribution of vector species and pathogens. Royal Society Open Science. 2019;**6**:1-12. DOI: 10.1098/rsos.190334

[13] Boussaa S et al. Species composition of sand flies and bionomics of Phlebotomus Papatasi and P. Sergenti (Diptera: Psychodidae) in cutaneous Leishmaniasis Endemic Foci, Morocco. Parasites and Vectors. 2016;**9**(1):1-11. DOI: 10.1186/s13071-016-1343-6

[14] Alvar J et al. Leishmaniasis worldwide and global estimates of its incidence. PLoS One. 2012;**7**(5):1-12

[15] Salam N, Al-shaqha WM, Azzi A. Leishmaniasis in the Middle East: Incidence and epidemiology. PLoS Neglected Tropical Diseases. 2014;**8**(10):1-8

[16] Alkulaibi MM, Suleiman AM, Khalil EAG, Al-Garadi MA. Prevalence of cutaneous leishmaniasis in Western Highlands in Yemen. Journal of Tropical Medicine. 2019;**2019**:1-7

[17] Ali MA et al. Epidemiological study of leishmaniasis in some Iraqi Provinces.

American Journal of Men's Health. 2018;**14**(4):18-24

[18] Galgamuwa LS, Dharmaratne SD, Iddawela D. Leishmaniasis in Sri Lanka: Spatial distribution and seasonal variations from 2009 to 2016. Parasites & Vectors. 2018;**11**(60):1-10. DOI: 10.1186/s13071-018-2647-5

[19] Khan NH, Llewellyn MS, Schonian G, Sutherland CJ. LSHTM variability of cutaneous Leishmaniasis lesions is not associated with genetic diversity of Leishmania tropica in Khyber Pakhtunkhwa Province of Pakistan. The American Journal of Tropical Medicine and Hygiene. 2017;**97**(5):1489-1497

[20] Abdellatif MZM, El-mabrouk K, Ewis AA. An epidemiological study of cutaneous leishmaniasis in Al-Jabal Al-Gharbi, Libya. The Korean Journal of Parasitology. 2013;**51**(1):75-84

[21] Khosravi A et al. The present status of cutaneous Leishmaniasis in a recently emerged focus in South-West of Kerman Province, Iran. Iranian Journal of Public Health. 2013;**42**(2):182-187

[22] Du R, Hotez PJ, Al-Salem WS, Acosta-Serrano A. Old world cutaneous Leishmaniasis and refugee crises in the Middle East and North Africa. PLOS Neglected Tropical Diseases. 2016;**10**(5): 1-11. DOI: 10.1371/journal.pntd.0004545

[23] Alsamarai AM, Alobaidi HS. Cutaneous leishmaniasis in Iraq. Journal of Infection in Developing Countries. 2009;**3**(2):123-129

[24] Al-Mayali HM. Evalution and Use of Some Immunological Tests in the Epidemiological Study of Leishmaniasis in Qadisiyah Governorate. Iraq: Al-Qadisiyah University; 2004

[25] Al-Obaidi MJ, Abd Al-Hussein MY, Al-Saqur IM. Survey study on the prevalence of cutaneous leishmaniasis in Iraq. Iraqi Journal of Science. 2016;**57**(3):2181-2187

[26] Flaih MH, Al-Abady FA, Hussein KR. Phylogenetic Analysis of Kinetoplast DNA: KDNA of Leishmania Tropica in Thi-Qar Province, Iraq. Comparative Immunology, Microbiology and Infectious Diseases. 2021;**78**:101696. Available from: https://linkinghub.elsevier.com/retrieve/pii/S0147957121000886

[27] Ramírez JD et al. Taxonomy, Diversity, Temporal and Geographical Distribution of Cutaneous Leishmaniasis in Colombia: A Retrospective Study. Scientific Reports. 2016;**6**(1):28266. Available from: http://www.nature.com/articles/srep28266

[28] Dayakar A, Chandrasekaran S, Kuchipudi SV, Kalangi SK. Cytokines: Key determinants of resistance or disease progression in visceral Leishmaniasis: Opportunities for novel diagnostics and immunotherapy. Frontiers in Immunology. 2019;**10**(670):1-23

[29] Saldanha MG et al. Characterization of the histopathologic features in patients in the early and late phases of cutaneous Leishmaniasis. The American Journal of Tropical Medicine and Hygiene. 2017;**96**(3):645-652

[30] Bilgic-Temel A, Murrell DF, Uzun S. Cutaneous Leishmaniasis: A neglected disfiguring disease for women. International Journal of Women's Dermatology. 2019;**5**(3):158-165. DOI: 10.1016/j.ijwd.2019.01.002

[31] Ahmed H et al. Cutaneous leishmaniasis pattern: A Pakistani perspective. Journal of Entomology and Zoology Studies. 2019;7(3):868-873

[32] Liu D, Uzonna JE. The early interaction of Leishmania with macrophages and dendritic cells and its

influence on the host immune response. Frontiers in Cellular and Infection Microbiology. 2012;**2**(83):1-8

[33] Sunter J, Gull K. Shape, form, function and Leishmania pathogenicity : From textbook descriptions to biological understanding. Open Biology. 2017;7:1-13. DOI: 10.1098/rsob.170165

[34] Alemayehu B, Alemayehu M. Leishmaniasis: A review on parasite, vector and reservoir host. Health Science Journal. 2017;**11**(4):1-6

[35] Söbirk SK. Leishmaniasis in Sweden Molecular, Diagnostic and Epidemiological Studies of the Parasite Leishmania in a Non- Endemic Country. Sweden: Lund University; 2019

[36] Martínez-lópez M, Soto M, Iborra S, Sancho D. Leishmania Hijacks Myeloid cells for immune escape. Frontiers in Microbiology. 2018;**9**:1-16

[37] Sarkar J, Pal S, Bhattacharya S, Biswas M. In vitro Antileishmanial activity of Pleumeria Pudica leaf extracts on Leishmania Donovani Promastigotes. American-Eurasian Journal of Scientific Research. 2013;**8**:68-71

[38] Banerjee A et al. Role of pro-inflammatory Cytokine IL-17 in Leishmania pathogenesis and in protective immunity by Leishmania vaccines. Cellular Immunology. 2016;**309**:37-41. DOI: 10.1016/j.cellimm.2016.07.004

[39] Olivier M, Gregory DJ, Forget G. Subversion mechanisms by which Leishmania parasites can escape the host immune response: A signaling point of view. Clinical Microbiology Reviews. 2005;**18**(2):293-305

[40] Sharma U, Singh S. Immunobiology of Leishmaniasis. Indian Journal of Experimental Biology. 2009;**47**(2009): 412-423

[41] Conceição-Silva F, Morgado FN. Leishmania Spp-Host interaction: There is always an onset, but is there an end? Frontiers in Cellular and Infection Microbiology. 2019;**9**(330):1-14

[42] AL-Atabi BAH. Epidemiological and Molecular Study of Cutaneous Leishmaniasis Using RT-PCR in Wasit Province – Iraq. Univer. Wasit. Colle. Scien; 2014

[43] Silva-almeida M et al. Proteinases as virulence factors in Leishmania Spp. infection in mammals. Parasites & Vectors. 2012;**5**(160):1-10

[44] Showler AJ, Boggild AK. Cutaneous Leishmaniasis in travellers: A focus on epidemiology and treatment in 2015. Current Infectious Disease Reports. 2015;**17**(7):2-12

[45] Casadevall A, Pirofski L. Virulence factors and their mechanisms of action: The view from a damage–Response framework. Journal of Water and Health. 2009;**7**(1):1-17

[46] Corrales RM, Sereno D, Mathieu-Daudé F. Deciphering the Leishmania exoproteome: What we know and what we can learn. FEMS Immunology and Medical Microbiology. 2010;**58**(1):27-38. DOI: 10.1111/j.1574-695X.2009.00608.x

[47] Forestier C, Gao Q, Boons G. Leishmania Lipophosphoglycan: How to establish structure-activity relationships for this highly complex and multifunctional glycoconjugate ? Cellular and Infection Microbiology. 2015;**4**:1-7

[48] Lima-junior DS, Beverley SM, Shao F, Zamboni DS. Leishmania Lipophosphoglycan triggers caspase- 11 and the non-canonical activation of the NLRP3 article Leishmania Lipophosphoglycan triggers caspase-11 and the non-canonical activation of the NLRP3 inflammasome. Cell Reports.

2019;**26**(2):429-437.e5. DOI: 10.1016/j.celrep.2018.12.047

[49] Prakash O et al. Identification of Leishmania major UDP-sugar Pyrophosphorylase inhibitors using biosensor-based small molecule fragment library screening. Molecules. 2019;**24**(996):1-16

[50] Atayde VD et al. Leishmania exosomes and other virulence factors : Impact on innate immune response and macrophage functions. Cellular Immunology. 2016;**309**:7-18. DOI: 10.1016/j.cellimm.2016.07.013

[51] Dostálová A, Volf P. Leishmania development in sand flies : parasite-vector interactions overview. Parasites & Vectors. 2012;**5**(276):1-12

[52] Franco LH, Beverley SM, Zamboni DS. Innate immune activation and subversion of mammalian functions by Leishmania Lipophosphoglycan. Parasitology Research. 2012;**2012**:1-11

[53] Aoki JI, Laranjeira-silva MF, Muxel SM, Floeter-winter LM. The impact of Arginase activity on virulence factors of Leishmania Amazonensis. Current Opinion in Microbiology. 2019;**52**:110-115. DOI: 10.1016/j.mib.2019.06.003

[54] Lázaro-Souza M et al. Leishmania infantum Lipophosphoglycan-deficient mutants: A tool to study host cell-parasite interplay. Frontiers in Microbiology. 2018;**9**(626):1-10. DOI: 10.3389/fmicb.2018.00626

[55] Dermine JF et al. Leishmania promastigotes require Lipophosphoglycan to actively modulate the fusion properties of phagosomes at an early step of phagocytosis. Cellular Microbiology. 2000;**2**:115-126

[56] Ant TH et al. Leishmania major glycosylation mutants require Phosphoglycans (Lpg 2 2) but not Lipophosphoglycan (Lpg1 2) for survival in permissive sand fly vectors. PLoS Neglected Tropical Diseases. 2010;**4**(1):1-7

[57] Rojas-Bernabe A et al. Leishmania Mexicana Lipophosphoglycan activates ERK and P38 MAP kinase and induces production of Proin Fl Ammatory Cytokines in human macrophages through TLR2 and TLR4. Parasitology. 2014;**141**:788-800

[58] Rossi M, Fasel N. How to master the host immune system? Leishmania parasites have the solutions! International Immunology. 2017;**30**(3):103-111

[59] Nogueira PM, Assis RR, Torrecilhas AC, Saraiva EM. Lipophosphoglycans from Leishmania Amazonensis strains display immunomodulatory properties via TLR4 and do not affect sand fly infection. PLoS Neglected Tropical Diseases. 2016:1-17

[60] Moradin N, Descoteaux A. Leishmania promastigotes : Building a safe Niche within macrophages. Cellular and Infection Microbiology. 2012;**2**:1-7

[61] Medina LS et al. The Gp63 gene cluster is highly polymorphic in natural Leishmania (Viannia) Braziliensis populations, but functional sites are conserved. PLOS ONE. 2016;**11**(9):1-13. DOI: 10.1371/journal.pone.0163284

[62] Ueno N, Wilson ME. Receptor-mediated phagocytosis of Leishmania: Implications for intracellular survival. Trends in Parasitology. 2012;**28**(8):335-344. DOI: 10.1016/j.pt.2012.05.002

[63] Hassani K et al. Absence of metalloprotease GP63 alters the protein content of Leishmania exosomes. PLoS One. 2014;**9**(4):1-14. DOI: 10.1371/journal.pone.0095007

[64] Yao C. Major surface protease of Trypanosomatids : One size fits all?

Infection and Immunity. 2010;**78**(1):22-31

[65] Isnard A, Shio MT, Olivier M, Bengoechea JA. Impact of Leishmania metalloprotease GP63 on macrophage signaling. Cellular and Infection Microbiology. 2012;**2**:1-9

[66] Murase LS et al. The role of metalloproteases in Leishmania species infection in the new world: A systematic review. Parasitology. 2019;**63**:1499-1509

[67] Leitherer S et al. Crossm characterization of the protein tyrosine phosphatase LmPRL-1 secreted by. Infection and Immunity. 2017;**85**(8):1-19

[68] Pandey S et al. Involvement of Leishmania Donovani major surface Glycoprotein Gp63 in Promastigote multiplication. Biosciences. 2004;**29**(1):15-22

[69] Rana S, Mahato JP, Kumar M, Sarsaiya S. Modeling and docking of cysteine Protease-A (CPA) of Leishmania Donovani. Journal of Applied Pharmaceutical Science. 2017;7(9):179-184

[70] Siqueira-neto JL et al. Cysteine proteases in Protozoan parasites. PLoS Neglected Tropical Diseases. 2018;**12**(8):1-20. DOI: 10.1371/journal.pntd.0006512

[71] Das P et al. Protease inhibitors in potential drug development for Leishmaniasis. Indian Journal of Biochemistry and Biophysics. 2013;**50**:363-376

[72] Buxbaum LU et al. Cysteine Protease B of Leishmania Mexicana inhibits host Th1 responses and protective immunity. The Journal of Immunology. 2003;**171**(7):3711-3717. DOI: 10.4049/jimmunol.171.7.3711

[73] Rafati S, Fasel N, Masina S. Leishmania cysteine proteinases : From gene to subunit vaccine. Current Genomics. 2003;**4**(3):109-121

[74] Scala A et al. Targeting of the Leishmania Mexicana cysteine protease CPB2.8DCTE by decorated fused Benzo[b] Thiophene Scaffol. The Royal Society of Chemistry. 2016;**6**:30628-30635

[75] Besteiro S, Coombs GH, Mottram JC. A potential role for ICP, a Leishmanial inhibitor of cysteine peptidases, in the interaction between host and parasite. Molecular Microbiology. 2004;**54**(5):1224-1236

[76] Saffari B, Mohabatkar H. Computational analysis of cysteine proteases (Clan CA, Family C1) of Leishmania major to find potential epitopic regions. Genomics, Proteomics & Bioinformatics. 2009;**7**(3):87-95. DOI: 10.1016/S1672-0229(08)60037-6

[77] Denise H et al. Studies on the CPA cysteine peptidase in the Leishmania infantum genome strain JPCM5. BMC Molecular Biology. 2006;**13**:1-13

[78] Williams RA, Tetley L, Mottram JC, Coombs GH. Cysteine peptidases CPA and CPB are vital for autophagy and differentiation in Leishmania Mexicana. Molecular Microbiology. 2006;**61**(3):655-674. DOI: 10.1111/j.1365-2958.2006.05274.x

[79] Paladi CS et al. In vitro and in vivo activity of a palladacycle complex on Leishmania (Leishmania) Amazonensis. PLoS Neglected Tropical Diseases. 2012;**6**(5):1-7

[80] Samant M et al. Immunization with the DNA-encoding N-terminal domain of proteophosphoglycan of Leishmania Donovani generates Th1-type immunoprotective response against experimental visceral Leishmaniasis. Immunology. 2009;**183**:470-479

[81] Kavoosi G et al. Leishmania major: Effects of proteophosphoglycan on

reactive oxygen species, IL-12, IFN-γ and IL-10 production in healthy individuals. Experimental Parasitology. 2008;**120**(1):62-66

[82] Mukbel RM. Leishmania Amazonensis and Macrophage Interactions: Immune Factors Necessary to Kill the Parasite. Graduate College. Iowa State University; 2005. Available from: https://dr.lib.iastate.edu/handle/20.500.12876/72308

[83] Mukhopadhyay S, Mandal C. Glycobiology of Leishmania Donovani. The Indian Journal of Medical Research. 2006;**123**:203-220

[84] Phillips MR. Characterization of Jabba, A Ricin - Resistant Mutant of Leishmania Donovani. University of Kentucky UKnowledge; 2014

[85] Montgomery J, Curtis J, Handman E. Genetic and structural heterogeneity of proteophosphoglycans in Leishmania. Molecular and Biochemical Parasitology. 2002;**121**:75-85

[86] Depledge DP et al. Comparative expression profiling of Leishmania : modulation in gene expression between species and in different host genetic backgrounds. PLoS Neglected Tropical Diseases. 2009;**3**(7):1-14

[87] Fernandez-prada C et al. High-Throughput Cos-Seq screen with intracellular Leishmania infantum for the discovery of novel drug-resistance mechanisms Christopher. Drugs and Drug Resistance. 2018;**8**(2):165-173. DOI: 10.1016/j.ijpddr.2018.03.004

[88] Samant M et al. Proteophosphoglycan is differentially expressed in sodium stibogluconate-sensitive and resistant Indian clinical isolates of Leishmania Donovani. Parasitology. 2007;**134**(9):1175-1184

[89] Giraud E, Martin O, Yakob L, Rogers M. Quantifying Leishmania metacyclic promastigotes from individual sandfly bites reveals the efficiency of vector transmission. Communications Biology. 2019;**2**(1):25-28. DOI: 10.1038/s42003-019-0323-8

[90] Ilg T, Montgomery J, Stierhof Y, Handman E. Molecular cloning and characterization of a novel repeat-containing Leishmania major gene, Ppg1, that encodes a membrane-associated form of proteophosphoglycan with a putative glycosylphosphatidylinositol anchor. Biological Chemistry. 1999;**274**(44):31410-31420

[91] Foth B et al. Leishmania major proteophosphoglycans exist as membrane-bound and soluble forms and localise to the cell membrane, the flagellar pocket and the lysosome. International Journal for Parasitology. 2002;**32**(14):1701-1708

Chapter 7

Geopolitical and Geospatial Conflicts Affecting Cutaneous Leishmaniasis: Iraqi Cases, 2014-2015

Karim Abdulkadim Muftin Al Zadawi

Abstract

In Iraq, increment of cutaneous leishmaniasis (CL) was reported, a zoonotic type caused by *Leishmania major* and an anthroponotic type caused by *Leishmania tropica*. This is attributed to environmental changes, irregular construction, increased waste, and stray dogs in the cities. Internal displacement, poverty, and malnutrition play a role in the occurrence of disease. *Iraq* has been exposed to wars, civil war, widespread violence, and terrorism, Internal displacement of population, unlawful housing, shortage of municipal services, and accumulation of garbage have been increasing in the cities since 2003. Reports from Iraqi MOH documented an increase in the rate of CL. Eventually, case investigation, vector, and reservoir controls were suspended. Geopolitical conflicts and geospatial health deterioration contributed to an increase in various dominant reservoir species in these areas, particularly for ZCL, and the activity of the sand flies. A sudden sharp increase in CL cases was observed during 2003–2015. In conclusion, ongoing crises exposed Iraq to deterioration, collapse, and destruction of health system infrastructure and uncontrolled urbanization, all of which can act as risk factors for Leishmaniasis.

Keywords: Iraq, cutaneous, leishmaniasis, conflicts, 2014, 2015

1. Introduction

1.1 Background

Leishmaniasis is one of the most common zoonotic infectious diseases worldwide. It is ranked second in mortality and fourth in morbidity among all tropical diseases [1].

According to the species of Leishmania parasite, there are three main forms: cutaneous leishmaniasis (CL), mucocutaneous leishmaniasis (MCL), and visceral leishmaniasis (VL) [2]. CL is the most common form of the disease and the skin is the most affected exposed part of the body characterized with symptoms such as skin sores or skin infection, which starting with small nodules that slowly enlarge, then ulcerate, and end within approximately 1 year with a characteristic permanent, depressed and disfiguring scar (**Figure 1**) [3].

Leishmaniasis is considered as an emerging and remerging disease and a major public health problem in some regions, mainly in developing countries [4–6]. This phenomenon is attributed to environmental changes, irregular construction,

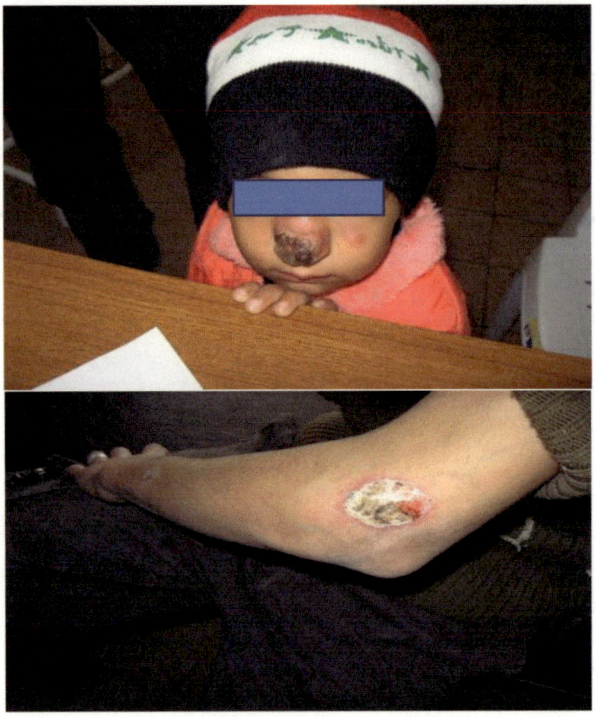

Figure 1.
Lesions affect exposed areas.

human activities, accumulation of waste, and increase in the number of stray dogs in the cities. Conflict, internal displacement, poverty, and malnutrition play a role in the CL occurrence and outbreak [3].

In 2012, the WHO estimated that about 350 million of the world population were at a risk of getting one form of leishmaniasis. Majority of cases (75%) are CL and MCL. Ninety-eight countries in four continents, including Latin America, Africa, Asia, and South Europe, reported cases of the disease [7, 8].

CL is endemic in Iraq and its neighboring countries; Syria, Saudi Arabia, and Turkey [9, 10]. In these countries, Sand-fly vectors and the reservoir for leishmaniasis species; dogs, foxes, rats, jerboas, and other small mammals have been described. Conflicts, violence, civil war, terrorism, limited funding, and internal displacement are *labeled* as predisposing factors to a reemergence of *the disease* in the Middle East [8, 11]. Consequently, the incidence of CL increases and becomes a public health problem, usually affecting poorer communities [12].

The epidemic of CL might occur when large numbers of nonimmune humans become exposed to infection for the first time. Travels from nonendemic areas to endemic areas during activities such as wars, military exercises, civilian works, and tourism may result in outbreak of the disease in certain populations [13].

In endemic areas, building mud houses near the natural habitats of the vector and the reservoir hosts increases human–sand fly contact and thus increases the risk for human Leishmaniasis [14].

2. Leishmaniasis in Iraq

Leishmaniasis is known to be endemic in Iraq since 3000–2000 B.C. and has been described for the first time by Abu Bakr Muhammad ibn Zakariya' al-Razi, one of the greatest names in medieval medicine, in 1500 A.D. [15, 16]. A common name of CL in Iraq is Baghdad boil, which suggests the disease has a long history in Iraq [17].

Two types of CL were reported in Iraq, a zoonotic type caused by *Leishmania major* and an anthroponotic type caused by *Leishmania tropica* [18]. Rural areas in Iraq are described as source of infection and endemicity because of the presence of animal reservoirs (rodents, dogs, and foxes) for ZCL and the use of clay to build some of the houses in villages in these areas [19, 20]. Underdeveloped clay buildings facilitate sand-fly breeding because they maintain a sufficient level of moisture which is important for the sand-fly a larval habitat. The human population in these regions more exposed to a sandfly bite due to their work mainly in the farms [18, 21, 22].

The incidence rate of disease is higher among males than females nearly in all age groups [23, 24]. Males were found to be more vulnerable to CL infection due to the nature of the Iraqi culture that they are mainly responsible for family finance and support, thus making them more exposed to the infectious agents and young males playing outdoors without clothes and swimming in the rivers or lakes due to constant power outage.

CL manifestations increase in October, peak in January, and then gradually decline, reaching their lowest level in August. Two-thirds of the cases were reported between December and March [25]. The difference in seasonal peak can be attrib uted to the presence of different types of reservoirs widespread in these areas, in particular for the ZCL, and to the activity of sandflies, which extends from April to November and reaches its peak in September to October [26].

Iraq has been exposed to wars, civil wars, widespread violence, and terrorism. Internal displacement of population, unlawful housing, shortage of municipal services, constant power outage, accumulation of waste, and uncontrolled stray dogs and animals in the cities since 2003 contributed to many CL outbreaks [9, 27] (**Figure 2**). In 2009, the Baghdad governorate reported CL outbreak with a high incidence of 45.5/100,000 population (**Figure 2**) [26, 28].

In 2014, the ISIS seized large areas of Iraqi lands that caused large internal displacement of the residents; they were mostly nonimmune and malnourished who moved to live in an endemic area with poor housing camps, lack of sanitation and water supply, and increased waste and garbage around their camps (**Figure 3**).

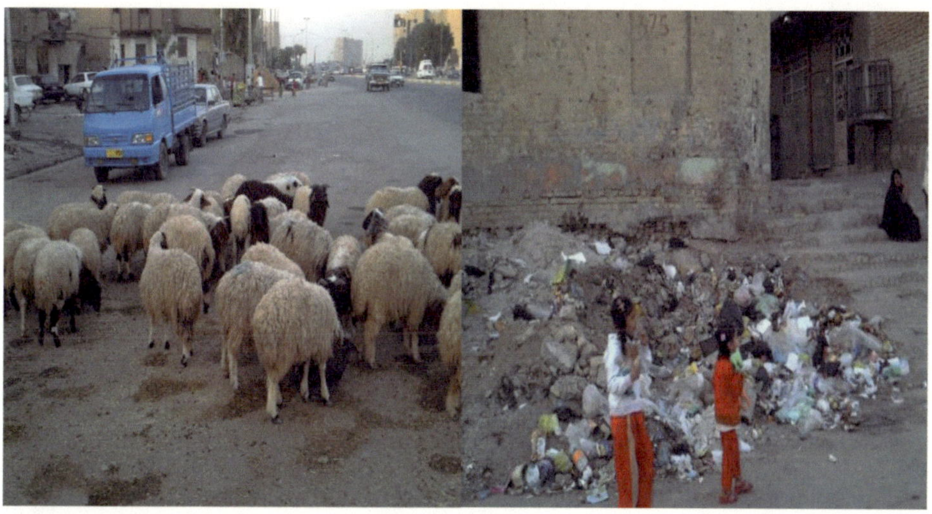

Figure 2.
Predisposing factors for CL occurrence.

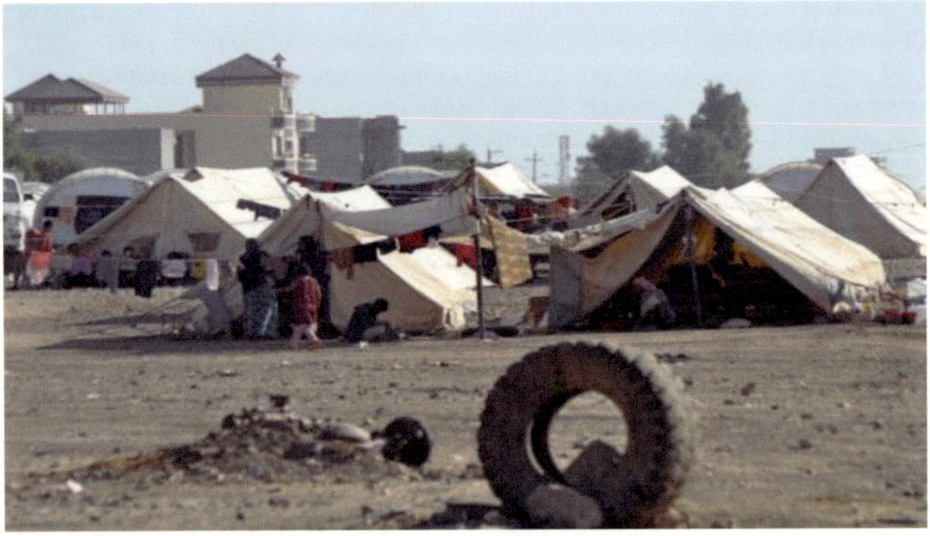

Figure 3.
IDPs camps.

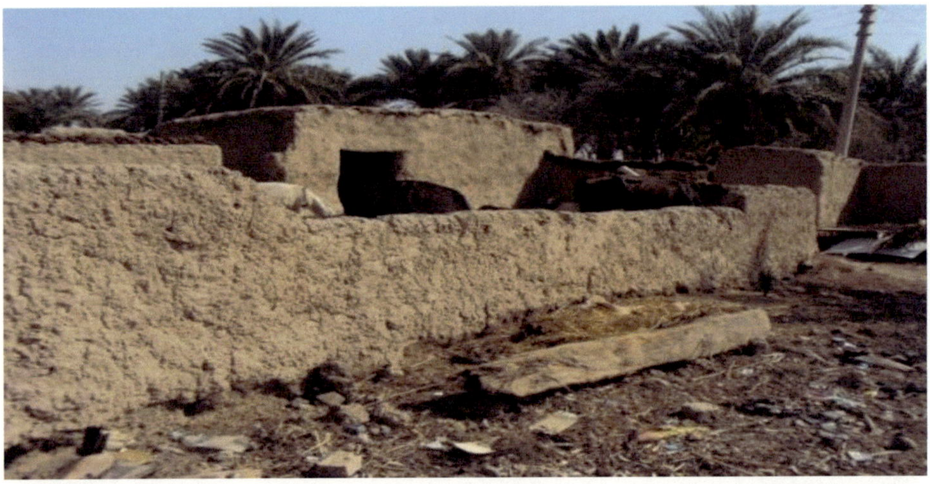

Figure 4.
Underdeveloped mud houses.

In addition, living in illegal underdeveloped mud houses with cracked walls, low socioeconomic status, and constant power outage may be playing as a risk factor for Leishmaniasis outbreak (**Figure 4**) [13, 29].

Sleeping without an insecticide-treated bed net outside the house due to a constant power outage and keeping domestic animals inside or around their houses are another risk factors for the transmission of the disease to human (**Figure 5**) [14, 30].

The conflicts had a negative impact on the health system in Iraq; many health programs were including the prevention and control measures of Leishmaniasis were affected. Eventually, an outbreak of Cutaneous Leishmaniasiss occurred in 2015 [9, 31].

Geopolitical conflicts and geospatial health deterioration contributed to an increase in various dominant reservoir species in Iraq, particularly for ZCL, and the activity of the sand flies [8]. There was a sudden, sharp increase in CL cases from 2671 cases in 2014 to 17,264 cases observed in 2015, and an outbreak was reported (**Figure 6**) [31].

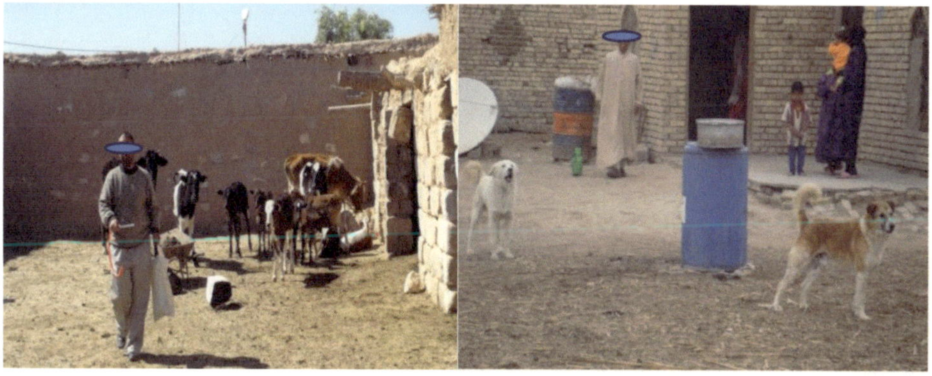

Figure 5.
Human behaviors.

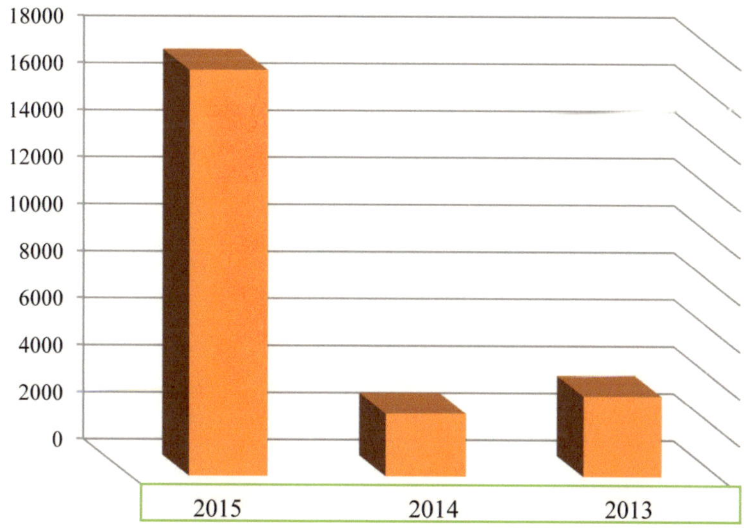

Figure 6.
Cutaneous leishmaniasis cases, Iraq, 2013–2014.

All Iraqi governorates reported CL cases during the CL outbreak in 2015, and the incidence rate was 49/100,000 population. The majority of cases, 4460 (25.8%), was observed in the Diyala governorate. Therefore, violence and conflicts had a negative impact on CL occurrence [11, 32].

3. Conclusion

An increment of CL was reported during the last years in Iraq. Violence, conflicts, internal displacement, bad socioeconomic status, and poor environmental sanitation play a big role in the proliferation of insect vectors and animal reservoir that lead to disease occurrence.

Acknowledgements

The authors are grateful to Professor Jawad K. Al-Diwan MB ChB, MSc, DCN, FIBMS, FFPH Community Medicine Department, College of Medicine, Baghdad University, Baghdad, Iraq.

Conflict of interest

The authors have no conflict of interests.

Abbreviations

CL	cutaneous leishmaniasis
MCL	mucocutaneous leishmaniasis
VL	visceral leishmaniasis
WHO	World Health Organization
PKDL	post kala-azar dermal Leishmaniasis
ZCL	zoonotic cutaneous leishmaniasis
ACL	anthroponotic cutaneous leishmaniasis
CDC	Center of Diseases Control in Atlanta
ISIS	Islamic State in Iraq and Syria
MoH	Ministry of Health
CDC/Baghdad	Communicable Diseases Center

Author details

Karim Abdulkadim Muftin Al Zadawi
The Arab Board of Health Specializations/Community Medicine, Baghdad, Iraq

*Address all correspondence to: karimmuftin@yahoo.com

References

[1] Mathers CD, Ezzati M, Lopez AD. Measuring the burden of neglected tropical diseases: The global burden of disease framework. PLoS Neglected Tropical Diseases. 2007;**1**:e114. DOI: 10.1371/journal.pntd.0000114

[2] Bailey F, Mondragon-Shem K, Hotez P, Ruiz-Postigo JA, Al-Salem W, Acosta-Serrano A, et al. A new perspective on cutaneous leishmaniasis—Implications for global prevalence and burden of disease estimates. PLoS Neglected Tropical Diseases. 2017;**1**(5). DOI: 10.1371/journal.pntd.0005739

[3] Khan SJ, Muneeb S. Cutaneous leishmaniasis in Pakistan. Dermatology Online Journal. 2005;**11**(1):4. DOI: 10.5070/D325b5x6b4

[4] Yamey G, Torreele E. The world's most neglected diseases. British Medical Journal. 2002;**325**:176-177. DOI: 10.1136/bmj.325.7357.176

[5] World Health Organization. WHO report on global surveillance of epidemic-prone infectious diseases leishmaniasis epidemic and pandemic alert and response (EPR). 2020. Available from: https://www.who.int/news-room/fact-sheets/detail/leishmaniasis [Accessed: 20 December 2012]

[6] Guessous-Idrissi N, Chiheb S, Hamdani A, Riyad M, Bichichi M, Hamdani S, et al. Cutaneous leishmaniasis: An emerging epidemic focus of *Leishmania tropica* in north Morocco. Transactions of the Royal Society of Tropical Medicine and Hygiene. 1997;**91**(6):660-663. DOI: 10.1016/S0035-9203(97)90511-3

[7] Alvar J, Vélez ID, Bern C, Herrero M, Desjeux P, Cano J, et al. Leishmaniasis worldwide and global estimates of its incidence. PLoS One. 2012;**7**(5):e35671. DOI: 10.1371/journal.pone.0035671

[8] Jacobson RL. Leishmaniasis in an era of conflict in the Middle East. Vector Borne and Zoonotic Diseases. 2011;**11**(3):247-258. DOI: 10.1089/vbz.2010.0068

[9] Salam N, Al-Shaqha WM, Azzi A. Leishmaniasis in the Middle East: Incidence and epidemiology. PLoS Neglected Tropical Diseases. 2014;**6**(7). DOI: 10.1371/journal.pntd.0003208

[10] WHO. Control of the Leishmaniasis: Report of a meeting of the WHO expert committee on the control of leishmaniasis. Geneva: WHO; 2010. Available from: https://apps.who.int/iris/handle/10665/44412

[11] World Health Organization. Report on the interregional meeting on leishmaniasis among neighbouring endemic countries in the Eastern Mediterranean, African and European regions, Amman, Jordan 23-25 September 2018. World Health Organization, Regional Office for the Eastern Mediterranean; 2019. Available from: https://creativecommons.org/licenses/by-nc-sa/3.0/igo

[12] Morsy TA, Naser AM, El Gibali MR, Anwar AM, El Said AM. Studies on zoonotic cutaneous leishmaniasis among a group of temporary workers in North Sinai Governorate, Egypt. Journal of the Egyptian Society of Parasitology. 1995;**25**(1):99. DOI: 10.4172/2329-891X.1000153

[13] Bailey MS, Lockwood DN. Cutaneous leishmaniasis. Clinics in Dermatology. 2007;**25**(2):203-211. DOI: 10.1016/j.clindermatol.2006.05.008

[14] Bern C, Courtenay O, Alvar J. Of cattle, sand flies, and men: A systematic review of risk factor analyses for South Asian visceral leishmaniasis and implications for elimination.

PLoS. Neglected Tropical Diseases. 2010;**2**(9). DOI: 10.1371/journal.pntd.0000599

[15] Abdulah SA, Abul-Hab J, El-Deen LD. Clinico-epidemiological study of cutaneous leishmaniasis in a sample of Iraqi Armed Forces. Iraqi Journal of Community Medicine. 2006;**19**(2):98-103

[16] Al-Yazachi M. New classification and treatment of cutaneous leishmaniasis. Journal of the Faculty of Medicine Baghdad. 1985;**27**:63-74

[17] Nazzaro G, Rovaris M, Veraldi S. Leishmaniasis: A disease with many names. JAMA Dermatology. 2014;**150**(11):1204. DOI: 10.1001/jamadermatol.2014.1015

[18] Al-Warid HS, Al-Saqur IM, Al-Tuwaijari SB, Zadawi KA. The distribution of cutaneous leishmaniasis in Iraq: Demographic and climate aspects. Asian Biomedicine. 2017;**11**(3):255-260. DOI: 10.5372/1905-7415.1103.556

[19] World Health Organization. Leishmaniasis: Background Information. A Brief History of the Disease. Geneva, Switzerland: World Health Organization; 2009

[20] Rahi AA. Cutaneous leishmaniasis at Wasit governorate. Baghdad Science Journal. 2011;**8**(2):286-288. DOI: 10.21123/bsj.2011.8.2.286-288

[21] Pringle G. Oriental sore in Iraq: Historical and epidemiological problems. Bulletin of Endemic Diseases. 1957;**2**(1/2):41-76

[22] Sharquie KE, Al-Talib KK, Chu AC. Intralesional therapy of cutaneous leishmaniasis with sodium stibogluconate antimony. British Journal of Dermatology. 1988;**119**(1):53-57. DOI: 10.1111/j.1365-2133.1988.tb07100

[23] World Health Organization. Country cooperation strategy for WHO and Iraq: 2012-2017 (No. WHO-EM/PME/004/E). Regional Office for the Eastern Mediterranean, World Health Organization; 2013. Available from: https://apps.who.int/iris/handle/10665/113230

[24] AL-Gorban HA. Comparison of the intralesional therapy of cutaneous leishmaniasis [dissertation]. College of Medicine, University of Tikrit. DOI:10.3855/jidc.59

[25] Hussian AK. Intra-lesional therapy of CL with hypertonic sodium chloride solution [diploma thesis]. Department of Dermatology & Venerology, College of Medicine, University of Baghdad; 1993. DOI:10.3855/jidc.59

[26] AlSamarai AM, AlObaidi HS. Cutaneous leishmaniasis in Iraq. The Journal of Infection in Developing Countries. 2009;**3**(2):123-129. DOI: 10.3855/jidc.59

[27] Majeed B, Sobel J, Nawar A, Badri S, Muslim H. The persisting burden of visceral leishmaniasis in Iraq: Data of the National Surveillance System, 1990-2009. Epidemiology and Infection. 2013;**141**(2):443-446. DOI: 10.1017/S0950268812000556

[28] WHO. Communicable Disease Working Group on Emergencies, HQ Division of Communicable Disease Control EMRO, WHO Office, Baghdad. Communicable Disease Toolkit, IRAQ Crisis. WHO; 2003. pp. 39-44. Available from: WHO/CDS/2003.17

[29] Ready PD. Leishmaniasis emergence and climate change. Revue Scientifique et Technique. 2008;**27**(2):399-412

[30] Saha S, Ramachandran R, Hutin YJ, Gupte MD. Visceral leishmaniasis is preventable in an endemic village in West Bengal, India. Transactions of the

Royal Society of Tropical Medicine and Hygiene. 2009;**103**(7):737-742. DOI: 10.1371/journal.pntd.0008132

[31] World Health Organization. Regional Office for the Eastern Mediterranean. Framework for action on cutaneous leishmaniasis in the Eastern Mediterranean Region 2014-2018. 2014. Available from: https://apps.who.int/iris/handle/10665/120003

[32] Alsamarai AM, Alobaidi AH, Aljumaili ZK, Jasim MM, Qatal S. Cutaneous leishmaniasis in Iraq: A continuing endemic disease. Journal of Drug Design and Research. 2016;**3**(1):1024

Section 3

New Drugs

Chapter 8

Use of Cell Biology to Identify Cellular Targets in Drug Development Process against *Leishmania* Sp.

Gabrielle dos Santos da Silva e Miranda, Joseane Lima Prado Godinho, Sara Teixeira de Macedo-Silva, Brunno Renato Farias Verçoza, Alisson Amaral da Rocha, Milena Barenco Pires de Abreu Sodré, Victor Feliciano dos Santos Ramos and Juliany Cola Fernandes Rodrigues

Abstract

Leishmaniasis is one of the most important neglected tropical diseases. The chemotherapy for its treatment uses very toxic compounds with a low efficacy rate. Thus, there is an urgent need to develop new chemotherapeutic agents to help countries control this devasting disease. In drug development, different approaches can be used to identify potential cellular targets that allow us to understand better the cell biology of eukaryotic cells. Several groups are dedicated to studying new molecules, searching for promising candidates against *Leishmania*. Different techniques have been used to characterize the cell biology, biochemistry, and molecular biology alterations induced by the treatments, trying to understand the mechanisms of action. The main goal of this chapter is to describe an overview of the literature exploring the several studies published about the chemotherapy of anti-*Leishmania* concerning the mechanisms of action of different classes of molecules or therapeutic alternatives.

Keywords: chemotherapy, drug development, cell biology, ergosterol, histone deacetylases, organometallic compounds, therapeutic combination, nanotechnology

1. Introduction

Leishmaniasis is a neglected tropical disease that comprises a large and complex group of infections caused by the *Leishmania* genus protozoan parasites. *Leishmania* parasites have intrinsic biological features that make chemotherapy challenging, presenting high adaptability and plasticity. Its life cycle has two different developmental stages: intracellular amastigotes that live in the mammalian host cells and promastigotes that develop in the insect vectors (**Figure 1**) [1].

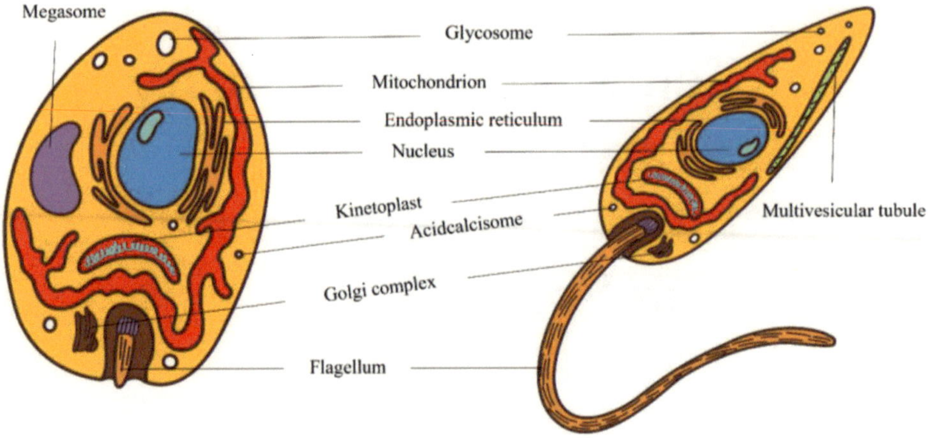

Figure 1.
Illustration of the amastigote (left) and promastigote (right) forms of Leishmania *sp. showing the main organelles and structures.*

The ultrastructure of *Leishmania* parasites (**Figure 2**) presents some conserved features and a classical internal organization of eukaryotic cells, with an individualized nuclear envelope, a single and ramified mitochondrion, endoplasmic reticulum, and Golgi complex, which can lead to difficulties in the development of *Leishmania*-specific drugs with low toxic side effects to mammalian hosts [1]. In addition, however, these protozoans have essential and exclusive organelles and structures such as acidocalcisomes, glycosomes, megasomes, and subpellicular microtubules (**Figure 1**) that can be exploited as drug targets [2].

The *Leishmania* plasma membrane comprises a lipid bilayer associated with proteins and a glycocalyx consisting of a myriad of glycoconjugates. The lipid bilayer has a trilaminar aspect with about 9 nm of thickness. The lipidic composition of the Trypanosomatidae family members is dependent on genus and species. In general, *Leishmania* has 24-methylated sterols, such as episterol, 5-dehydroepisterol, and traces of ergosterol as the major endogenous sterols' constituents, which are absent in mammalian host cells, where cholesterol is the main source of membrane sterols [3]. This divergence in sterol profiles has been exploited to develop drugs that affect the sterols biosynthesis pathway, including azoles,

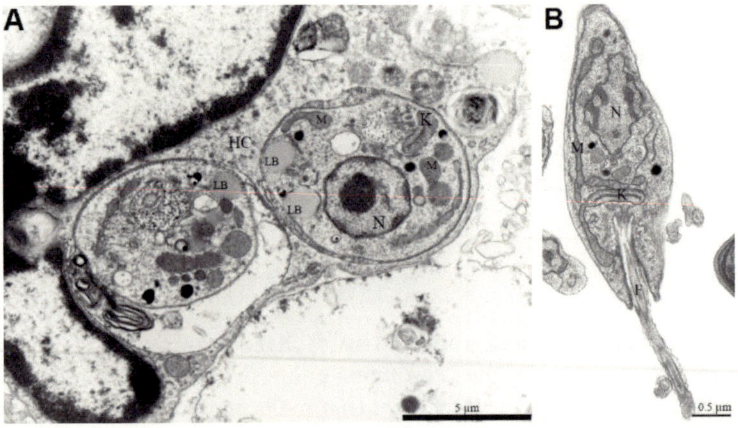

Figure 2.
Ultrathin sections of L. amazonensis *amastigotes (A) and promastigote (B). F, flagellum; HC, host cell; K, kinetoplast; LB, lipid body; M, mitochondrion; N, nucleus.*

azasterols, and others [2]. In addition, many attempts to develop drugs targeting *Leishmania* glycocalyx have also been performed [4].

Leishmania parasites present a single and ramified mitochondrion frequently associated with the plasma membrane, subpellicular microtubules, and endoplasmic reticulum. As well as in other eukaryotes, *Leishmania* mitochondrion operates in energetic metabolism, compartmentalizing the Krebs cycle and performing cellular respiration. The amphotericin B and pentamidine, two of the currently used drugs for the treatment of leishmaniasis, target mitochondria, resulting in a decrease of the mitochondrial membrane potential. Moreover, other drugs targeting mitochondria, such as hydroxynaphthoquinones, have been evaluated against *Leishmania* [5].

To maintain its morphological structure, *Leishmania* has a cytoskeleton composed mainly of subpellicular microtubules, which are filaments finely associated to plasma membrane inner leaflet, regularly spaced, and longitudinally oriented throughout the parasite's cellular body. Despite the phylogenetic conservation of α and β-tubulins, structural divergences in specific tubulin drug binding sites have suggested these proteins as a potential target, as described for podophyllotoxin derivatives and others [6, 7].

In the Medicinal Chemistry field, several approaches have been attempted, trying to find potential cellular targets for developing anti-*Leishmania* drugs. First, nanotechnology-based drug delivery systems have been applied, improving efficacy and enhancing pharmacokinetics properties of currently available drugs [8]. Second, molecular hybridization techniques can combine two drugs or chemical groups with previously known biological activity, producing a single and novel molecule with increased activity [9]. Finally, another alternative is the transposition of a drug already used to treat another disease; it is the case of miltefosine, the last treatment included in the arsenal of chemotherapeutic agents against leishmaniasis. Miltefosine was initially designed as an anticancer medicine, and in 2002 it was registered as first-line treatment, mainly for visceral leishmaniasis (VL), in Asia, Africa, and some regions of Europe.

2. Challenging the target: phospholipid and ergosterol biosynthesis

The first metabolically stable analogs derived from lysophosphatidylcholine were synthesized in the late 1960s. Two decades later, Eibl and Unger synthesized the first alkyl phospholipids (APLs), also called miltefosine, first administrated by an intravenous route to treat systemic tumors [10]. However, the treatment failed, and miltefosine was evaluated against topical cutaneous metastases from breast cancer [11]. In the late 1990s, miltefosine was assessed *in vitro* against the *Leishmania* genus [12, 13] and in murine models infected with *L. donovani* and *L. infantum* [14]. More recently, miltefosine was also evaluated against murine models of cutaneous leishmaniasis, alone or in combination with paromomycin [15–17].

After the evidence of the excellent anti-*Leishmania* activity of miltefosine demonstrated *in vitro* and *in vivo*, clinical tests began to be carried out immediately. Thus, miltefosine was the first oral drug approved for the treatment of visceral leishmaniasis, and for several years it was used as the first choice for the treatment of visceral leishmaniasis (VL), mainly in India [13, 18].

Miltefosine was also evaluated in patients infected with cutaneous leishmaniasis in Colombia, Guatemala, and Brazil [19, 20]. The efficacy in this clinical manifestation was variable, depending on the species. For patients infected with *L. panamensis* in Colombia, the cure rate was 91%, while in Guatemala, the cure rate was 53% for infections with *L. braziliensis* and *L. mexicana* [19]. Furthermore, in Brazil, in patients infected with *L. braziliensis*, the cure rate was 75%, compared to 53% cure achieved with pentavalent antimonials [20].

Several studies have demonstrated that the primary target of miltefosine is the cell membranes, affecting cellular processes such as signal transduction, lipid metabolism, and calcium homeostasis [21]. The selectivity for the plasma membrane is related to its chemical structure formed by a polar choline head bound to a long non-polar hydrocarbon chain, which easily inserts into the lipid bilayer, presenting detergent properties that lead to cell lysis in high concentrations [10]. In *L. donovani* and *T. cruzi*, miltefosine inhibits the phosphatidylcholine biosynthesis pathway (Greenberg pathway), being more selective for the protozoan parasites than mammalian cells, where the main route for phospholipid synthesis is the Kennedy pathway [22, 23]. Miltefosine also interfered with the ergosterol biosynthesis and promoted a disturbance in GPI synthesis [21, 24–26], leading to membrane permeability and fluidity changes. In addition, miltefosine interfered with the host immune response by inducing the production of interferon γ cytokine, leading to a biased immune response towards Th1, which would be a beneficial outcome for immunosuppressed patients [26, 27]. About the ultrastructure of *Leishmania* treated with miltefosine (**Figure 3A**), some studies revealed that it induced several alterations, mainly observed in the mitochondrion, in the plasma membrane, an increase of autophagic structures and phenotypes related to cell cycle arrest and apoptosis-like cell death [26, 28, 29].

With the success of miltefosine, several groups worldwide began to study new chemical routes to synthesize ether phospholipid derivatives in searching for novel molecules more active and selective against *Leishmania* [30]. Our group studied a novel hybrid derivative called alkyl phosphocholine-dinitroaniline, which presented a potent effect against *L. amazonensis* at least around 15-times better than miltefosine [31].

Another essential metabolic route for *Leishmania* and other protozoan parasites is the biosynthesis of ergosterol (or 24-methyl sterols) [32]. *Leishmania* has in these cell membranes three major sterol components that are absent in mammalian cells, 5-dehydroepisterol, episterol, and ergosterol. In mammals, cholesterol is the principal sterol present in cell membranes. Thus, the differences between some steps and enzymes in the biosynthetic route of the protozoan parasites and mammalian host cells have been exploited as targets to develop novel drugs as candidates to chemotherapeutic agents [32].

At least 20 metabolic steps are necessary to synthesize ergosterol, and several enzymes participate in these reaction sequences [32–34]. Furthermore, several works have shown that multiple classes of compounds targeting 24-methyl sterol biosynthesis exhibit suitable anti-trypanosomatid activities *in vitro* (**Figure 3B, C**) and *in vivo* [33–39].

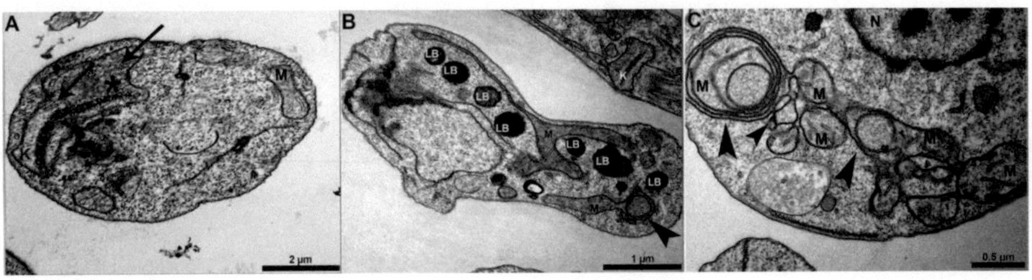

Figure 3.
Ultrathin sections of L. amazonensis *promastigotes treated with miltefosine and two ergosterol biosynthesis inhibitors. (A) 30 µM miltefosine for 72 h; (B) 3 µM ravuconazole for 48 h; (C) 1 µM posaconazole for 48 h. Mitochondrion was the organelle more affected in all treatments, presenting alterations in the cristae and kDNA structure (asterisk, thin arrow, and arrowheads) and mitochondrial swelling and disorganization of its ultrastructure. In panel C, several lipid bodies appeared after treatment. K, kinetoplast; LB, lipid body; M, mitochondrion; N, nucleus.*

More than 30 drugs have been studied in the last 30 years. These drugs are included in large classes of inhibitors, such as 1) Statins, which inhibit the enzyme 3-hydroxy-3-methyl-glutaryl-CoA reductase (HMG-CoA reductase), also evaluated as cholesterol-lowering drugs; 2) Bisphosphonates that act in the enzyme farnesyl pyrophosphate synthase and inhibit the isoprenoid pathway, mainly used to treat hypercalcemia; 3) Quinuclidines and zaragozic acid, developed to inhibit the squalene synthase, the enzyme that catalyzes the first committed step in the sterol biosynthesis pathway. This class of drugs was developed as an alternative to statin use because they do not inhibit the synthesis of the isoprenoids. 4) Allylamines, which include the known antifungal terbinafine that inhibits the squalene epoxidase; 5) Azoles, which are essential medicines to treat many fungal diseases and inhibit the C14α-demethylase. Several azoles were developed, always trying to find new tolerate and efficacy drugs, also searching to novel molecules to solve the problems with antifungal resistance; finally, 6) Azasterols, which inhibit the enzyme $\Delta^{24,25}$ sterol methyltransferase absent in mammalian cells, one enzyme that catalyzes the methylation of steroid nucleus of sterols, producing 24-methyl sterols, essential for *Leishmania*, *T. cruzi* and fungi (Reviewed in [32]).

In summary, several works have pointed to the importance of looking for the biochemical properties of each enzyme involved in the pathway and its relevance as an essential target for the parasite viability; this feature characterizes the enzyme as a promising target for the development of potential chemotherapeutic candidates for the treatment of leishmaniasis.

3. Challenging the target: histone deacetylases

Histone deacetylase (HDACs) inhibitors are a relatively new class of potential agents in treating neurodegenerative diseases, various types of cancer, and parasitic infections. HDACs have broad importance in the cellular environment. They regulate histone and non-histone proteins affecting the cell cycle, energy metabolism, and inducing cell death. Some HDAC inhibitors were already approved by the FDA (Food and Drug Administration) to treat lymphoma and myeloma, such as vorinostat, romidepsin, belinostat, and panobinostat, in combination with bortezomib and dexamethasone [40]. Given the results obtained *in vitro* and *in vivo* in several disease models, the advancement of clinical trials in tumors, and the transposition of drugs as an old ally in the treatment of leishmaniasis, HDAC inhibitors are a promising approach in the understanding of cell biology of the parasite, especially concerning its chemotherapy.

There are 18 histone deacetylases in humans, which can be grouped according to cell location and the molecule used as a cofactor for its enzymatic action. These HDACs are divided into 1) zinc-dependent HDACs, also called "classical" histone deacetylases; and 2) nicotinamide and adenine dinucleotide [NAD^+]-dependent HDACs. The first one comprises class I (HDACs 1–3, 8), IIa (HDACs 4, 5, 7, and 9), IIb (HDACs 6 and 10), and IV (HDAC 11). While the second one, the NAD^+-HDAC, belongs to class III and is also known as sirtuins (SIRT 1–7). HDACs are still poorly understood and characterized in *Leishmania*. So far, four Zn^{2+}-dependent histones deacetylases and three NAD^+-dependent histones deacetylases were discovered in the parasite [41, 42]. Although four homologs of classical HDACs were identified, none was functionally characterized. Among the information in the literature, a *L. major* HDAC (gene LmjF21.0680) was shown to be expressed during the differentiation of promastigotes to amastigotes, with a possible role in chromatin structure and impacts on gene transcription [43]. Furthermore, Prasanna et al. [44] managed to isolate, express, and purify an *L. donovani* histone deacetylase

(LD_HDAC), with less than 40% identity with class I human HDACs. Information about classical HDACs in the *Leishmania* genus is still very early and deserves further development.

Unlike classical HDACs, there are several studies about NAD^+-dependent HDACs in the *Leishmania* genus. Three sirtuins were already found in *Leishmania*, SIR2RP1, SIR2RP2, and SIR2RP3 [45]. These sirtuins were not found in the nucleus, as described for *Saccharomyces cerevisiae* [45]. SIR2RP1 is expressed from a single copy gene in *L. amazonensis* (LaSIR2RP1), resulting in a monomeric protein with NAD^+-dependent deacetylase action immunodetected in its glycosylated form [46]. LaSIR2RP1 has dispersed localization in the cytosol or cytoplasmic granules [47] and is secreted in lesions derived from intracellular amastigotes [48]. In addition, the *L. donovani* SIR2RP1 was 46% similar to the human SIRT2 [49]. In *L. infantum* and *L. major*, the SIR2RP1 proteins present two functional sites for NAD^+-dependent deacetylation activity and ADP-ribosyl transferase activity [49].

In *L. major* SIR2RP1, removing the acetyl group of lysine 40 from α-tubulin was demonstrated *in vitro* and *in vivo* [50]. However, in these parasites, the ribosylation function of α-tubulin ADP was also shown, resulting in its depolymerization or even inhibiting its assembly [51]. Thus, sirtuins in *Leishmania* have demonstrated an essential role in cytoskeleton dynamics and may have significant implications for remodeling the parasite's morphology and its interaction with the host cell. LmSIR2RP1 also showed a close relationship with the HSP83 protein, an orthologous chaperone of the human HSP90 chaperone, although the intracellular levels of LmSIR2RP1 do not influence the acetylation status of HSP83 [52]. The use of geldanamycin, an HSP90 inhibitor, induced alterations in the cytodifferentiation of promastigotes to intracellular amastigotes [53]; the same was observed for protozoa overexpressing or knockout for the LmSIR2RP1 gene [52]. This study confirms that the SIR2RP1/HSP83 interaction may play an essential role in the differentiation of the parasite.

The work in [54] demonstrated that *L. major* sirtuins may be related to the success of infection through interaction with macrophage surface proteins and, therefore, play a regulatory role in immune responses [55]. This work also showed the capacity of *L. major* sirtuins to trigger the effector response of B cells, promoting a robust humoral response with the secretion of specific antibodies, such as IgG1 and IgG2a [55]. Meanwhile, the overexpression of *L. major* sirtuin, also observed for *L. infantum* sirtuin [48], revealed that it would be involved in the proliferation rate, besides participating in the regulation of death factors, thus preventing death by apoptosis.

The SIR2RP2 present in *L. infantum* mitochondrion is related to the growth rates of promastigote forms with a direct relationship with NAD^+ homeostasis [56]. In 2017, a study revealed that the *L. donovani* SIR2RP2 also has a mitochondrial location [49]. The deletion of this gene led to a reduction in the proliferation rate, further resulting in the interruption of the cell cycle in the G2/M phase. Furthermore, the deletion of LdSIR2RP2 resulted in greater susceptibility of the parasite to commercially available sirtuin inhibitors and a reduction in the mitochondrial membrane potential, resulting in a low concentration of ATP in the mitochondrion. Interestingly, in this SIR2RP2 knockout *Leishmania*, there was an intensification of glycolysis that could be an attempt to compensate for the disbalance of the mitochondrial metabolism. LdSIR2RP2 showed NAD^+-dependent ADP-ribosyl transferase activity with 39% similarity to SIRT4 from humans [49].

The third sirtuin, SIR2RP3, still has few descriptions in the literature. The *L. donovani* SIR2RP3 was 37% similar to the human SIRT5 [49], so that molecular coupling assays, using known inhibitors and SIR2RP3, revealed a strong analogy with SIRT5, which refers to the form of interaction with inhibitors. However, the interaction of these inhibitors with SIR2RP3 also demonstrated significant molecular differences compared to SIRT5 in humans, which could act as selective targets for the treatment of leishmaniasis [57].

A recent study with a histone deacetylase inhibitor *in L. amazonensis* revealed the sirtuins' potential to develop novel molecules with anti-*Leishmania* activity [58]. Furthermore, this study from our group demonstrated the potent inhibition of parasite proliferation that is probably related to essential functions for HDACs in *Leishmania*, which include the control of the cell cycle and the induction of cell death [58]. Other effects already observed with HDAC inhibitors are different levels of chromatin compaction, increased number of lipid bodies randomly distributed throughout the cytosol, increased production of reactive oxygen species, changes in *Leishmania* morphology, and increased expression of acetylated α-tubulin (**Figure 4**) [58].

However, the parasite's ability to modulate the histone deacetylases of the mammalian host to establish the infection has already been observed. For example, the upregulation of the macrophage HDAC1 was observed during infection with *L. amazonensis*, resulting in deacetylation of the histone tail of the gene's promoter region responsible for producing nitric oxide. This deacetylation prevents the access of transcription factors, which culminates in the repression of nitric oxide production, which allows the establishment of intracellular amastigote forms in the parasitophorous vacuole [59].

Besides, HDAC inhibitors have also been used in combination therapy to treat antimony-resistant *L. donovani* infection, where the upregulation of the multiresistant protein depends on IL-10 production. Thus, the imipramine antidepressant positively regulates HDAC11, inhibiting the acetylation of the IL-10 promoter, which leads to a decrease in its production [60]. This imipramine-mediated lowering of the IL-10 level reduces MDR-1 expression and aids in the elimination of the parasite.

Thus, histone deacetylase inhibitors belong to a class of compounds with potential application to develop novel molecules with anti-*Leishmania* activity and for the treatment of leishmaniasis, alone or in combination with other medications already established. Furthermore, the World Health Organization (WHO) has already recommended the therapeutic combination to reduce the doses and toxicity and develop a more effective and safe treatment. Finally, HDAC inhibitors seem to be an exciting tool for a better understanding of the Cell Biology of *Leishmania* and enabling the knowledge of new routes for the development of novel drug candidates.

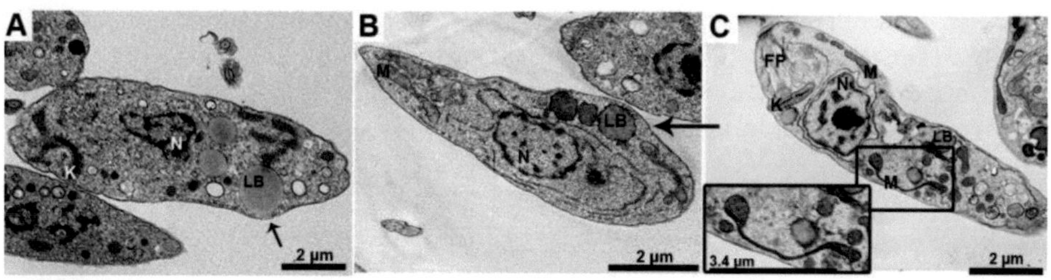

Figure 4.
Ultrathin sections of L. amazonensis *promastigotes treated with HDAC inhibitors for 48 h. (A) 1.5 µM NIH119; (B) 1 µM NIH119; (C) 15 µM tubastina A. NIH119 and tubastatin a induced different ultrastructural alterations such as 1) increase in the number of lipid bodies, some of them presenting different morphologies (A, B); 2) presence of membrane protrusions (A, B – Arrow); 3) alterations in the kinetoplast (A); 4) decondensation of chromatin (B, C); and, 5) changes in mitochondrial ultrastructure. FP, flagellar pocket; K, kinetoplast; LB, lipid body; M, mitochondrion; N, nucleus.*

4. Challenging the target: organometallic compounds

Although metals have been used in Medicine for centuries, most compounds produced by the pharmaceutical industry are still based on organic molecules. Nevertheless, new perspectives about metal-based drugs and their therapeutic potential against cancer, bacteria, virus, and even trypanosomatid infections have emerged in the last few years. In this context, *Leishmania* infections have been treated with pentavalent antimonials since the 1940s [1], which indicates that new compounds containing other kinds of metals may present anti-*Leishmania* activity, thus opening the possibility to reduce the toxicity based on the metal-drug synergism.

Platinum-derived metals are well known to have antitumor effects due to their ability to bind to DNA molecules. So, since tumor cells and kinetoplastid parasites present similar metabolic pathways [61], the coordination of these metals to organic compounds might be efficient in treating *Leishmania* infections. For example, the (2,2′:6′2″-terpyridine)platinum(II) complexes can inhibit 100% of the growth of *L. donovani* amastigotes at a concentration of 1 μM through the intercalation of terpyridine and platinum(II) into the DNA, probably binding to guanine bases or some enzyme active sites [62]. More recently, cisplatin-derived complexes (*cis*-diamminedichloroplatinum(II)), an anticancer drug, were tested on *L. infantum* promastigotes and amastigotes, revealing a remarkable anti-*Leishmania* activity with IC_{50} values of 1.03 μM and 0.10 μM, respectively. Furthermore, the treatment with *cis*-DDP induced loss of mitochondrial transmembrane potential and DNA fragmentation, thus leading to apoptosis-like death [63].

In addition to platinum and its derivatives, other transition metals have been widely studied in terms of antiprotozoal activity. For example, organometallic complexes containing ruthenium(II) and anti-inflammatories were evaluated active against *L. amazonensis* and *L. infantum* promastigotes, presenting IC_{50} values comparable to the meglumine antimoniate, one of the first-line drugs for *Leishmania* infections [64]. Moreover, the coordination of gold compounds with organic ligands was efficient against *L. amazonensis* and *L. braziliensis* promastigotes while presenting low toxicity to host cells [65]. Thus, the therapeutic mechanism of these organometallic molecules may be related to induction of oxidative damage and alterations in the membrane permeabilization by the inhibition of specific membrane protein channels and zinc-binding proteins. These alterations can lead to parasite cell death by apoptosis-like and necrosis.

Among transition metals, the essential ones, such as zinc and copper, are present in cell structures and involved in many cellular processes, becoming indispensable for host–parasite interactions. Zinc regulates gene transcription processes and cell signaling, while copper is also a critical enzymatic cofactor for organ functioning and multiple metabolic processes [66]. Therefore, the coordination of organic molecules to essential metals regarding new antiprotozoal treatments might increase the drug uptake and contribute to the parasite's elimination. The zinc(II)-dipicolylamine (ZnDPA) coordination complexes were active against *L. major* promastigotes *in vitro* with IC_{50} values between 12.7 μM and 0.3 μM and minimal mammalian cell toxicity. The compounds also showed *in vivo* activity, with a high affinity for intracellular amastigotes and low toxicity to mice [67]. The effects of a copper dimethoxy bipyridine (CuDMOBP) complex were also investigated against *L. major*; the complex presented significant *in vitro* activity with high selectivity index [68]. Results from quantitative real-time PCR also indicate a significant reduction in cellular expression of IL-10 and TNF-α in macrophages treated with CuDMOBP, probably due to a reduction of the parasite population.

Metals have also been combined with ergosterol biosynthesis inhibitors, including the azoles family of drugs, which are used to treat fungal infections and present activity against protozoan parasites. For example, a recent study from our group revealed the potent effect of the combination of itraconazole (ITZ) with zinc (Zn) against *L. amazonensis* promastigotes (**Figure 5B**) and intracellular amastigotes [69]. The biological effects were significantly increased when the itraconazole was coupled with zinc, resulting in IC_{50} values in nanomolar ranges and cell death of parasites in low concentrations [69]. Likewise, the coordination of clotrimazole, ketoconazole (**Figure 5A**), and miconazole to manganese (Mn) provide novel molecules with better activity against *L. major* when compared to the original organic antifungals [70].

Despite Medicine's advances in the past decades, information about organometallic drugs is still lacking. More profound studies must be done to understand the role of metals in host–parasite interactions, thereby better comprising the mechanisms of organometallics drugs against the parasites and mammalian host cells. Nevertheless, the literature available indicates that organometallics are a promising class of drugs for treating leishmaniasis.

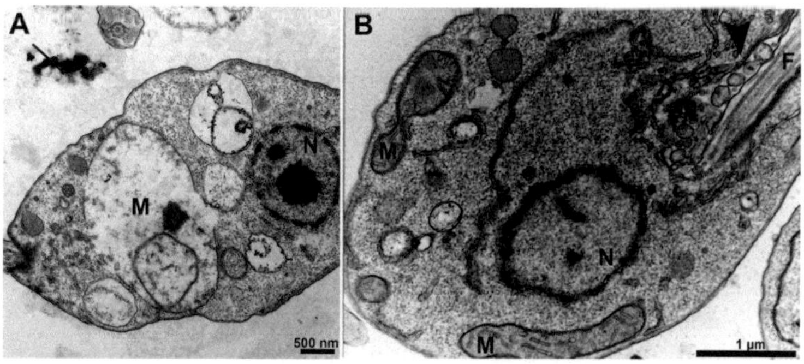

Figure 5.
Ultrathin sections of L. amazonensis *promastigotes treated with organometallic compounds. (A) Treatment with 300 nM ketoconazole-ruthenium induced alterations in the mitochondria, such as swelling and loss of the mitochondrial matrix and the formation of large autophagic vacuoles. (B) Treatment with 0.5 µM itraconazole-zinc resulted in mitochondrial alterations and an increase in the secretion of vesicles (arrowhead) at the flagellar pocket. In both panels, the nuclear chromatin appeared altered. F, flagellum; M, mitochondrion; N, nucleus.*

5. Therapeutic combination: what do we know?

There are many strategies to treat leishmaniasis; however, several studies have shown the numerous advantages of therapeutic combination, like observing for other diseases. For example, combining drugs from different chemical classes could reduce the total drug doses or treatment duration. These aspects are important to minimize toxic side effects, submission at treatment, less load on the public health system and reduce cases of drug resistance. Also, the therapeutic combination could improve treatment efficacy for refractory or complicated cases, such as in patients coinfected with HIV. A successful study conducted by the Drugs for Neglected Diseases initiative (DNDi), in partnership with Médicins Sans Frontières (MSF) and other institutions, pointed to evidence of the high efficacy of the combination therapy to treat patients with visceral leishmaniasis (VL) in coinfection with HIV [71]. Although the current WHO guidelines recommend the treatment of HIV/VL coinfection with liposomal amphotericin B (AmBisome®), this work strongly supports a change in the treatment recommendations, from AmBisome monotherapy to combination therapy as the first-line treatment. Moreover, they suggest the combination with miltefosine once this combination therapy has a good safety profile and is highly efficacious [71].

Nowadays, combination therapy is an efficient tool to treat many microbial infections such as AIDS, tuberculosis, malaria, and several other diseases. Recent works have shown that combination therapy for leishmaniasis has progressively been recommended to increase treatment tolerance and efficacy, reduce cost and treatment duration, and limit the growth of drug resistance [72–75]. For the treatment of leishmaniasis, WHO has recommended combination therapy based on many studies showing the efficacy of this therapeutic tool; the combinations include novel synthesized drugs, nanoparticles developed for drug delivery, repositioned drugs, old medicines, and immunomodulatory agents [76–79]. Indeed, several studies have reported the superior efficacies of combination therapies against leishmaniasis. Some of them demonstrated the synergic effects of combinations between amphotericin B with other available medicines, such as meglumine antimoniate, miltefosine, paromomycin, or azithromycin [80–82].

Analysis of drug interactions aimed to show if the interaction between them is classified as synergistic, antagonistic, or indifferent. *In vitro* data are based on an extended ratio and concentration range. However, *in vivo* combinations are more complex and less defined, with the number of doses limited. The synergy between two (or more drugs) occurs when their combined activities are improved over the sum of their separate individual effects. Synergistic drug combinations provide lower concentrations of both compounds, enhancing therapy outcomes by increasing efficacy and reducing side effects. Moreover, synergistic combinations could reintroduce those that have lost activity against drug-resistant strains. The FICI (fractional inhibitory concentration index) value is considered the standard reference parameter to quantify interactions between pairs of drugs. Odds in 2003 [83] established more restrictive criteria to analyze experiments and defined "synergy" as a $\geq$ 4-fold reduction in the MICs of both compounds in combination when compared to their MICs alone, where the FICI value must be $\leq$0.5. MIC means the minimum inhibitory concentration, i.e., the lowest drug concentration with no visible cell growth.

In vitro studies against *L. amazonensis* suggest that combinations between compounds that act in different biosynthetic pathways of the parasite, such as sterol biosynthesis, are promising [32]. Interestingly, a recent study showed that sterol biosynthesis inhibitors and alkylphosphocholine analogs, combined with medicines available to treat other diseases, are efficient against trypanosomatids [32, 36, 78, 84]. Besides, another study showed the *in vivo* efficacy of the combination therapy between miltefosine, an alkylphosphocholine, and amphotericin B or paromomycin [85], a therapeutic alternative to treat antimony-resistant VL cases in India. Furthermore, topical treatment against cutaneous leishmaniasis might be effective when amphotericin B and miltefosine are co-loaded at second-generation ultra-deformable liposomes since *in vivo* studies displayed a significant reduction in the parasitic burden [86]. However, a Brazilian survey against *L. infantum* revealed a decrease of the miltefosine concentration when combined with lopinavir (anti-HIV drug); yet, the synergistic effect was not evidenced [87]. Unexpectedly, the combination of nelfinavir with miltefosine presented better results, with FICI $\leq$0.5. Thus, this study also concluded that the combination might be helpful to treat patients with visceral leishmaniasis who also are infected with HIV [88].

Combination therapy is a promising strategy to treat several diseases. Therefore, it is urgent to investigate synergistic and other drug combinations to increase novel probabilities of therapeutic protocols to treat leishmaniasis. The discovery and the analysis of drug combinations can be facilitated by the collective use of different approaches and methods. Drug combinations have proved to be a successful strategy to shorten the course of therapy and reduce toxicity through lower dosage administration; these strategies should reduce the appearance of new resistant parasites. Thus, recent proposals of combinations have been suggested as state-of-the-art for the treatment of leishmaniasis. In the short run, combination therapy is an interesting way to improve the treatment for leishmaniasis.

6. Where are we going? Nanotechnology

Recent advances in Nanotechnology have had a profound impact on health sciences, especially Medicine, because of the development of different nanomaterials designed as intracellular carriers to deliver drugs and genes. The development and use of nanocarriers have also been established in the field of Pharmaceutical Sciences by enabling the encapsulation of drugs creating stable and controlled environments, and improving the biocompatibility of these drugs in various biological systems. These nanocarriers were developed to improve the solubility of poorly soluble drugs, control or maintain their release, and protect them from degradation. These characteristics increase drug bioavailability, reduce systemic side effects, and increase drug specificity for biological targets. For these reasons, Nanotechnology is a new field that allows the construction of versatile diagnostic and therapeutic platforms using nanocarriers as molecular machinery for different clinical applications.

The development of nanocarriers began in the 1960s to always seek to improve biocompatibility and reduce the toxicity of nanomaterials. The second generation of nanocarriers was developed around the 1980s and sought to improve the surface of these materials by increasing their stability, stealth, and targeting ability. The third generation of nanocarrier introduced the idea of intelligent nanomedication to enhance the targeting mechanisms and theranostic capabilities of these nanomaterials [89]. The word *nanoparticle* has been widely applied to describe numerous pharmaceutical carriers or imaging systems based on nanoscale materials. Nanoparticles are particulate materials in their solid or dispersed state present in a size scale between 10 nm and 100 nm (ISO/TS 80.004–1:2015). Due to the great diversity of these nanomaterials, the scientific community elaborates a classification based on their characteristics and properties.

Initially, the nanomaterials are divided into two classes: inorganic and organic. However, they are divided into three subgroups, according to some of their characteristics. The first would concentrate single-chain polymer-drug conjugates, polymeric colloids prepared by techniques such as emulsion polymerization, cross-linked nanogel matrices, dendrimers, and carbon nanotubes, where the nanocarrier is a single synthetic molecule with covalent bonds and a relatively large molar mass. The second subgroup of nanocarriers would comprise self-assembly of smaller molecules such as 1) liposomes and polyplexes, the most studied members of this group of nanoparticles; 2) polymersomes and other sets of block copolymers; 3) colloidosomal aggregates of latex particles and sets of proteins or peptides. In this case, the dynamic nature of these types of systems depends on intermolecular forces and biological conditions. Finally, the last subgroup of nanocarriers would include complexes based on fullerenes, silica, colloidal gold, gold nanoshells, quantum dots, and superparamagnetic particles.

Another critical point in developing nanocarriers is the synthesis, which can be rationally divided into two fundamental stages: nucleation and growth. Understanding and manipulating these two steps have created new possibilities allowing researchers to easily control the synthesis of nanoparticles in terms of size, morphology, and monodispersity. The choice of the synthesis route provides a characteristic set of advantages and disadvantages in nanomaterial production.

In *Leishmania* sp., the use of nanocarriers has been studied since the late 1970s with the development of liposomal amphotericin B [90, 91]. Since its development, liposomal amphotericin B has become more efficient and bioavailable, less toxic, and better tolerated by patients [92, 93]. This formulation also has a broad and rapid biodistribution reaching steady-state plasma concentrations faster with higher total plasma concentration when compared to its deoxycholate form. Furthermore, liposomal amphotericin B is probably inactive because it is fixed to the liposome; thus, the biologically active drug is released only after direct contact with protozoa or fungal cell walls [94]. In 2010, the WHO proposed the administration of liposomal amphotericin B.

The success achieved by the liposomal formulation of amphotericin B is related to its properties as a nanocarrier system, which has numerous advantages. However, despite these advantages, this system has some disadvantages, including its high cost, limiting its use [94]. Thus, the development of new, cheaper, and more efficient nanoformulations is necessary. Furthermore, different nanocarriers have been developed in recent decades, searching for new therapeutic alternatives to treat leishmaniasis, including nanoparticles based on liposomal, lipid, polymeric, and metallic nanomaterials [8, 95–98]. Therefore, choosing the correct nanocarriers is crucial to define properties and characteristics for this proposed new therapeutic approach. Thereby, this enormous diversity of available nanoparticles makes the development of nanocarriers for the treatment of leishmaniasis very promising since each of these carrier systems has advantages and limitations over each other [8].

Some nanoparticles have been generating significant repercussions for presenting theranostic properties, thus allowing them to be used simultaneously for diagnosis and therapy. Superparamagnetic iron oxide nanoparticles (SPIONs) are one example of this type of nanomaterials. SPIONs have excellent biocompatibility, degradability in moderate acid conditions, magnetic properties, and the ability to generate heat when subjected to an alternating current magnetic field [99, 100]. In addition, this type of nanomaterial still has a large surface area presenting great chemical diversity, which can increase the efficacy of the treatment. Finally, these nanomaterials can also be conjugated to specific molecules to facilitate selective and efficient drug delivery to a diseased tissue or organ [101]. The application of this type of nanomaterial for the treatment of leishmaniasis has been studied by different groups and has shown promising results over the past few years (**Figure 6**) [102–105].

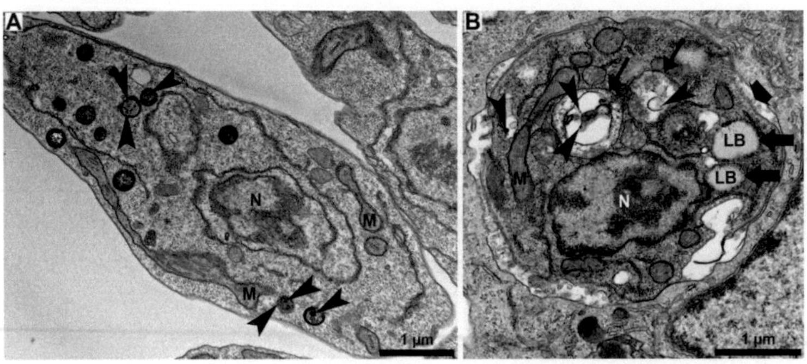

Figure 6.
Ultrathin sections of L. amazonensis *promastigotes (A) and amastigotes (B) after treatment with 100 µg/mL SPIONs for 24 h. In both developmental stages, SPIONs were found inside membrane-bound structures (arrowheads). Some alterations were also observed in the treated parasites, such as increased number of lipid bodies (arrows), presence of autophagosome (thin arrows), and secretion of extracellular vesicles (large arrow).*

In summary, Nanotechnology and the use of nanoparticles inaugurated a new field in health science called Nanomedicine, one of the most promising branches of contemporary Medicine. Thus, the development of new nanomaterials to treat leishmaniasis significantly increases the possibility of finding novel therapeutic alternatives, mainly considering the great diversity of clinical manifestations. An excellent example of this is the use of nanoparticles to develop a topical treatment that can revolutionize the treatment of cutaneous leishmaniasis.

7. Conclusions and perspectives

The treatment of infectious diseases depends on a better understanding of Cell Biology, mainly for parasites that are intracellular obligate eukaryotes, such as *Leishmania*. The knowledge about these parasites allows the identification of essential metabolic pathways and the mechanisms of action involved in drug inhibition, enabling the application of new treatments and conventional treatments combined with new therapies, also using Nanotechnology. Thus, the improvement of tested molecules associated with drug delivery techniques is the path to success for novel leishmaniasis treatments.

Acknowledgements

We acknowledge the Brazilian funding agencies Coordenação de Aperfeiçoamento de Pessoal de Nível Superior (CAPES), Conselho Nacional de Desenvolvimento e Pesquisa (CNPq), and Fundação Carlos Chagas Filho de Amparo à Pesquisa do Estado do Rio de Janeiro (FAPERJ) for financial support.

Author details

Gabrielle dos Santos da Silva e Miranda[1], Joseane Lima Prado Godinho[1,2], Sara Teixeira de Macedo-Silva[3], Brunno Renato Farias Verçoza[1], Alisson Amaral da Rocha[1], Milena Barenco Pires de Abreu Sodré[1], Victor Feliciano dos Santos Ramos[1] and Juliany Cola Fernandes Rodrigues[1*]

1 Federal University of Rio de Janeiro, Campus UFRJ Duque de Caxias Prof. Geraldo Cidade, Duque de Caxias, Brazil

2 Graduate Program in Public Health, Federal University of Maranhão, Maranhão, Brazil

3 CENABIO - Advanced Microscopy Unit, Federal University of Rio de Janeiro, Rio de Janeiro, Brazil

*Address all correspondence to: juliany.rodrigues@xerem.ufrj.br

References

[1] Rodrigues JCF, Godinho JLP, de Souza W. Biology of human pathogenic trypanosomatids: Epidemiology, lifecycle and ultrastructure. Subcellular Biochemistry. 2014;**74**:1-42

[2] Chawla B, Madhubala R. Drug targets in *Leishmania*. Journal of Parasitic Diseases. 2010;**34**(1):1-13

[3] de Souza W, Rodrigues JCF. Sterol biosynthesis pathway as target for anti-trypanosomatid drugs. Interdisciplinary Perspectives on Infectious Diseases. 2009;**2009**:1-19

[4] Cabezas Y, Legentil L, Robert-Gangneux F, Daligault F, Belaz S, Nugier-Chauvin C, et al. *Leishmania* cell wall as a potent target for antiparasitic drugs. A focus on the glycoconjugates. Organic and Biomolecular Chemistry. 2015;**13**(31): 8393-8404

[5] Fidalgo LM, Gille L. Mitochondria and trypanosomatids: Targets and drugs. Pharmaceutical Research. 2011;**28**(11):2758-2770

[6] Escudero-Martínez JM, Pérez-Pertejo Y, Reguera RM, Castro MÁ, Rojo MV, Santiago C, et al. Antileishmanial activity and tubulin polymerization inhibition of podophyllotoxin derivatives on *Leishmania infantum*. International Journal for Parasitology: Drugs and Drug Resistance. 2017;7(3):272-285

[7] Chatterji BP, Jindal B, Srivastava S, Panda D. Microtubules as antifungal and antiparasitic drug targets. Expert Opinion on Therapeutic Patents. 2011;**21**(2):167-186

[8] Saleem K, Khursheed Z, Hano C, Anjum I, Anjum S. Applications of nanomaterials in leishmaniasis: A focus on recent advances and challenges. Nanomaterials. 2019;**9**(12):1-18

[9] Walsh J, Bell A. Hybrid drugs for malaria. Current Pharmaceutical Design. 2009;**15**(25):2970-2985

[10] van Blitterswijk W, Verheij M. Anticancer alkylphospholipids: mechanisms of action, cellular sensitivity and resistance, and clinical prospects. Current Pharmaceutical Design. 2008;**14**(21):2061-2074

[11] Leonard R, Hardy J, van Tienhoven G, Houston S, Simmonds P, David M, et al. Randomized double-blind, placebo-controlled, multicenter trial of 6% miltefosine solution, a topical chemotherapy in cutaneous metastases from breast cancer. Journal of Clinical Oncology. 2001;**19**(21): 4150-4159

[12] Achterberg V, Gercken G. Cytotoxicity of ester and ether lysophospholipids on *Leishmania donovani* promastigotes. Molecular and Biochemical Parasitology. 1987;**23**(2): 117-122

[13] Croft SL, Neal RA, Pendergast W, Chan JH. The activity of alkyl phosphorylcholines and related derivatives against *Leishmania donovani*. Biochemical Pharmacology. 1987; **36**(16):2633-2636

[14] Kuhlencord A, Maniera T, Eibl H, Unger C. Allgemeine Hygiene I. Hexadecylphosphocholine: Oral treatment of visceral leishmaniasis in mice. Antimicrobial Agents and Chemotherapy. 1992;**36**(8):1630-1634

[15] Aguiar MG, Pereira AMM, Fernandes AP, Ferreira LAM. Reductions in skin and systemic parasite burdens as a combined effect of topical paromomycin and oral miltefosine treatment of mice experimentally infected with *Leishmania* (*Leishmania*) *amazonensis*. Antimicrobial Agents and Chemotherapy. 2010;**54**(11):4699-4704

[16] Aguiar MG, Silva DL, Nunan FA, Nunan EA, Fernandes AP, Ferreira LAM. Combined topical paromomycin and oral miltefosine treatment of mice experimentally infected with *Leishmania* (*Leishmania*) *major* leads to reduction in both lesion size and systemic parasite burdens. Journal of Antimicrobial Chemotherapy. 2009;**64**(6):1234-1240

[17] Godinho JLP, Simas-Rodrigues C, Silva R, Ürmenyi TP, de Souza W, Rodrigues JCF. Efficacy of miltefosine treatment in *Leishmania amazonensis*-infected BALB/c mice. International Journal of Antimicrobial Agents. 2012;**39**(4):326-331

[18] Sundar S, Jha TK, Thakur CP, Engel J, Sindermann H, Fischer C, et al. Oral miltefosine for indian visceral leishmaniasis. New England Journal of Medicine. 2002;**347**(22):1739-1746

[19] Soto J, Arana BA, Tolado J, Rizzo N, Vega JC, Diaz A, et al. Miltefosine for new world cutaneous leishmaniasis. Clinical Infectious Diseases. 2004;**38**(9): 1266-1272

[20] Machado PR, Ampuero J, Guimarães LH, Villasboas L, Rocha AT, Schriefer A, et al. Miltefosine in the treatment of cutaneous leishmaniasis caused by *Leishmania braziliensis* in Brazil: A randomized and controlled trial. PLoS Neglected Tropical Diseases. 2010;**4**(12):1-6

[21] Rakotomanga M, Blanc S, Gaudin K, Chaminade P, Loiseau PM. Miltefosine affects lipid metabolism in *Leishmania donovani* promastigotes. Antimicrobial Agents and Chemotherapy. 2007;**51**(4): 1425-1430

[22] Lira R, Contreras LM, Santa Rita RM, Urbina JA. Mechanism of action of anti-proliferative lysophospholipid analogues against the protozoan parasite *Trypanosoma cruzi*: Potentiation of *in vitro* activity by the sterol biosynthesis inhibitor ketoconazole. Journal of Antimicrobial Chemotherapy. 2001;**47**(5):537-546

[23] Saraiva VB, Gibaldi D, Previato JO, Mendonça-Previato L, Bozza MT, Freire-de-Lima CG, et al. Proinflammatory and cytotoxic effects of hexadecylphosphocholine (miltefosine) against drug-resistant strains of *Trypanosoma cruzi*. Antimicrobial Agents and Chemotherapy. 2002;**46**(11):3472-3477

[24] Seifert K. Structures, targets and recent approaches in anti-leishmanial drug discovery and development. The Open Medicinal Chemistry Journal. 2011;**5**:31-39

[25] Ouellette M, Drummelsmith J, Papadopoulou B. Leishmaniasis: Drugs in the clinic, resistance and new developments. Drug Resistance Updates. 2004;**7**(4-5):257-266

[26] Dorlo TPC, Balasegaram M, Beijnen JH, de vries PJ. Miltefosine: A review of its pharmacology and therapeutic efficacy in the treatment of leishmaniasis. Journal of Antimicrobial Chemotherapy. 2012;**67**(11):2576-2597

[27] Maltezou HC. Drug resistance in visceral leishmaniasis. Journal of Biomedicine and Biotechnology. 2010;**2010**:1-8

[28] Santa-Rita RM, Henriques-Pons A, Barbosa HS, de Castro SL. Effect of the lysophospholipid analogues edelfosine, ilmofosine and miltefosine against *Leishmania amazonensis*. Journal of Antimicrobial Chemotherapy. 2004;**54**(4):704-710

[29] Verma NK, Singh G, Dey CS. Miltefosine induces apoptosis in arsenite-resistant *Leishmania donovani* promastigotes through mitochondrial dysfunction. Experimental Parasitology. 2007;**116**(1):1-13

[30] Calogeropoulou T, Angelou P, Detsi A, Fragiadaki I, Scoulica E. Design and synthesis of potent antileishmanial cycloalkylidene-substituted ether phospholipid derivatives. Journal of Medicinal Chemistry. 2008;**51**(4): 897-908

[31] Godinho JLP, Georgikopoulou K, Calogeropoulou T, de Souza W, Rodrigues JCF. A novel alkyl phosphocholine-dinitroaniline hybrid molecule exhibits biological activity *in vitro* against *Leishmania amazonensis*. Experimental Parasitology. 2013;**135**(1): 153-165

[32] de Macedo-Silva S, Souza W, Rodrigues J. Sterol biosynthesis pathway as an alternative for the anti-protozoan parasite chemotherapy. Current Medicinal Chemistry. 2015;**22**(18): 2186-2198

[33] Rodrigues JCF, Attias M, Rodriguez C, Urbina JA, de Souza W. Ultrastructural and biochemical alterations induced by promastigote and amastigote forms of *Leishmania amazonensis*. Antimicrobial Agents and Chemotherapy. 2002;**46**(2):487-499

[34] Emami S, Tavangar P, Keighobadi M. An overview of azoles targeting sterol 14α-demethylase for antileishmanial therapy. European Journal of Medicinal Chemistry. 2017;**135**:241-259

[35] Urbina JA, Docampo R. Specific chemotherapy of Chagas disease: Controversies and advances. Trends in Parasitology. 2003;**19**(11):495-501

[36] Benaim G, Sanders JM, Garcia-Marchán Y, Colina C, Lira R, Caldera AR, et al. Amiodarone has intrinsic anti-*Trypanosoma cruzi* activity and acts synergistically with posaconazole. Journal of Medicinal Chemistry. 2006;**49**(3):892-899

[37] de Macedo-Silva ST, Urbina JA, de Souza W, Rodrigues JCF. *In vitro* activity of the antifungal azoles itraconazole and posaconazole against *Leishmania amazonensis*. PLoS One. 2013;**8**(12): e83247

[38] Mukherjee S, Basu S, Zhang K. Farnesyl pyrophosphate synthase is essential for the promastigote and amastigote stages in *Leishmania major*. Molecular and Biochemical Parasitology. 2019;**230**:8-15

[39] Gadelha APR, Brigagao CM, da Silva MB, Rodrigues ABM, Guimarães ACR, Paiva F, et al. Insights about the structure of farnesyl diphosphate synthase (FPPS) and the activity of bisphosphonates on the proliferation and ultrastructure of *Leishmania* and *Giardia*. Parasites and Vectors. 2020;**13**(1):1-18

[40] Shah RR. Safety and tolerability of histone deacetylase (HDAC) inhibitors in oncology. Drug Safety. 2019;**42**(2):235-245

[41] Andrews KT, Haque A, Jones MK. HDAC inhibitors in parasitic diseases. Immunology and Cell Biology. 2012; **90**(1):66-77

[42] Kumar D, Rajanala K, Minocha N, Saha S. Histone H4 lysine 14 acetylation in *Leishmania donovani* is mediated by the MYST-family protein HAT4. Microbiology. 2012;**158**(2):328-337

[43] Saxena A, Lahav T, Holland N, Aggarwal G, Anupama A, Huang Y, et al. Analysis of the *Leishmania donovani* transcriptome reveals an ordered progression of transient and permanent changes in gene expression during differentiation. Molecular and Biochemical Parasitology. 2007;**152**(1): 53-65

[44] Prasanna P, Kumar R, Singh VK, Upadhyay A. Cloning, purification, and homology modeling of histone deacetylase in *Leishmania donovani*. Infection, Genetics and Evolution. 2021;**89**:1-6

[45] Yahiaoui B, Taibi A, Ouaissi A. A *Leishmania major* protein with extensive homology to silent information regulator 2 of *Saccharomyces cerevisiae*. Gene. 1996;**169**(1):115-118

[46] Ritagliati C, Alonso VL, Manarin R, Cribb P, Serra EC. Overexpression of cytoplasmic TcSIR2RP1 and mitochondrial TcSIR2RP3 impacts on *Trypanosoma cruzi* growth and cell invasion. PLoS Neglected Tropical Diseases. 2015;**9**(4):1-22

[47] Vergnes B, Sereno D, Madjidian-Sereno N, Lemesre JL, Ouaissi A. Cytoplasmic SIR2 homologue overexpression promotes survival of *Leishmania* parasites by preventing programmed cell death. Gene. 2002;**296**(1-2):139-150

[48] Vergnes B, Sereno D, Tavares J, Cordeiro-Da-Silva A, Vanhille L, Madjidian-Sereno N, et al. Targeted disruption of cytosolic SIR2 deacetylase discloses its essential role in *Leishmania* survival and proliferation. Gene. 2005;**363**(1-2):85-96

[49] Mittal N, Muthuswami R, Madhubala R. The mitochondrial SIR2 related protein 2 (SIR2RP2) impacts *Leishmania donovani* growth and infectivity. PLoS Neglected Tropical Diseases. 2017;**11**(5):e0005590

[50] North BJ, Marshall BL, Borra MT, Denu JM, Verdin E. The human Sir2 ortholog, SIRT2, is an NAD^+-dependent tubulin deacetylase. Molecular Cell. 2003;**11**(2):437-444

[51] Tavares J, Ouaissi A, Santarém N, Sereno D, Vergnes B, Sampaio P, et al. The *Leishmania infantum* cytosolic SIR2-related protein 1 (LiSIR2RP1) is an NAD^+-dependent deacetylase and ADP-ribosyltransferase. Biochemical Journal. 2008;**415**(3):377-386

[52] Adriano MA, Vergnes B, Poncet J, Mathieu-Daude F, da Silva AC, Ouaissi A, et al. Proof of interaction between *Leishmania* SIR2RP1 deacetylase and chaperone HSP83. Parasitology Research. 2007;**100**(4):811-818

[53] Wiesgigl M, Clos J. Heat shock protein 90 homeostasis controls stage differentiation in *Leishmania donovani*. Molecular Biology of the Cell. 2001;**12**:3307-3316

[54] Zemzoumi K, Sereno D, François C, Guilvard E, Lemesre JL, Ouaissi A. *Leishmania major*: Cell type dependent distribution of a 43 kDa antigen related to silent information regulatory-2 protein family. Biology of the Cell. 1998;**90**(3):239-245

[55] Silvestre R, Cordeiro-Da-Silva A, Tavares J, Sereno D, Ouaissi A. *Leishmania* cytosolic silent information regulatory protein 2 deacetylase induces murine B-cell differentiation and *in vivo* production of specific antibodies. Immunology. 2006;**119**(4):529-540

[56] Vergnes B, Gazanion E, Grentzinger T. Functional divergence of SIR2 orthologs between trypanosomatid parasites. Molecular and Biochemical Parasitology. 2016;**207**(2):96-101

[57] Sacconnay L, Smirlis D, Queiroz EF, Wolfender JL, Soares MBP, Carrupt PA, et al. Structural insights of SIR2rp3 proteins as promising biotargets to fight against Chagas disease and leishmaniasis. Molecular BioSystems. 2013;**9**(9):2223-2230

[58] Verçoza BRF, Godinho JLP, de Macedo-Silva ST, Huber K, Bracher F, de Souza W, et al. KH-TFMDI, a novel sirtuin inhibitor, alters the cytoskeleton and mitochondrial metabolism promoting cell death in *Leishmania amazonensis*. Apoptosis. 2017;**22**(9): 1169-1188

[59] Calegari-Silva TC, Vivarini ÁC, Pereira R de MS, Dias-Teixeira KL,

Rath CT, Pacheco ASS, et al. *Leishmania amazonensis* downregulates macrophage iNOS expression via Histone Deacetylase 1 (HDAC1): A novel parasite evasion mechanism. European Journal of Immunology. 2018;**48**(7):1188-1198

[60] Mukherjee S, Mukherjee B, Mukhopadhyay R, Naskar K, Sundar S, Dujardin J-C, et al. Imipramine exploits histone deacetylase 11 to increase the IL-12/IL-10 ratio in macrophages infected with antimony-resistant *Leishmania donovani* and clears organ parasites in experimental infection. The Journal of Immunology. 2014;**193**(8):4083-4094

[61] Perez J, Fuertes M, Nguewa P, Castilla J, Alonso C. Anticancer compounds as leishmanicidal drugs: Challenges in chemotherapy and future perspectives. Current Medicinal Chemistry. 2008;**15**(5):433-439

[62] Lowe G, Droz AS, Vilaivan T, Weaver GW, Tweedale L, Pratt JM, et al. Cytotoxicity of (2,2′,6′,2″-Terpyridine) platinum(II) Complexes to *Leishmania donovani*, *Trypanosoma cruzi*, and *Trypanosoma brucei*. Journal of Medicinal Chemistry. 1999;**42**(6):999-1006

[63] Tavares J, Ouaissi M, Ouaissi A, Cordeiro-da-Silva A. Characterization of the anti-*Leishmania* effect induced by cisplatin, an anticancer drug. Acta Tropica. 2007;**103**(2):133-141

[64] Miranda VM, Costa MS, Guilardi S, Machado AEH, Ellena JA, Tudini KAG, et al. *In vitro* leishmanicidal activity and theoretical insights into biological action of ruthenium(II) organometallic complexes containing anti-inflammatories. Biometals. 2018;**31**(6):1003-1017

[65] Minori K, Rosa LB, Bonsignore R, Casini A, Miguel DC. Comparing the antileishmanial activity of gold(I) and gold(III) compounds in *L. amazonensis* and *L. braziliensis in vitro*. ChemMedChem. 2020;**15**(22):2146-2150

[66] Morey JR, McDevitt CA, Kehl-Fie TE. Host-imposed manganese starvation of invading pathogens: Two routes to the same destination. Biometals. 2015;**28**(3):509-519

[67] Rice DR, Vacchina P, Norris-Mullins B, Morales MA, Smith BD. Zinc(II)-dipicolylamine coordination complexes as targeting and chemotherapeutic agents for *Leishmania major*. Antimicrobial Agents and Chemotherapy. 2016;**60**(5):2932-2940

[68] Mirzaei M, Nadushan AS, Nooshadokht M, Abiri A, Anjomshoa M, Sharifi I, et al. *In silico* and *in vitro* inhibitory potential of an organometallic Cu (II) complex on *Leishmania major* stages. Annals of Parasitology. 2021;**67**(1):45-54

[69] de Azevedo-França JA, Granado R, de Macedo Silva ST, dos Santos-Silva G, Scapin S, Borba-Santos LP, et al. Synthesis and biological activity of novel zinc-itraconazole complexes in protozoan parasites and *Sporothrix* spp. Antimicrobial Agents and Chemotherapy. 2020;**64**(5):e01980-e01919

[70] Ravera M, Moreno-Viguri E, Paucar R, Pérez-Silanes S, Gabano E. Organometallic compounds in the discovery of new agents against kinetoplastid-caused diseases. European Journal of Medicinal Chemistry. 2018;**155**:459-482

[71] Diro E, Blesson S, Edwards T, Ritmeijer K, Fikre H, Admassu H, et al. A randomized trial of AmBisome monotherapy and AmBisome and miltefosine combination to treat visceral leishmaniasis in HIV co-infected patients in Ethiopia. PLoS Neglected Tropical Diseases. 2019;**13**(1):1-19

[72] Miret JA, Moreno J, Nieto J, Carter KC, Mullen AB, Ambros L, et al.

Antileishmanial efficacy and tolerability of combined treatment with non-ionic surfactant vesicle formulations of sodium stibogluconate and paromomycin in dogs. Experimental Parasitology. 2021;**220**:108033

[73] Rashid HU, Ullah I, Adeeb H, Zeb M, Mohammad A, Rehman N. Synergistic effect of oral allopurinol and intralesional sodium stibogluconate in the treatment of cutaneous leishmaniasis. Journal of Ayub Medical College, Abbottabad : JAMC. 2020;**32**(4):558-561

[74] Brustolin AÁ, Ramos-Milaré ÁCFH, de Castro KR, Mota CA, Pelloso SM, Silveira TGV. Successful combined therapy with Glucantime™ and pentoxifylline for the nasal mucosal lesion recently developed in a leishmaniasis patient having untreated cutaneous lesion for seven decades. Parasitology International. 2021; **85**:102422

[75] van Griensven J, Balasegaram M, Meheus F, Alvar J, Lynen L, Boelaert M. Combination therapy for visceral leishmaniasis. The Lancet Infectious Diseases. 2010;**10**(3):184-194

[76] Kar A, Jayaraman A, Charan Raja MR, Srinivasan S, Debnath J, Mahapatra SK. Synergic effect of eugenol oleate with amphotericin B augments anti-leishmanial immune response in experimental visceral leishmaniasis *in vitro* and *in vivo*. International Immunopharmacology. 2021;**91**:107291

[77] Albalawi AE, Abdel-Shafy S, Khalaf AK, Alanazi AD, Baharvand P, Ebrahimi K, et al. Therapeutic potential of green synthesized copper nanoparticles alone or combined with meglumine antimoniate (Glucantime®) in cutaneous leishmaniasis. Nanomaterials. 2021;**11**(4):891

[78] Bahrami S, Oryan A, Bemani E. Efficacy of amiodarone and voriconazole combination therapy in cutaneous leishmaniasis in the mice experimentally infected with *Leishmania major*. Journal of Infection and Chemotherapy. 2021;**27**(7):984-990

[79] Caridha D, Sciotti RJ, Sousa J, Vesely B, Teshome T, Bonkoungou G, et al. Combination of subtherapeutic doses of tretazicar and liposomal amphotericin B suppresses and cures *Leishmania major*-induced cutaneous lesions in murine models. ACS Infectious Diseases. 2021;**7**(2):506-517

[80] de Morais-Teixeira E, Gallupo MK, Rodrigues LF, Romanha á lvaro J, Rabello A. *In vitro* interaction between paromomycin sulphate and four drugs with leishmanicidal activity against three New World *Leishmania* species. Journal of Antimicrobial Chemotherapy. 2014;**69**(1):150-154

[81] Sundar S, Rai M, Chakravarty J, Agarwal D, Agrawal N, Vaillant M, et al. New treatment approach in Indian visceral leishmaniasis: Single-dose liposomal amphotericin b followed by short-course oral miltefosine. Clinical Infectious Diseases. 2008;**47**(8): 1000-1006

[82] Singh N, Kumar M, Singh RK. Leishmaniasis: Current status of available drugs and new potential drug targets. Asian Pacific Journal of Tropical Medicine. 2012;**5**(6):485-497

[83] Odds FC. Synergy, antagonism, and what the chequerboard puts between them. Journal of Antimicrobial Chemotherapy. 2003;**52**(1):1

[84] Ahmed H, Curtis CR, Tur-Gracia S, Olatunji TO, Carter KC, Williams RAM. Drug combinations as effective anti-leishmanials against drug resistant: *Leishmania mexicana*. RSC Medicinal Chemistry. 2020;**11**(8):905-912

[85] Seifert K, Croft SL. *In vitro* and *in vivo* interactions between miltefosine

and other antileishmanial drugs. Antimicrobial Agents and Chemotherapy. 2006;**50**(1):73-79

[86] Dar MJ, Khalid S, McElroy CA, Satoskar AR, Khan GM. Topical treatment of cutaneous leishmaniasis with novel amphotericin B-miltefosine co-incorporated second generation ultra-deformable liposomes. International Journal of Pharmaceutics. 2020;**573**:118900

[87] Rebello KM, Andrade-Neto VV, Gomes CRB, de Souza MVN, Branquinha MH, Santos ALS, et al. Miltefosine-lopinavir combination therapy against *leishmania infantum* infection: *In vitro* and *in vivo* approaches. Frontiers in Cellular and Infection Microbiology. 2019;**9**:1-8

[88] Valdivieso E, Mejías F, Carrillo E, Sánchez C, Moreno J. Potentiation of the leishmanicidal activity of nelfinavir in combination with miltefosine or amphotericin B. International Journal of Antimicrobial Agents. 2018;**52**(5): 682-687

[89] Banik BL, Fattahi P, Brown JL. Polymeric nanoparticles: The future of nanomedicine. Wiley Interdisciplinary Reviews: Nanomedicine and Nanobiotechnology. 2016;**8**(2):271-299

[90] Black CDV, Watson GJ, Ward RJ. The use of pentostam liposomes in the chemotherapy of experimental leishmaniasis. Transactions of the Royal Society of Tropical Medicine and Hygiene. 1977;**71**(6):550-552

[91] Alving CR, Steck EA, Chapman WL, Waits VB, Hendricks LD, Swartz GM, et al. Therapy of leishmaniasis: Superior efficacies of liposome encapsulated drugs. Proceedings of the National Academy of Sciences of the United States of America. 1978;**75**(6):2959-2963

[92] Müller RH, Jacobs C, Kayser O. Nanosuspensions as particulate drug formulations in therapy: Rationale for development and what we can expect for the future. Advanced Drug Delivery Reviews. 2001;**47**(1):3-19

[93] Brown M, Noursadeghi M, Boyle J, Davidson RN. Successful liposomal amphotericin B treatment of *Leishmania braziliensis* cutaneous leishmaniasis. British Journal of Dermatology. 2005;**153**(1):203-205

[94] Shirzadi MR. Lipsosomal amphotericin B: A review of its properties, function, and use for treatment of cutaneous leishmaniasis. Research and Reports in Tropical Medicine. 2019;**10**:11-18

[95] Gutiérrez V, Seabra AB, Reguera RM, Khandare J, Calderón M. New approaches from nanomedicine for treating leishmaniasis. Chemical Society Reviews. 2016;**45**(1):152-168

[96] Akbari M, Oryan A, Hatam G. Application of nanotechnology in treatment of leishmaniasis: A Review. Acta Tropica. 2017;**172**:86-90

[97] de Souza A, Marins DSS, Mathias SL, Monteiro LM, Yukuyama MN, Scarim CB, et al. Promising nanotherapy in treating leishmaniasis. International Journal of Pharmaceutics. 2018;**547**(1-2):421-431

[98] Nafari A, Cheraghipour K, Sepahvand M, Shahrokhi G, Gabal E, Mahmoudvand H. Nanoparticles: New agents toward treatment of leishmaniasis. Parasite Epidemiology and Control. 2020;**10**:e00156

[99] Barick KC, Aslam M, Lin YP, Bahadur D, Prasad VP, Dravid VP. Novel and efficient MR active aqueous colloidal Fe_3O_4 nanoassemblies. Journal of Materials Chemistry. 2009;**19**(38): 7023-7029

[100] Lee JH, Jang JT, Choi JS, Moon SH, Noh SH, Kim JW, et al.

Exchange-coupled magnetic nanoparticles for efficient heat induction. Nature Nanotechnology. 2011;**6**(7):418-422

[101] Barick KC, Singh S, Jadhav NV, Bahadur D, Pandey BN, Hassan PA. PH-responsive peptide mimic shell cross-linked magnetic nanocarriers for combination therapy. Advanced Functional Materials. 2012;**22**(23): 4975-4984

[102] Kumar R, Pandey K, Sahoo GC, Das S, Das VNR, Topno RK, et al. Development of high efficacy peptide coated iron oxide nanoparticles encapsulated amphotericin B drug delivery system against visceral leishmaniasis. Materials Science and Engineering C. 2017;**75**:1465-1471

[103] Abazari R, Mahjoub AR, Molaie S, Ghaffarifar F, Ghasemi E, Slawin AMZ, et al. The effect of different parameters under ultrasound irradiation for synthesis of new nanostructured Fe_3O_4@bio-MOF as an efficient anti-leishmanial *in vitro* and *in vivo* conditions. Ultrasonics Sonochemistry. 2018;**43**:248-261

[104] Zomorodian K, Veisi H, Mousavi SM, Ataabadi MS, Yazdanpanah S, Bagheri J, et al. Modified magnetic nanoparticles by PEG-400-immobilized ag nanoparticles (Fe3O4@PEG–Ag) as a core/shell nanocomposite and evaluation of its antimicrobial activity. International Journal of Nanomedicine. 2018; **13**:3965-3973

[105] Berry SL, Walker K, Hoskins C, Telling ND, Price HP. Nanoparticle-mediated magnetic hyperthermia is an effective method for killing the human-infective protozoan parasite *Leishmania mexicana in vitro*. Scientific Reports. 2019;**9**(1):1-9

Chapter 9

Toward New Antileishmanial Compounds: Molecular Targets for Leishmaniasis Treatment

Huseyin Istanbullu and Gulsah Bayraktar

Abstract

The leishmaniases are a group of diseases caused by protozoan parasites—*Leishmania* sp. Leishmaniasis is classified among the 20 neglected diseases by WHO. Although the disease has been known for more than 120 years, the number of drugs used for the treatment is still limited to 5–6. The first-line drugs against leishmaniasis are pentavalent antimonials, which were introduced to the treatment 70 years ago—despite all their side effects. Molecular targets are becoming increasingly important for efficacy and selectivity in postgenomic drug research studies. In this chapter, we have discussed potential therapeutic targets of antileishmanial drug discovery such as pteridine reductase (PTR1), trypanothione reductase (TR), N-myristoyltransferase (NMT), trypanothione synthetase (TryS), IU-nucleoside hydrolase, and topoisomerases, enzymes and their inhibitors reported in the literature.

Keywords: antileishmanial compounds, molecular target, pteridine reductase, N-myristoyltransferase, inhibitors

1. Introduction

Leishmaniasis is a parasitic disease that occurs in the tropic and subtropics regions, and the parts of southern Europe. The disease is classified among neglected tropical diseases (NTDs) [1]. Leishmaniasis is spread by the bite of phlebotomine sand flies that causes the infection with *Leishmania* parasites. There are three main forms of the disease—cutaneous leishmaniasis (CL) known as the most common form, that causes skin sores; visceral leishmaniasis (VL; kala-azar) is the most severe form, that affects several internal organs; and mucocutaneous leishmaniasis (MCL) that has a chronic and metastatic behavior [2, 3].

Although the disease has been known for more than 120 years, the number of drugs used for the treatment is still limited to 5–6. The first-line drugs used against leishmaniasis are pentavalent antimony (Sb^V) compounds namely sodium stibogluconate (Pentostam®) and meglumine antimonate (Glucantime®), which was introduced into treatment more than 70 years ago, despite all their side effects. Neither their mechanism of action nor their chemical structures have been clarified/verified yet in spite of their wide use for a long time. Other drugs used in *Leishmania* infections are liposomal amphotericin B (L-AmB), miltefosine, paromomycin (aminosidine), and azole-derived antifungals; ketoconazole, itraconazole, and fluconazole.

The need for effective, safe, and selective chemotherapeutics against leishmaniasis increases every day. Targeting distinct molecular pathways is a widely used strategy in rational drug design and discovery for developing such agents to treat leishmaniasis. In this chapter, we would like to focus on enzymes which being targeted by the researcher for antileishmanial studies.

2. Potential molecular targets for the treatment of leishmaniasis

2.1 Pteridine reductase (PTR1, Pteridine reductase 1, EC 1.5.1.33)

PTR1 enzyme is an NADPH-dependent, short-chained reductase enzyme family member [4]. It is broadly active and can reduce a variety of unconjugated pteridines, as well as folates [5]. This enzyme has been investigated in studies of resistance to the dihydrofolate reductase inhibitor methotrexate (MTX) [6, 7]. After finding the missing link of resistance, researchers have suggested that inhibition of PTR1 may be a rational target for chemotherapy [4]. Since trypanosomatids are auxotrophic for folates and pterins, the inhibition of the PTR1 enzyme may also lead to selectivity. Therefore, PTR1 appears to be a rational target for antileishmanial drug development.

The first reported PTR1 inhibitors are pteridine analogs (diaminopteridines and quinazolines) and their activity was tested against purified *Leishmania major* pteridine reductase (*Lm*PTR1) [8]. The structure of *Lm*PTR1 in complex with NADPH and the inhibitor 2,4,6-triaminoquinazoline (TAQ) were reported in 2004 [9]. Based on its crystal structure, Cavazzutti *et al.* analyzed a library of 440 synthetic folate-like compounds and tested selected compounds on *Lm*PTR1 among other enzymes such as DHFR [10]. In this study compound, 6b was found to be the most promising compound with a Ki value of 37 nM toward LmPTR1. Then, the crystal structure of the *Lm*PTR1:NADPH:6b ternary complex revealed a substrate-like binding mode (**Figure 1**) [10].

It was reported that pteridine, pyrrolopyrimidine, and 2,4-diaminopyrimidine scaffold as PTR1 inhibitors with a structure-based approach by Tulloch et al. [11]. Among the tested compounds, compounds 11 and 13 bearings pyrrolopyrimidine core were reported with a modest ED50 value and a good lethality to the parasites. Additionally, a combination of MTX and compound 13 resulted in an improvement in efficacy [11]. Based on these hit molecules, TbPTR1 inhibitors were developed for the treatment of human African trypanosomiasis (**Figure 1**) [12].

Also, nonfolate scaffolds with *Lm*PTR1 inhibition activity were reported. After three rounds of election considering computational and experimental results, 18 compounds were selected, and among them, compound 28b and compound 5c known CNS active drug, showed promising activity with their IC50 values of 93 μM and 50 μM, Ki values of 7 μM and 4 μM, respectively (**Figure 1**) [13]. Moreover, 5c in combination with pyrimethamine showed antileishmanial activity on promastigotes with no hDHFR inhibition [14]. Another nonfolate scaffold, hexahydro pyrimido pyrimidinone, was introduced with potential antileishmanial activity in a virtual screening study. Compound 7 was reported as a potent *Ld*PTR1 enzyme inhibitor (Ki of 0.72 μM) and showed promising *Leishmania donovani* amastigote and *Labrus donovani promastigote* activity with the IC50 value of 3 μM and 29 μM, respectively [15].

Apart from the compounds summed up so far, thianthrene [16], dihydropyrimidines [17], benzothiazoles [18], thiazolidinedione [19, 20], thienopyrimidine [21], thiazolopyrimidine [22], and natural products such as flavanone derivatives

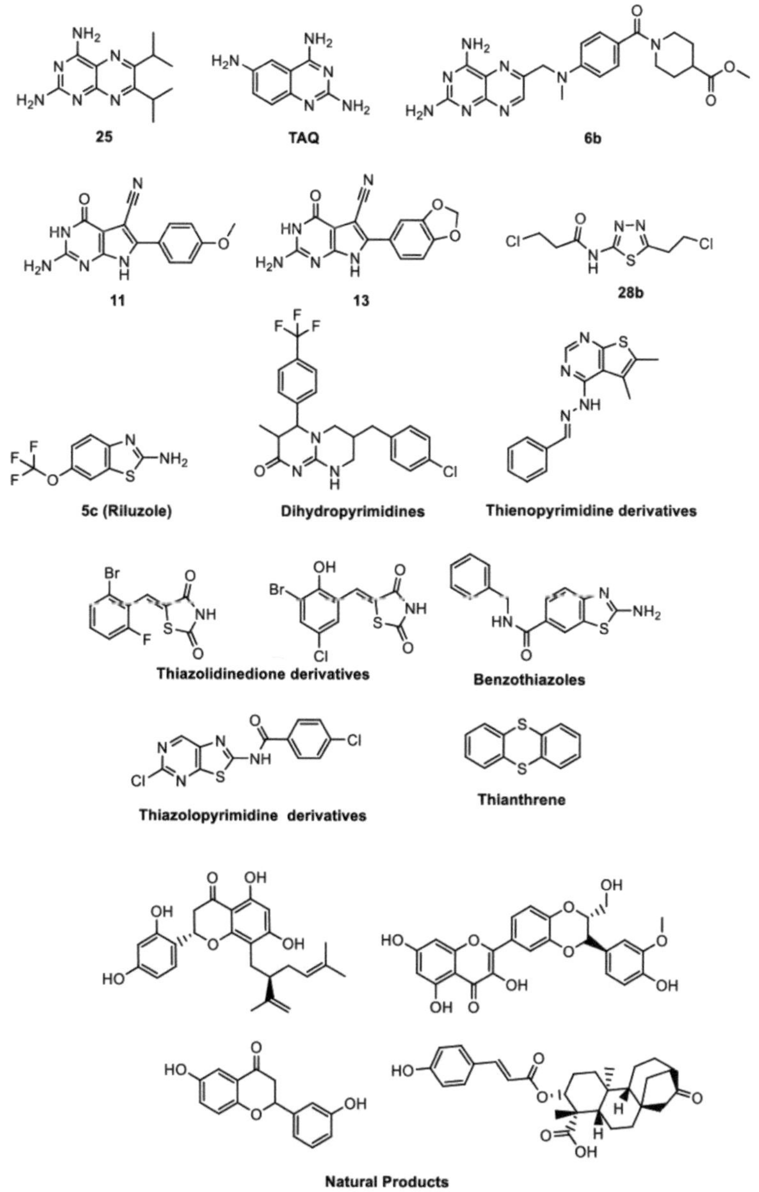

Figure 1.
Examples of PTR1 inhibitor structures with antileishmanial activity.

[23], 2,3-dehydrosilybin A, and sophoraflavanone G [24], kaurane-type diterpenes [25] were reported as PTR1 inhibitors with antileishmanial properties in the literature (**Figure 1**).

2.2 *N*-Myristoyltransferase (glycylpeptide N-tetradecanoyltransferase, NMT; EC 2.3.1.97)

NMT catalyzes the co- and post-translational addition of myristic acid (saturated, 14-carbon fatty acid) onto the N-terminal glycine of specific proteins in eukaryotes (**Figure 2**). This physiological pathway, *N*-myristoylation, plays an important role in the correct cellular localization and biological functions. NMT enzyme was purified and characterized from yeasts for the first time and it is thought to be a target for development of a new class of antifungal drugs [26]. The presence of NMT in *L. major* was verified in 1997 [27]. Later, NMT enzyme activity was proven essential for viability in *Leishmania sp*. then, it attracted attention as a potential drug target in kinetoplastid parasites [28]. The validation of this enzyme as a target for antitrypanosomal and antileishmanial drug discovery was not until 2010 (**Figure 2**) [29, 30].

A group of antifungal agents was tested to identify the first NMT inhibitors by Panethymitaki et al. in 2006 [31]. Although some of the tested compounds were found to be NMP inhibitors in a low μM concentration range, their antileishmanial activity has not been reported [31].

In an HTS campaign led by Pfizer, around 150.000 compounds from the Pfizer Global Diverse Representative Set were screened against protozoan NMTs. Four different scaffolds, namely aminoacylpyrrolidine (PF-03402623 IC_{50} of 0.093 μM), piperidinylindole (PF-03393842 IC50 of 0.102 μM), thienopyrimidine (PF-00349412 (IC50 of 0.482 μM), and biphenyl (PF-00075634 (IC50 of 0.158 μM) derivatives were identified as novel inhibitors of *Labrus donovani* NMP (**Figure 3**) [32].

Following the previous study, the crystal structures of PF-03393842 and PF-03402623 with the enzyme, the initial hits selected in the HTS campaign, were elucidated. Based on this data, a fused hybrid compound **43** was developed as a highly potent *L. donovani* NMT inhibitor (Ki of 1.6 nM) with good selectivity over the human isoform of the enzyme (Ki 27 nM) (**Figure 3**) [33]. Although the lack of cell activity of 43 attributed to its poor uptake, the HTS campaign, and hybridization of the hit compounds have resulted in the discovery of a new scaffold [33].

Another HTS assay dedicated to identifying novel *Leishmania sp.* NMT inhibitors was focused on a set of 1600 pyrazolyl sulfonamide compounds [34]. Interestingly, no correlation between the enzyme potency of these inhibitors and their cellular activity against *L. donovani* axenic amastigotes was observed. This might be rationalized by the fact that poor cellular uptake considering the basicity of the compounds. The most potent inhibitor of *Lm*NMT (compound 2, Ki of 0.34 nM) exhibited modest activity against *L. donovani* intracellular amastigotes

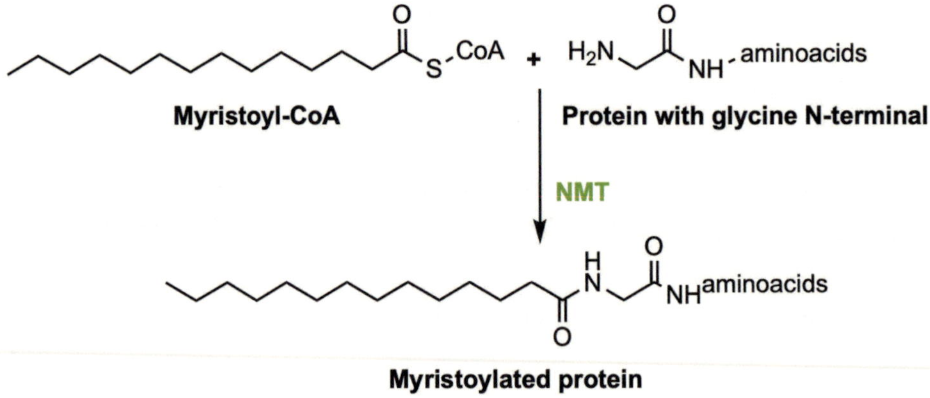

Figure 2.
Myristoylated proteins with NMT.

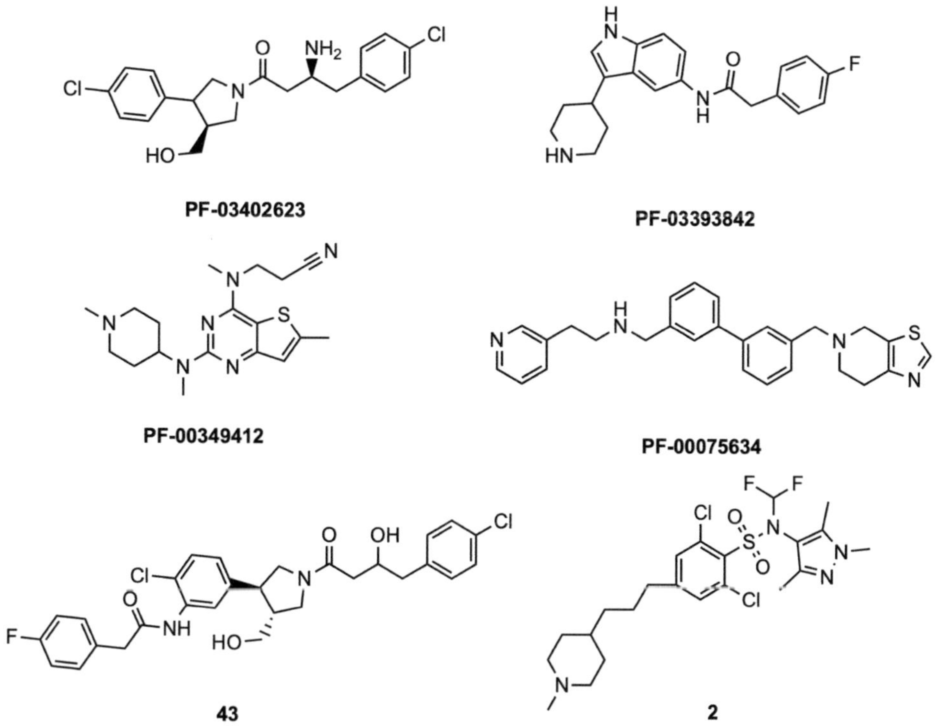

Figure 3.
Examples of NMT inhibitor structures with antileishmanial activity.

(EC50 of 2.4 μM). Yet, advanced studies on compound 2 confirmed the on-target mechanism. Moreover, oral use of compound 2 resulted in a 52% reduction in parasite burden in the mouse model of VL (**Figure 3**) [34].

Other NMT inhibitors as potential antileishmanial compounds were reported in a few publications and patents. In these studies, pyrrolidines, piperidinylindoles, azetidinopyrimidines, aminomethylindazoles, benzimidazoles, thienopyrimidines, biphenyl derivatives, benzofuranes, benzothiophenes, oxadiazoles, (pyrazolomethyl)-1,3,4-oxadiazoles and thienopyrimidine scaffolds, and peptidomimetic inhibitors were reported with their NMT inhibitory properties [35–38].

2.3 Inosine-uridine (IU) nucleoside hydrolase (IU-NH, EC:3.2.2.2)

The nucleoside hydrolase enzyme is an important target for the development of antiparasitic drugs due to its role in the purine salvage pathway. The amino acid sequence and X-ray structure of the enzyme from *L. major* were revealed in 1999 [39]. IU-NH enzyme establishes a homolog in *Leishmania* species.

In contrast to these facts, there is no study on IU-NH enzyme inhibitors possessing *in vitro/in vivo* antileishmanial activity up to our knowledge. Yet, few inhibitors of *Leishmania* IU-nucleoside hydrolase were reported.

Fuernaux et al. reported transition state analogs of nucleosides with IU-NH inhibitory activity [40]. Later, Berg et al. reported iminoribitol derivatives and evaluated their not only *Tabanus vivax*-NH activity but also human purine nucleoside phosphorylase to determine selectivity [41]. In other studies, two ribose-quinolone derivatives were tested against *Ld*NH [42] and Casanova et al. reported proanthocyanidins with *Ld*NH activity [43].

2.4 Enzymes Involved in Polyamine metabolism in *Leishmania*

In *Leishmania* parasites (and other members of the trypanosomatids), polyamine pathways can be considered as a unique pathway; most enzymes are essential for parasitic survival and infectivity (**Figure 4**).

2.4.1 Arginase (L-arginine amidinohydrolase, ARG, E.C. 3.5.3.1)

Arg is an enzyme that catalyzes the conversion of L-arginine amino acid to L-ornithine and urea.

The expression of the *Leishmania amazonensis* ARG in a bacterial host was done [44]. da Silva et al. expressed the recombinant enzyme in *E. coli* and performed biochemical and biophysical characterization studies [45].

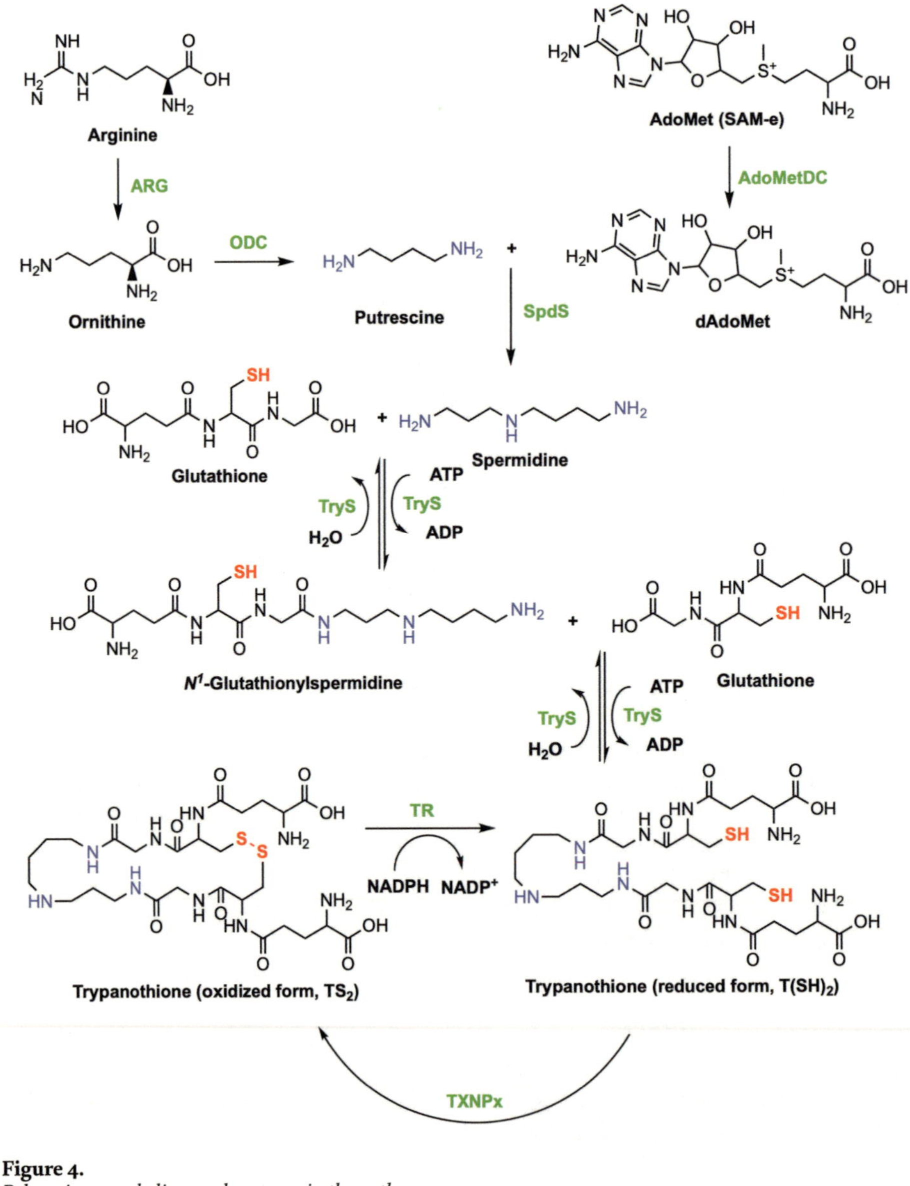

Figure 4.
Polyamine metabolism and enzymes in the pathway.

Reguera et al. suggest that broad inhibition of ARG activity alone will be insufficient to achieve therapeutically useful control of leishmaniasis, but combined inhibition of ARG with downstream enzymes leading to polyamine synthesis could result in improved therapeutic responses [46]. 3′-methoxy-cinnamoyl-1,3,4-thiadiazolium-2-phenylamine, an ARG inhibitory compound, exhibited moderate antileishmanial activity upon amastigotes of *L. amazonensis* [47].

[1,2,4]triazolo[1,5-a]pyrimidine derivatives [48], pyrazolo[3,4-d]pyrimidine derivatives [49], α,α-difluorohydrazide derivatives [50], chalcone derivatives [51], cinnamide derivatives [52], and 7,8-dihydroxyflavone—gold nanoparticles [53] were also studied as antileishmanial compounds with the mechanism of ARG inhibition.

On the other hand, antileishmanial natural products exhibiting ARG inhibitor activity with antileishmanial properties were reported—flavonoid and quercetin derivative [54], orientin and isovitexin [55], verbascoside [56], fisetin [57], rosmarinic acid, and caffeic acid [58].

2.4.2 Ornithine decarboxylase (ODC, EC 4.1.1.17)

ODC metabolizes ornithine to the diamine putrescine by its catalytic action [59]. Although alpha-difluoromethylornithine (DFMO) is an irreversible inhibitor of ODC, DFMO has not shown any antileishmanial activity [60]. Therefore, inhibition of ODC serves as a promising therapeutic paradigm for the treatment of leishmaniasis [61].

3-aminooxy-1-aminopropane was reported as a selective ODC inhibitor with potent antileishmanial activity against *Labrus donovani* (*L. donovani* promastigotes IC50 of 42 μM and *L. donovani* amastigotes IC50 of 5 μM) [62].

Gama-guanidinooxypropylamine [63], diospyrin [64], oxochromen, xanthone, and azaspirodecene derivatives [65] are reported in the literature with their ability to inhibit ODC enzyme and antileishmanial activity.

2.4.3 Spermidine synthase (SpdSyn, SpdS, EC 2.5.1.16)

SpdS catalyzes the conversion of putrescine to spermidine, a crucial polyamine for parasite proliferation. Genetic studies proved that SpdS is an essential gene in *L.donovani* [66]. Additionally, it was demonstrated that *L. donovani* amastigotes require SpdS activity to sustain a robust infection in mice; which is required for virulence [67].

Up to our knowledge, the only reported SpdS inhibitor with antileishmanial properties is natural compound hypericin [68].

2.4.4 S-Adenosylmethionine decarboxylase (AdoMetDC, EC 4.1.1.50)

AdoMetDC is involved in the synthesis of spermidine and spermine, an essential polyamine for *Leishmania*. Therefore, AdoMetDC may be a potential therapeutic target for leishmaniasis [69].

CGP40215A, a specific AdoMetDC inhibitor, was also reported with the antileishmanial effect that verified the potential of AdoMetDC enzyme inhibition strategy [70].

2.4.5 Trypanothione synthetase (Trypanothione synthase, TryS; EC 6.3.1.9)

TryS bifunctionally catalyzes both biosynthesis and hydrolysis of the glutathione-spermidine adduct trypanothione, which is the main regulator in intracellular

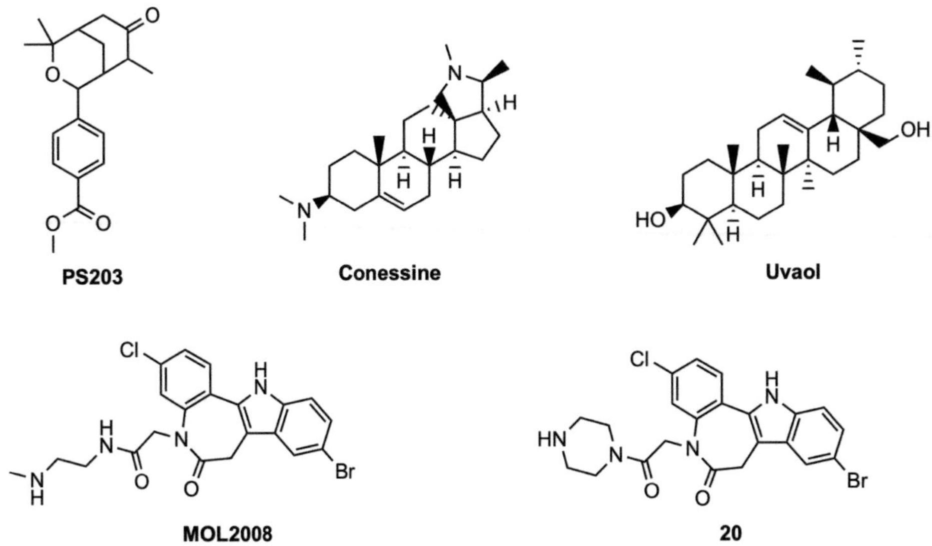

Figure 5.
Examples of TryS inhibitor structures with antileishmanial activity.

thiol-redox metabolite for parasitic trypanosomatids. As TryS is absent in humans, targeting this enzyme provides selectivity. Inhibition of TryS results in controlling relative levels of the critical metabolites, trypanothione, glutathionylspermidine, and spermidine in *Leishmania* [71]. Genetic and chemical analyses reveal that TryS is essential for *Leishmania infantum* [72].

In a computational screening campaign, oxabicyclo[3.3.1]nonanone skeleton was identified not only as a TryS inhibitor but also with TR inhibitory properties. A modest antileishmanial activity was reported for compound PS203 upon *L. donovani* promastigotes (**Figure 5**) [73]. In another study, TryS from *L. donovani* was characterized and inhibition studies with the natural compounds selected from an earlier Micro Source discovery natural product data set were performed [74]. Among the tested natural compounds, conessine and uvaol showed good TryS inhibition (Ki of 3.12 μM and 3.55 μM, respectively) with significant antileishmanial activity on *L. donovani* promastigotes (IC50 of 13,42 μM and 11,23 μM, respectively) (**Figure 5**) [74].

About 144 compounds belonging to seven different scaffolds were tested for TyrS inhibitory properties in a study by Benitez et al. One of the most promising inhibitors (IC50 of 0.15 μM) namely MOL2008, an N^5-substituted paullone derivative was evaluated upon *L. infantum* promastigotes (EC50 of 12.6 μM) (**Figure 5**) [75]. Following these results, 36 different derivatives of MOL2008 were developed by the same group [76]. Based on intriguing TyrS inhibition of compound 20 (IC50 0.3 μM), it was tested on both *L. infantum* promastigotes and *L. infantum* amastigotes. The metabolic changes exerted by 20 in both promastigote form and amastigote form of *L. infantum* are compatible with TryS inhibition (**Figure 5**) [76].

2.4.6 Trypanothione reductase (TR, TryR, Trypanothione-disulfide reductase 1, EC 1.8.1.12)

One of the main strategies of the host organism to overcome the infection is oxidative stress. TR has been purified from *T.cruzi* [77], first, and then from *Labrus donovani* [78]. TR enzyme is responsible for keeping trypanothione in the reduced state that is a variant of glutathione in *Leishmania* parasites. These enzyme inhibitors have been investigated in antileishmanial drug discovery as the enzyme is essential for the parasite survival and its absence in the host, in which glutathione reductase (GR) is found, provides selectivity [79]. Although both TR and GR are inhibited by trivalent antimonials, TR is considerably more sensitive [80]. TR enzyme is also a target for anti-Chagas compounds and antimalarials. The main limitation of TR becoming a target in antileishmanial drug discovery is that in order to obtain a considerable effect in parasites' redox state, a minimum of *85%* inhibition is required [81]. Additionally, GR should be considered as an off-target for TR inhibitors and the selectivity over TR enzyme of the compounds may be presented. Apart from being an interesting target for antileishmanial drug design, it is also a popular target for antimalarial compounds.

The early discovery of tricyclic inhibitors that are specific for TR over GR led to the design and synthesis of a group of phenothiazine derivatives and their opened-ring analogs.

The first rational drugs with TR inhibitor activity over GR inhibition are tricyclic structures like phenothiazine and imipramine. Based on this, among several of quaternary phenothiazines, [3-(2-chloro-4a,10a-dihydrophenothiazin-10-yl) propyl] - (3,4-dichlorobenzyl) dimethylammonium derivative (Ki 0.12 μM) was reported possessing improved activity up to 2-fold compared to chlorpromazine on *L. donovani* species [82]. Compound **10**, an opened ring analog of phenothiazine, showed antileishmanial activity upon *L. donovani* (IC50 of 3.9 μg/mL). Expectedly, it was one of the most active compounds for TR enzyme with the Ki value of 6.5 μM [83].

A series of bis (2-amino diphenyl sulfides) were designed and synthesized to inhibit TR [84]. Among them, compound **15** was found to be the most active with the IC50 value of 200 nM. Although there was no correlation between TR inhibition and antileishmanial activity, the compounds showed activity upon *L. infantum* amastigotes (**Figure 6**) [84]. Sulfonamide and urea derivatives of quinacrine with varying methylene spacer lengths were designed as TR inhibitors and their antiprotozoal activities were evaluated [85]. Compound **2b** (TR IC50 of 3.3 μM and GR IC50 of 27.2 μM) was also one of the most active compounds upon *L. donovani* among with *Trypanosoma cruzi and Trypanosoma brucei* [85] (**Figure 6**).

In the pursuit of discovering novel lead heteroaromatic frameworks, harmaline, pyrimidobenzothiazine, and aspidospermine scaffolds were tested against TR inhibition (Ki of 35.1 μM, Ki of 26.9 and Ki of 64.6 μM, respectively) and *L. amazonensis* promastigote toxicity. Moreover, compounds have not exhibited any GR inhibitory activity [86]. Interestingly, Blackie et al. has introduced ferrocenic 4-aminoquinoline urea compounds with TR inhibitory and antileishmanial properties to the literature [87]. Although compounds inhibited TR in a low μM range with good selectivity over GR and showed antileishmanial activity on *L. donovani* amastigotes, unfortunately, these compounds were found to be toxic to macrophages (**Figure 6**) [87].

In an HTS campaign, 100,000 lead-like compounds were evaluated for their TR inhibition. As our focus on antileishmanial compounds, 2 series of compounds namely, nitrogenous heterocycles (triazine and pyrimidine derivatives) and conjugated indole derivatives took our interest in their potential on *L. donovani* amastigotes (**Figure 6**) [88].

Various chemical structures were reported with TR inhibitor activity and leishmaniacidal activity to the literature: Ag(0) nanoparticles encapsulated by ferritin molecules [89], Cu(II) diketonates [90], oxabicyclo[3.3.1]nonanones [73], azole-based compounds – e. pyrrole [91], β-carboline–quinazolinone hybrid [92], phenothiazine and phenoxazine derived chloroacetamides [93], selenocyanates and diselenide compounds [94, 95], iminodibenzyl derivatives with ethylenediamine,

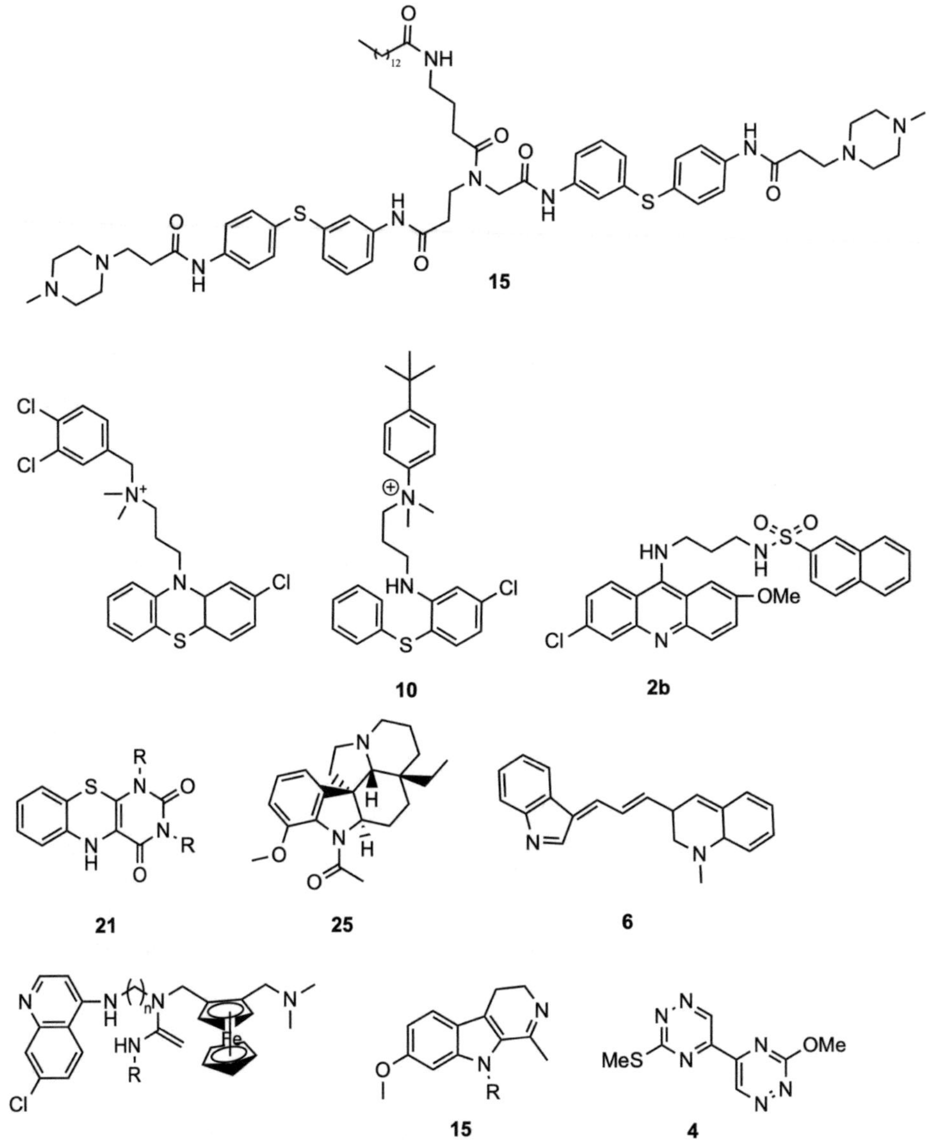

Figure 6.
Examples of TR inhibitor structures with antileishmanial activity.

ethanolamine and diethylenetriamine and their copper(II) complexes [96], diaryl sulfide derivatives [97], ammonium trichloro [1,2-ethanediolato-*O,O′*]-tellurat [98], all-hydrocarbon stapled peptides [99] chalcone derivatives [100], thiophene derivatives [101], imidazole-phenyl-thiazole compounds [102], isothiocyanate derivatives [103], (phenylthio)pyrimidin-4-amine derivatives [104], ferrocenylquinoline derivatives [105], triazole-phenyl-thiazoles derivatives [106], fluorene derivatives [107], adamantan derivatives, and their gold complexes [108] and natural products [109, 110] (**Figure 6**).

2.4.7 Tryparedoxin peroxidase (TryPI, TXNPx, EC 1.11.1.15)

Crystal structures of the tryparedoxin-tryparedoxin (TXN-TXNPx) peroxidase couple were reported but there is no study that targeted this system with antileishmanial activity [111].

2.5 Phosphotidylinositol-3-kinase (PI3K, EC 2.7.1.137)

The discovery of apoptotic pathways regulated by intracellular protozoan parasites and inhibit apoptosis, studies on signaling pathways have accelerated [112–114]. Interestingly, it was reported that there is an *L. major* PI3K mediated negative feedback mechanism for IL-12 production and PI3K/Akt signaling in *Leishmania* promastigotes [115].

Various heterocyclic compounds (quinoline, quinazoline, purine, thiazolopyrimidine scaffolds, etc.) as PI3K inhibitors were reported for treatment of several diseases alongside *Leishmania* [116, 117]. Later, Khadem et al. showed idelalisib—known PI3K inhibitor—and ampB combination therapy resulted in the reduction in parasite burden and moderate immune response [117]. A recent study showed that PI3K/mTOR inhibitor Torin2, Dactolisib, and NVP-BGT226 also possess good antileishmanial activity [118].

Imidazo[1,2-b]pyridazin scaffold was designed to inhibit various eukaryotic kinases by Bendjeddou et al. [119]. In this study, some of the compounds were tested against *L. amazonensis* parasites. The compounds showed antileishmanial activity at rather high concentrations (10 μM) although the compounds have not exhibited any toxicity at cell viability assays regarding concentrations [119].

Because of *Leishmania* parasite has a life cycle in the mammalian host, inhibition of signal transduction protein kinases for antileishmanial activities was investigated. Polyfluoroalkyl sp^2-glycolipid compounds were reported with antileishmanial properties by binding p38a-MAPK [120]. Purine derivatives, benzopyrroles, and benzopyrrolidines exhibited CRK3 cyclin-dependent kinase inhibitory properties and showed antileishmanial activity upon *Labrus donovani* amastigotes [121]. Lastly, a chemical inhibitor of heat shock protein 78 (HSP78), namely Ap5A reported with antileishmanial activity [122].

2.6 Topoisomerase I and II (TOPI, EC 5.6.2.1; TOPII, EC 5.6.2.2)

Topoisomerases are enzymes that modulate DNA topology. Firstly, topoisomerase II and then topoisomerase I enzymes were reported in *Leishmania* species [123, 124].

Different classes of TOP inhibitors show activity against *L. donovani* parasites by the means of DNA TOPI catalytic activity. The most important point is providing selectivity over parasite-human topoisomerase enzymes [125]. Pentostam's one of the proposed modes of action is inhibition of TOPI of *L. donovani* [126]. Werbovetz et al. tested known TOPII inhibitors, acridine derivatives, against *L. chagasi* and *L. donovani*, therefore, it was suggested that TOPII could serve as a useful target for parasite chemotherapy [127].

16-phenyl-6-hexadecynoic acid and 16-phenylhexadecanoic acid derivatives were synthesized by Carballeira et al. [128]. Compounds 1 and 2 showed promising activity on *L. donovani* TOPIB (EC50 14 μM and 36 μM, respectively). Moreover, compounds 1 and 2 showed cytotoxicity toward L. infantum amastigotes (IC50 of 3–6 μM) and L. infantum promastigotes (IC50 of 60–70 μM) [128].

In another study, compounds bearing 1,5-naphthyridine scaffold were reported [129]. Compound 22 was found to be one of the promising ones with the IC50 value (0.58 ± 0.03 μM) against L. infantum amastigotes similar to the standard drug amphotericin B (0.32 ± 0.05 μM) and selectivity over host murine splenocytes. Additionally, this compound showed remarkable inhibition on leishmanial TopIB [129].

Three compounds were identified in a very recent virtual screening campaign with a significant *Ld*TopIB activity (IC50of LRL-TP-85: 1.3 μM; LRL-TP-94: 2.9 μM;

and LRL-TP-101: 35.3 μM) [130]. Further studies showed that compounds were selective for *Ld*TopIB over *Homo sapiens* (Hs) TopIB. After that, compounds were evaluated for their in extracellular promastigote (4.9 μM, 1.4 μM, and 27.8 μM, respectively) and intracellular amastigote (34.0 μM, 53.7 μM, and 11.4 μM, respectively) activities [130].

Apart from these recent advances, several scaffolds such as bis-naphtoquinone [131, 132] betulinic acid derivatives [133], bisbenzimidazoles [134] and protoberberine alkaloids [135], and 1,3,4-thiadiazole derivatives [136] were identified with TOP inhibitor activity as potential antileishmanial compounds. Additionally, acetylenic fatty acids, 6-heptadecynoic acid, and 6-icosynoic acid derivatives [137], 2-octadecynoic acid [138], 3,3′-diindolylmethane derivatives [139], bis-lawsone analogs [140], spirooxindole derivatives [141], indeno-1,5-naphthyridines [142], diamidine derivatives [143], and copper salisylaldoxime [144] compounds are other reported topoisomerase inhibitors with antileishmanial activity.

2.7 Cysteine synthase (CS, O-acetylserine sulfhydrylase, OASS, EC 2.5.1.47)

Cysteine biosynthesis is a potential target for antileishmanial drug development. The structure of *L. major* cysteine synthase was revealed in 2012 by Fyfe et al. [145]. Cyclic imide derivatives were identified with a multitarget profile including TOPOI, *N*-myristoyltransferase, cyclophilin, and CS enzymes using *in silico* approach and *L. amazonensis* activity of the compounds were reported [146].

2.8 Oligopeptidase B (OPB, EC 3.4.21.83)

It was found out that a high level of serine protease activity was expressed by *L. donovani*, which was explained by an increase in OPB enzyme activity [147]. The crystal structure of *L. major* OPB was revealed in 2010 by McLuskey et al. [148]. Epoxy-α-lapachone was shown activity on both promastigote and amastigote forms of *L. amazonensis* in a study exploring natural compounds as potential antileishmanial agents. Moreover, this activity was associated with serine proteinase inhibitory activity of epoxy-α-lapachone in the same study [149]. Peptidic structure ShPI-I (Kunitz-type protease inhibitor from the sea anemone *Stichodactyla helianthus*) was shown to be a potent inhibitor of *L. amazonensis* serine proteases [150].

2.9 Superoxide dismutase (SOD, EC 1.15.1.1)

SOD enzyme was found in *L. tropica* by Meshnick and Eaton and it was suggested that the enzyme may be containing iron (Fe) which causes a difference from its host's enzymes which is linked to a copper or zinc atom [151]. Later, molecular isolation and characterization of Fe containing SOD cDNAs of *L. chagasi* were reported in 1997 [152] and the 3D structure of Fe-dependent superoxide dismutases (FeSODs) from *L. major* was reported [153].

In a study, imidazole-containing phthalazine derivatives were found to be potent inhibitors of Fe-SOD with antileishmanial properties. Additionally, the tested compounds were selective toward parasite Fe-SOD over human CuZn-SOD [154]. Arylamine Mannich base derivatives, known to be effective against *Trypanosoma cruzi*, were exhibited remarkable activity against *Leishmania* species. The mechanism of action of these compounds was linked to their potent Fe-SOD inhibition [155].

2-Iminothiazole derivatives [156], scorpiand-like azamacrocycles [157, 158], pyrazole-containing polyamine macrocycles [159], natural product momordicatin [ethyl 2-(4-hydroxybutyl)benzoate] [160], imidazole or pyrazole-based benzo [g] phthalazine derivatives [161], triphenyl tin salicylanilide thiosemicarbazone [162], Se containing aromatics and heteroaromatic compounds [163], ruthenium complexes with purine analogs [164], fisetin—a flavanoid anolog [57] and dialkyl pyrazole-3,5-dicarboxylates [165] were reported as SOD inhibitors exhibiting antileishmanial activity in the literature.

2.10 Nitroreductases (NTR, EC 1.7.1.16)

Nitroreductase enzymes catalyze the reduction of nitro/nitroaromatic compounds. Based on oxygen sensitivity, NTRs are divided into two groups: NTR1 is oxygen-insensitive and functions via a series of two-electron reductions, NTR2 is oxygen-sensitive and mediated a one-electron reduction [166]. NTR1 enzyme is found mainly in bacteria and absent in most eukaryotes. Keeping this in mind, *L. major* NTR1 (*Lm*NTR) was characterized and identified as a potential drug target for leishmaniasis [167].

It was reported that aziridinyl nitrobenzamide compounds [168], nitroquinolinone derivatives [169], 3-nitro-2-(phenylsulfonylmethyl) imidazo[1,2-a]pyridine derivatives [170], and nitro-heteroaryl nitrone derivatives [172] are NTR inhibitors with antileishmanial effects.

2.11 Nucleoside hydrolases (NH, EC 3.2.2.1)

Koszalka and Krenitsky, separated and purified three nucleoside hydrolases from promastigotes of *L. donovani*—purine 2′-deoxyribonucleosidase, purine ribonucleosidase, and pyrimidine ribonucleosidase [172]. Then, the X-Ray structure and amino acid sequence of nucleoside hydrolase from *L. major* was revealed alongside its several nanomolar transition state inhibitors [39].

Augustyns's research group design and synthesize various compounds and tested against IAG-NH (inosine-adenosine-guanosine nucleoside hydrolase) from *Tabanus vivax*. In contrast to promising enzyme activity of the compounds, antileishmanial activity of the compounds hasn't been investigated [41, 173, 174]. Freitas et al. also tested immucillin derivatives against *L. donovani*, *L. inf. Chagasi* and *L. amazonensis* parasites [175].

It was found out that hydroxychromenone and tetrahydrocyclohexanecarboxylic acid fragments could bind to the enzyme in a fragment-based analysis on *Ld*NH using saturation transfer difference (STD) NMR spectroscopy [176].

In a recent study, a natural product from Brazilian flora, flavonoids, and proanthocyanidins, with antileishmanial activity screened against *Ld*NH and described as an inhibitor of *Ld*NH [43, 177].

Interestingly, *Ld*NH (NH36) is the main area of interest for human recombinant vaccine-based studies and phase I trial of nucleoside hydrolase NH36 of *L. donovani*, the main antigen of the Leishmune® vaccine, and the sterol 24-c-methyltransferase (SMT) from *L. infantum* is in progress [178].

2.12 Cysteine proteases

There are two cysteine protease genes from *L. major*—one is structurally similar to the cathepsin L (CatL) family and the other is similar to the cathepsin B (CatB) family of cysteine proteases. These cysteine protease enzymes were isolated and sequenced by Sakanari et al. [179].

It is reported that aziridine-2,3-dicarboxylate [180], natural products flavone derivatives [181], trans-aziridine-2,3-dicarboxylate derivatives [182] organotellurane RF07 and palladacycle complex [183–185], and dipeptidyl enoates [186] exhibit antileishmanial effect and inhibit cysteine proteases.

2.13 Glyceraldehyde-3-phosphate dehydrogenase (GAPDH, EC 1.2.1.12)

GAPDH activity was detected in two cell compartments of *Leishmania mexicana* promastigotes [187]. Then, the crystal structure of *L. mexicana* GAPDH in complex with inhibitors was reported to the literature [188].

Although GAPDH enzyme is found in *Leishmania sp.*, it is an attractive target for the development of novel antitrypanosomatid agents rather than antileishmanial compounds.

2.14 Dihydroorotate dehydrogenase (DHODH, EC 1.3.5.2)

DHODH enzyme catalyzes the stereoselective oxidation of (S)-dihydroorotate (DHO) to orotate (ORO) in the *de novo* pyrimidine biosynthetic pathway. The structure of *L. major* DHODH was revealed by X-ray diffraction analysis [189]. It was reported that natural compounds from Asteraceae species could inhibit *Lm*DHODH by Chibli et al., though the antileishmanial effect of the compounds has not been evaluated [190].

2.15 Methionyl-tRNA synthetase (MetRS, EC 6.1.1.10)

Considering the structure of *L. major* MetRS, the difference in human cytosolic and mitochondrial MetRS and near the ATP- and methionine-binding regions of *Lm*MetRS promises selectivity for MetRS inhibitors [191].

DDD806905, a known *Tb*MetRS inhibitor, tested against *Ld*MetRS and showed antileishmanial effect upon *Leishmania* axenic amastigote yet, it has not shown efficacy in an animal model of leishmaniasis due to high protein binding as well as sequestration of this dibasic compound into acidic compartments [192]. Researchers have characterized a new series of *Ld*MetRS inhibitors bearing 4,6-diamino-substituted pyrazolopyrimidine core that target a previously undefined, allosteric binding site in the enzyme recently [193].

2.16 Phosphodiesterases (PDE, EC 3.1.4.17)

Phosphodiesterases control the cellular concentration of the second messengers cAMP and cGMP that are key regulators of several physiological processes.

A correlation between cAMP concentration in *Leishmania* cells and proliferation and transformation is demonstrated. By the addition of phosphodiesterase inhibitors to the culture medium, the intracellular level of cAMP was increased [194].

Crystal structure of the *L. major* phosphodiesterase *Lmj*PDEB1, one of the five PDE encoding genes, was reported in 2007 [195].

Isoxazolo[3,4-d]pyridazinone analogs were reported to inhibit PDE extracted from *L. mexicana* [196]. Later, it was reported that triphenyl-substituted imidazole compound exhibits *in vitro* antileishmanial and PDE inhibitor activity. Moreover, there was a correlation between *in vitro* antileishmanial activity and cAMP content [197].

2.17 Squalene synthase (SQS, SSN, E.C. 2.5.1.21)

SQS enzyme catalyzes the first step in sterol biosynthesis. Cloning, expression, and purification of a catalytically active recombinant squalene synthase of *L. donovani* (*Ld*SSN) [198].

Biphenylazabicyclooctanol, biphenylquiniclidine, and quiniclidine derivatives possessing *Lm*SQS inhibitory activity have shown antileishmanial effects against

L. amazonensis, therefore, SQS might serve as a potential target for antileishmanial drug discovery [199–201].

2.18 Uridinediphosphate-glucose pyrophosphorylase (UGPase, EC 2.7.7.9)

UGPase enzyme catalyzes the reaction of UTP and glucose-1-phosphate to 3-UDP-glucose and PPi in the presence of Mg^2 *in vivo*. It was reported that protozoan UGP differed from its mammalian counterparts which might provide selectivity [202]. *L. major* UGPase three-dimensional structure was reported but there has not been any reported *in vitro/in vivo* inhibitor of the enzyme yet although virtual screening campaigns have been applied to the enzyme [203].

2.19 Deoxyuridine 5′-triphosphate nucleotidohydrolase (dUTPase, EC 3.6.1.23)

The levels of dUTP are kept low by the action of dUTPase, a ubiquitous enzyme that catalyzes the hydrolysis of dUTP to PPi and dUMP, a substrate for thymidylate synthase (TS) [204]. The purification and characterization of *L. major* dUTPase were reported alongside its crystal structure [205, 206].

Deoxyuridine derivatives were shown to inhibit *L. major*, and human dUTPase enzymes exhibited moderate activity against *L. donovani* [207].

2.20 γ-Glutamylcysteine synthetase (Gcs, EC 6.3.2.2)

Gcs is an essential protein of the trypanothione biosynthesis pathway, which catalyzes ATP-dependent ligation of L-cysteine to L-glutamate. Characterization of *L. donovani* Gcs was reported to the literature in 2016 [208]. Agnihotri et al. identified carbamate, urea, and purine derivatives as Gcs inhibitors using *in silico* tools, then antileishmanial effect of the compounds was reported *in vitro* [209].

2.21 Cyclophilin (Cyp, Peptidylprolyl isomerase, EC 5.2.1.8)

Cyclophilins are a ubiquitous class of proteins with peptidylprolyl *cis-trans* isomerase activity. The structure of cyclophilin from *L. donovani* bound to cyclosporin was reported in 2009 [210]. Interestingly, a recent study showed that cyclosporin A, cyclophilin A modulator, does not express any significant inhibitory effect on intracellular *L. donovani* amastigotes, therefore, further studies are needed to validate this enzyme [211].

2.22 Other *Leishmania sp.* enzymes

We have summarized the validated targets for antileishmanial drug discovery and tried to give examples of potential modulators of these targets so far. Up to our knowledge, there are several other enzymes involved in kinetoplastids' physiological pathways which might serve as a potential target and provide selectivity, such as NDKb (nucleoside diphosphate kinase B, C 2.7.4.6), GPD (glycerol-3-phosphate dehydrogenase, EC 1.1.1.8), PGI (glucose-6-phosphate isomerase, EC 5.3.1.9), GspS (glutathionylspermidine synthetase, EC 6.3.1.8), PMM (phosphomannomutase, EC 5.4.2.8), PyK (pyruvate kinase, EC 2.7.1.40), TIM (triosephosphate isomerase, EC 5.3.1.1.), DHS (deoxyhypusine synthase, EC 2.5.1.46), and DOHH (deoxyhypusine hydroxylase, EC 1.14.99.29). Yet, the antileishmanial effect by the modulation of these targets has not been reported therefore further studies on these targets are needed.

3. Conclusion

Leishmaniasis treatment research has long been neglected. In this postgenomic era, work on leishmaniasis has accelerated, but great challenges still remain for medicinal chemists and chemical biologists—selectivity over human enzymes and efficacy over parasite life cycles. This chapter will be useful for researchers who will do *in silico* and *in vitro* studies.

Author details

Huseyin Istanbullu[1*] and Gulsah Bayraktar[2]

1 Department of Pharmaceutical Chemistry, Faculty of Pharmacy, Izmir Katip Celebi University, Izmir, Turkey

2 Department of Pharmaceutical Chemistry, Faculty of Pharmacy, Ege University, Izmir, Turkey

*Address all correspondence to: huseyin.istanbullu@ikc.edu.tr

References

[1] Leishmaniasis. Available from: https://www.cdc.gov/parasites/leishmaniasis/index.html [Page last reviewed: February 14, 2020 Accessed: August 5, 2021]

[2] Ronet C, Beverley SM, Fasel N. Muco-cutaneous leishmaniasis in the New World. Virulence. 2011;**2**:547-552. DOI: 10.4161/viru.2.6.17839

[3] Leishmaniasis. Available from: https://www.who.int/health-topics/leishmaniasis#tab=tab_1 [Accessed: August 5, 2021]

[4] Bello AR, Nare B, Feedman D, Hardy L, Beverley SM. PTR1: A reductase mediating salvage of oxidized pteridines and methotrexate resistance in the protozoan parasite *Leishmania major*. Proceedings of the National Academy of Sciences of the United States of America. 1994;**91**:11442-11446. DOI: 10.1073/pnas.91.24.11442

[5] Nare B, Hardy LW, Beverley SM. The roles of pteridine reductase 1 and dihydrofolate reductase-thymidylate synthase in pteridine metabolism in the protozoan parasite *Leishmania major*. The Journal of Biological Chemistry. 1997;**272**:13883-13891. DOI: 10.1074/jbc.272.21.13883

[6] Callahan HL, Beverley SM. A member of the aldoketo reductase family confers methotrexate resistance in Leishmania. The Journal of Biological Chemistry. 1992;**267**:24165-24168

[7] Papadopoulou B, Roy G, Ouellette M. A novel antifolate resistance gene on the amplified H circle of Leishmania. The EMBO Journal. 1992;**11**:3601-3608. DOI: 10.1002/j.1460-2075.1992.tb05444.x

[8] Hardy LW, Matthews W, Nare B, Beverley SM. Biochemical and genetic tests for inhibitors of Leishmania Pteridine pathways. Experimental Parasitology. 1997;**87**:157-169. DOI: 10.1006/expr.1997.4207

[9] McLuskey K, Gibellini F, Carvalho P, Avery MA, Hunter WN. Inhibition of Leishmania major pteridine reductase by 2,4,6-triaminoquinazoline: Structure of the NADPH ternary complex. Acta Crystallographica. Section D, Biological Crystallography. 2004;**60**:1780-1785. DOI: 10.1107/S0907444904018955

[10] Cavazzuti A, Paglietti G, Hunter WN, Gamarro F, Piras S, Loriga M, et al. Discovery of potent pteridine reductase inhibitors to guide antiparasite drug development. Proceedings of the National Academy of Sciences of the United States of America. 2008;**105**:1448-1453. DOI: 10.1073/pnas. 0704384105

[11] Tulloch LB, Martini VP, Iulek J, Huggan JK, Lee JH, Gibson CL, et al. Structure-based design of pteridine reductase inhibitors targeting African sleeping sickness and the Leishmaniases. Journal of Medicinal Chemistry. 2010;**53**:221-229. DOI: 10.1021/jm901059x

[12] Khalaf AI, Huggan JK, Suckling CJ, Gibson CL, Stewart K, Giordani F, et al. Structure-based design and synthesis of antiparasitic pyrrolopyrimidines targeting pteridine reductase 1. Journal of Medicinal Chemistry. 2014;**57**:6479-6494. DOI: 10.1021/jm500483b

[13] Ferrari S, Morandi F, Motiejunas D, Nerini E, Henrich S, Luciani R, et al. Virtual screening identification of nonfolate compounds, including a CNS drug, as antiparasitic agents inhibiting pteridine reductase. Journal of Medicinal Chemistry. 2011;**54**:211-221. DOI: 10.1021/jm1010572

[14] Guerrieri D, Ferrari S, Costi MP, Michels PAM. Biochemical effects of riluzole on Leishmania parasites. Experimental Parasitology. 2013;**133**:250-254. DOI: 10.1016/j.exppara.2012.11.013

[15] Kaur J, Kumar P, Tyagi S, Pathak R, Batra S, Singh P, et al. *In Silico* screening, structure-activity relationship, and biologic evaluation of selective pteridine reductase inhibitors targeting visceral Leishmaniasis. Antimicrobial Agents and Chemotherapy. 2011;**55**:659-666. DOI: 10.1128/AAC.00436-10

[16] Kaur J, Dube D, Ramachandran R, Singh P, Singh N. Thianthrene is a novel inhibitor of Leishmania donovani pteridine reductase 1 (PTR1). Journal of Molecular Biochemistry. 2012;**1**:68-75

[17] Rashid U, Sultana R, Shaheen N, Hassan SF, Yaqoob F, Ahmad MJ, et al. Structure based medicinal chemistry-driven strategy to design substituted dihydropyrimidines as potential antileishmanial agents. European Journal of Medicinal Chemistry. 2016;**115**:230-244. DOI: 10.1016/j.ejmech.2016.03.022

[18] Linciano P, Pozzi C, Iacono LD, di Pisa F, Landi G, Bonucci A, et al. Enhancement of benzothiazoles as Pteridine Reductase-1 (PTR1) inhibitors for the treatment of Trypanosomatidic infections. Journal of Medicinal Chemistry. 2019;**62**:3989-4012. DOI: 10.1021/acs.jmedchem.8b02021

[19] Neri FSM, Junior DBC, Froes TQ, da Silva PBG, do Egito MS, POL M, et al. Antileishmanial activity evaluation of thiazolidine-2,4-dione against *Leishmania infantum* and *Leishmania braziliensis*. Parasitology Research. 2020;**119**:2263-2274. DOI: 10.1007/s00436-020-06706-3

[20] Leite FHA, Santiago PBGS, Froes TQ, Filho JS, da Silva SG, Ximenes RM, et al. Structure-guided discovery of thiazolidine-2,4-dione derivatives as a novel class of *Leishmania major* pteridine reductase 1 inhibitors. European Journal of Medicinal Chemistry. 2016;**123**:639-648. DOI: 10.1016/j.ejmech.2016.07.060

[21] Leite FHA, Froes TQ, da Silva SG, de Souza EIM, Vital-Fujii DG, Trossini GHG, et al. An integrated approach towards the discovery of novel non-nucleoside *Leishmania major* pteridine reductase 1 inhibitors. European Journal of Medicinal Chemistry. 2017;**132**:322-332. DOI: 10.1016/j.ejmech.2017.03.043

[22] Istanbullu H, Bayraktar G, Akbaba H, Cavus I, Coban G, Debelec-Butuner B, et al. Design, synthesis, and in vitro biological evaluation of novel thiazolopyrimidine derivatives as antileishmanial compounds. Archiv der Pharmazie. 2020;**353**:1900325. DOI: 10.1002/ardp.201900325

[23] di Pisa F, Landi G, Iacono LD, Pozzi C, Borsari C, Ferrari S, et al. Chroman-4-one derivatives targeting pteridine reductase 1 and showing anti-parasitic activity. Molecules. 2017;**22**:426. DOI: 10.3390/molecules22030426

[24] Herrmann FC, Sivakumar N, Jose J, Costi MP, Pozzi C, Schmidt TJ. In silico identification and in vitro evaluation of natural inhibitors of *Leishmania major* pteridine reductase I. Molecules. 2017;**22**:2166. DOI: 10.3390/molecules22122166

[25] Herrera-Acevedo C, Flores-Gaspar A, Scotti L, Mendonca-Junior FJB, Scotti MT, Coy-Barrera E. Identification of Kaurane-type diterpenes as inhibitors of Leishmania pteridine reductase I. Molecules. 2021;**26**:3076. DOI: 10.3390/molecules26113076

[26] Duronio RJ, Towler DA, Heuckeroth RO, Gordon JI. Disruption of the yeast N-myristoyl transferase gene causes recessive lethality. Science. 1989;**243**:796-800. DOI: 10.1126/science.2644694

[27] McKean PG, Delahay R, Pimena PFP, Smith DF. Characterisation of a second protein encoded by the differentially regulated LmcDNA16 gene family of *Leishmania major*. Molecular and Biochemical Parasitology. 1997;**85**:221-231. DOI: 10.1016/S0166-6851(97)02829-6

[28] Price HP, Menon MR, Panethymitaki C, Goulding D, McKean PG, Smith DF. Myristoyl-CoA:protein N-myristoyltransferase, an essential enzyme and potential drug target in kinetoplastid parasites. Journal of Biological Chemistry. 2003;**278**:7206-7214. DOI: 10.1074/jbc.M211391200

[29] Price HP, Güther MLS, Ferguson MAJ, Smith DF. Myristoyl-CoA:protein N-myristoyltransferase depletion in trypanosomes causes avirulence and endocytic defects. Molecular and Biochemical Parasitology. 2010;**169**:55-58. DOI: 10.1016/j.molbiopara.2009.09.006

[30] Branningan JA, Smith BA, Yu Z, Brzozowski AM, Hodgkinson MR, Maroof A, et al. *N*-Myristoyltransferase from *Leishmania donovani*: Structural and functional characterisation of a potential drug target for visceral Leishmaniasis. Journal of Molecular Biology. 2010;**396**:985-999. DOI: 10.1016/j.jmb.2009.12.032

[31] Panethymitaki C, Bowyer PW, Price HP, Leatherbarrow RJ, Brown KA, Smith DF. Characterization and selective inhibition of myristoyl-CoA:protein *N*-myristoyltransferase from *Trypanosoma brucei* and *Leishmania major*. The Biochemical Journal. 2006;**396**:277-285. DOI: 10.1042/BJ20051886

[32] Bell AS, Mills JE, Williams GP, Brannigan JA, Wilkinson AJ, Parkinson T, et al. Selective inhibitors of protozoan protein *N*-myristoyltransferases as starting points for tropical disease medicinal chemistry programs. PLoS Neglected Tropical Diseases. 2012;**6**:e1625. DOI: 10.1371/journal.pntd.0001625

[33] Hutton JA, Goncalves V, Brannigan JA, Paape D, Wright MH, Waugh TM, et al. Structure-based design of potent and selective *Leishmania N*-myristoyltransferase inhibitors. Journal of Medicinal Chemistry. 2014;**57**:8664-8670. DOI: 10.1021/jm5011397

[34] Corpas-Lopez V, Moniz S, Thomas M, Wall RJ, Torrie LS, Zander-Dinse D, et al. Pharmacological validation of *N*-myristoyltransferase as a drug target in *Leishmania donovani*. ACS Infectious Diseases. 2019;**5**:111-122. DOI: 10.1021/acsinfecdis.8b00226

[35] Leatherbarrow R, Tate EW, Yu Z, Rackham M. Novel Compounds and Their Use in Therapy. 2013. WO 2013/083991 A1

[36] Rackham MD, Yu Z, Brannigan JA, Heal WP, Paape D, Barker KV, et al. Discovery of high affinity inhibitors of *Leishmania donovani N*-myristoyltransferase. Medicinal Chemistry Communications. 2015;**6**:1761-1766. DOI: 10.1039/C5MD00241A

[37] Bell AS, Yu Z, Hutton JA, Wright MH, Brannigan JA, Paape D, et al. Novel thienopyrimidine inhibitors of *Leishmania N*-myristoyltransferase with on-target activity in intracellular amastigotes. Journal of Medicinal Chemistry. 2020;**63**:7740-7765. DOI: 10.1021/acs.jmedchem.0c00570

[38] Olalye TO, Brannigan JA, Roberts SM, Leatherbarrow RJ, Wilkinson AJ, Tate EW. Peptidomimetic inhibitors of *N*-myristoyltransferase from human malaria and leishmaniasis parasites. Organic & Biomolecular Chemistry. 2014;**12**:8132-8137. DOI: 10.1039/C4OB01669F

[39] Shi W, Schramm VL, Almo SC. Nucleoside hydrolase from *Leishmania major:* Cloning, expression, catalytic properties, transition state inhibitors, and the 2.5-Å crystal structure. Journal of Biological Chemistry. 1999;**274**:21114-21120. DOI: 10.1074/jbc.274.30.21114

[40] Furneaux RH, Schramm VL, Tyler PC. Transition state analogue inhibitors of protozoan nucleoside hydrolases. Bioorganic & Medicinal Chemistry. 1999;**7**:2599-2606. DOI: 10.1016/S0968-0896(99)00210-2

[41] Berg M, Bal G, Goeminne A, der Veken PV, Versees W, Steuaert J, et al. Synthesis of bicyclic N-arylmethyl-substituted iminoribitol derivatives as selective nucleoside hydrolase inhibitors. ChemMedChem. 2009;**4**:249-260. DOI: 10.1002/cmdc.200800231

[42] Renno MN, Franca TCC, Nico D, Palatnik-de-Sousa CB, Tinoco LW, Figueroa-Villar JD. Kinetics and docking studies of two potential new inhibitors of the nucleoside hydrolase from *Leishmania donovani*. European Journal of Medicinal Chemistry. 2012;**56**:301-307. DOI: 10.1016/j.ejmech.2012.07.052

[43] Casanova LM, Rodrigues LM, de Aguiar PF, Tinoco LW. An NMR-based chemometric strategy to identify *Leishmania donovani* nucleoside hydrolase inhibitors from the Brazilian tree *Ormosia arborea*. Journal of Natural Products. 2020;**83**:243-254. DOI: 10.1021/acs.jnatprod.9b00622

[44] da Silva ER, Castilho TM, Pioker FC, Silva CHTP, Floeter-Winter LM. Genomic organisation and transcription characterisation of the gene encoding *Leishmania (Leishmania) amazonensis* arginase and its protein structure prediction. International Journal of Parasitology. 2002;**32**:727-737. DOI: 10.1016/S0020-7519(02)00002-4

[45] da Silva ER, da Silva MFL, Fischer H, Mortara RA, Mayer MG, Framesqui K, et al. Biochemical and biophysical properties of a highly active recombinant arginase from *Leishmania (Leishmania) amazonensis* and subcellular localization of native enzyme. Molecular and Biochemical Parasitology. 2008;**159**:104-111. DOI: 10.1016/j.molbiopara.2008.02.011

[46] Reguera RM, Balana-Fouce R, Showalter M, Hickerson S, Beverley SM. *Leishmania major* lacking arginase (ARG) are auxotrophic for polyamines but retain infectivity to susceptible BALB/c mice. Molecular and Biochemical Parasitology. 2009;**165**:48-56. DOI: 10.1016/j.molbiopara.2009.01.001

[47] Soares-Bezerra RJ, da Silva EF, Echevarria A, Gomes-da-Silva L, Cysne-Finkelstein L, Monteiro FP, et al. Effect of mesoionic 4-phenyl-5-(cinnamoyl)-1,3,4-thiadiazolium-2-phenylamine chloride derivative salts on the activities of the nitric oxide synthase and arginase of *Leishmania amazonensis*. Journal of Enzyme Inhibition and Medicinal Chemistry. 2008;**23**:328-333. DOI: 10.1080/14756360701585619

[48] da Silva ER, Boechat N, Pinheiro LCS, Bastos MM, Costa CCP, Bartholomeu JC, et al. Novel selective inhibitor of *Leishmania (Leishmania) amazonensis* Arginase. Chemical Biology & Drug Design. 2015;**86**:969-978. DOI: 10.1111/cbdd.12566

[49] Feitosa LM, da Silva ER, Hoelz LVB, Souza DL, Come JAASS, Cardoso-Santos C, et al. New pyrazolopyrimidine derivatives as *Leishmania amazonensis* arginase inhibitors. Bioorganic & Medicinal Chemistry. 2019;**27**:3061-3069. DOI: 10.1016/j.bmc.2019.05.026

[50] de Lima EC, Castelo-Branco FS, Maquiaveli CC, Farias AB, Renno MN, Boechat N, et al. Phenylhydrazides as

inhibitors of *Leishmania amazonensis* arginase and antileishmanial activity. Bioorganic & Medicinal Chemistry. 2019;**27**:3853-3859. DOI: 10.1016/j.bmc.2019.07.022

[51] Garcia AR, Oliveira DMP, Jesus JB, Souza AMT, Sodera ACR, Vermelho AB, et al. Identification of chalcone derivatives as inhibitors of *Leishmania infantum* arginase and promising antileishmanial agents. Frontiers in Chemistry. 2021;**8**:624678. DOI: 10.3389/fchem.2020.624678

[52] da Silva ER, Come JAASS, Brogi S, Calderone V, Chemi G, Campiani G, et al. Cinnamides target *Leishmania amazonensis* arginase selectively. Molecules. 2020;**25**:5271. DOI: 10.3390/molecules25225271

[53] Prasanna P, Kumar P, Mandal S, Payal T, Kumar S, Hossain SU, et al. 7,8-dihydroxyflavone-functionalized gold nanoparticles target the arginase enzyme of *Leishmania donovani*. Nanomedicine. 2021;**16**:1887-1903. DOI: 10.2217/nnm-2021-0161

[54] da Silva ER, Maquiaveli CC, Magalhaes PP. The leishmanicidal flavonols quercetin and quercitrin target *Leishmania (Leishmania) amazonensis* arginase. Experimental Parasitology. 2012;**130**:183-188. DOI: 10.1016/j.exppara.2012.01.015

[55] Cruz EM, da Silva ER, Maquiaveli CC, Alves ESS, Lucon-Junior JF, dos Reis MBG, et al. Leishmanicidal activity of *Cecropia pachystachya* flavonoids: Arginase inhibition and altered mitochondrial DNA arrangement. Phytochemistry. 2013;**89**:71-77. DOI: 10.1016/j.phytochem.2013.01.014

[56] Maquiaveli CC, Lucon-Junior JF, Brogi S, Campiani G, Gemma S, Vieira P, et al. Verbascoside inhibits promastigote growth and arginase activity of *Leishmania amazonensis*. Journal of Natural Products. 2016;**79**:1459-1463. DOI: 10.1021/acs.jnatprod.5b00875

[57] Adinehbeigi K, Jalali MHR, Shahriari A, Bahrami S. *In vitro* antileishmanial activity of fisetin flavonoid via inhibition of glutathione biosynthesis and arginase activity in *Leishmania infantum*. Pathogens and Global Health. 2017;**111**:176-185. DOI: 10.1080/20477724.2017.1312777

[58] Garcia AR, Oliveira DMP, Amaral ACF, Jesus JB, Sodero ACR, Souza AMT, et al. *Leishmania infantum* arginase: Biochemical characterization and inhibition by naturally occurring phenolic substances. Journal of Enzyme Inhibition and Medicinal Chemistry. 2019;**34**:1100-1109. DOI: 10.1080/14756366.2019.1616182

[59] Perdeh J, Berioso B, Love Q, LoGiudice N, Le TL, Harrelson JP, et al. Critical functions of the polyamine putrescine for proliferation and viability of *Leishmania donovani* parasites. Amino Acids. 2020;**52**:261-274. DOI: 10.1007/s00726-019-02736-z

[60] Kaur K, Emmett K, McCann PP, Sjoerdsma A, Ullman B. Effects of DL-Alpha-Difluoromethylornithine on *Leishmania donovani* promastigotes. Eukaryotic Microbiology. 1986;**33**:518-521. DOI: 10.1111/j.1550-7408.1986.tb05654.x

[61] Boitz JM, Yates PA, Kline C, Gaur U, Wilson ME, Ullman B, et al. *Leishmania donovani* ornithine decarboxylase is indispensable for parasite survival in the mammalian host. Infection and Immunity. 2009;**77**:756-763. DOI: 10.1128/IAI.01236-08

[62] Singh S, Mukherjee A, Khomutov AR, Persson L, Heby O, Chatterjee M, et al. Antileishmanial effect of 3-aminooxy-1-aminopropane is due to polyamine depletion. Antimicrobial Agents and

Chemotherapy. 2007;**51**:528-534. DOI: 10.1128/AAC.01055-06

[63] Singh S, Jhingran A, Sharma A, Simonian AR, Soininen P, Vepsalainen J, et al. Novel agmatine analogue, g-guanidinooxypropylamine (GAPA) efficiently inhibits proliferation of *Leishmania donovani* by depletion of intracellular polyamine levels. Biochemical and Biophysical Research Communications. 2008;**375**:168-172. DOI: 10.1016/j.bbrc.2008.07.143

[64] Hazra S, Ghosh S, Sarma MD, Sharma A, Das M, Saudagar P, et al. Evaluation of a diospyrin derivative as antileishmanial agent and potential modulator of ornithine decarboxylase of *Leishmania donovani*. Experimental Parasitology. 2013;**135**:407-413. DOI: 10.1016/j.exppara.2013.07.021

[65] Das M, Singh S, Dubey VK. Novel inhibitors of ornithine decarboxylase of *Leishmania* parasite (*Ld*ODC): The parasite resists *Ld*ODC inhibition by overexpression of spermidine synthase. Chemical Biology & Drug Design. 2016;**87**:352-360. DOI: 10.1111/cbdd.12665

[66] SC R, Jiang Y, Jardim A, Carter NS, Heby O, Ullman B. Genetic analysis of spermidine synthase from *Leishmania donovani*. Molecular and Biochemical Parasitology. 2001;**115**:217-226. DOI: 10.1016/S0166-6851(01)00293-6

[67] Gilroy C, Olenyik T, Roberts SC, Ullman B. Spermidine synthase is required for virulence of *Leishmania donovani*. Infection and Immunity. 2011;**79**:2764-2769. DOI: 10.1128/IAI.00073-11

[68] Singh S, Sarma S, Katiyar SP, Das M, Bhardwaj R, Sundar D, et al. Probing the molecular mechanism of hypericin-induced parasite death provides insight into the role of spermidine beyond redox metabolism in *Leishmania donovani*. Antimicrobial Agents and Chemotherapy. 2015;**59**:15-24. DOI: 10.1128/AAC.04169-14

[69] Roberts SC, Scott J, Gasteier JE, Jiang Y, Brooks B, Jardim A, et al. S-adenosylmethionine decarboxylase from *Leishmania donovani*. Journal of Biological Chemistry. 2002;**277**:5902-5909. DOI: 10.1074/jbc.M110118200

[70] Mukhopadhyay R, Kapoor P, Madhubala R. Antileishmanial effect of a potent S-Adenosylmethionine decarboxylase inhibitor: CGP 40215A. Pharmacological Research. 1996;**33**:67-70. DOI: 10.1006/phrs.1996.0011

[71] Fyfe PK, Oza SL, Fairlamb AH, Hunter WN. *Leishmania* trypanothione synthetase-amidase structure reveals a basis for regulation of conflicting synthetic and hydrolytic activities. Journal of Biological Chemistry. 2008;**283**:17672-17680. DOI: 10.1074/jbc.M801850200

[72] Sousa AF, Gomes-Alves AS, Benitez D, Comini MA, Flohe L, Jaeger T, et al. Genetic and chemical analyses reveal that trypanothione synthetase but not glutathionylspermidine synthetase is essential for *Leishmania infantum*. Free Radical Biology and Medicine. 2014;**73**:229-238. DOI: 10.1016/j.freeradbiomed.2014.05.007

[73] Saudagar P, Saha P, Saikia AK, Dubey VK. Molecular mechanism underlying antileishmanial effect of oxabicyclo[3.3.1]nonanones: Inhibition of key redox enzymes of the pathogen. European Journal of Pharmaceutics and Biopharmaceutics. 2013;**85**:569-577. DOI: 10.1016/j.ejpb.2013.08.014

[74] Saudagar P, Dubey VK. Cloning, expression, characterization and inhibition studies on trypanothione synthetase, a drug target enzyme, from *Leishmania donovani*. Biological Chemistry. 2011;**392**:1113-1122. DOI: 10.1515/BC.2011.222

[75] Benitez D, Medeiros A, Fiestas L, Panozzo-Zenere EA, Maiwald F, Prousis KC, et al. Identification of novel chemical scaffolds inhibiting trypanothione synthetase from pathogenic trypanosomatids. PLoS Neglected Tropical Diseases. 2016;**10**:e0004617. DOI: 10.1371/journal.pntd.0004617

[76] Mederios A, Benitez D, Korn RS, Ferreira VC, Barrera E, Carrion F. Mechanistic and biological characterisation of novel N^5-substituted paullones targeting the biosynthesis of trypanothione in *Leishmania*. Journal of Enzyme Inhibition and Medicinal Chemistry. 2020;**35**:1345-1358. DOI: 10.1080/14756366.2020.1780227

[77] Krauth-Siegel RL, Enders B, Henderson GB, Fairlamb AH, Schirmer RH. Trypanothione reductase from *Trypanosoma cruzi* Purification and characterization of the crystalline enzyme. The FEBS Journal. 1987;**164**:123-128. DOI: 10.1111/j.1432-1033.1987.tb11002.x

[78] Cunningham ML, Fairlamb AH. Trypanothione reductase from *Leishmania donovani*. The FEBS Journal. 1995;**230**:460-468. DOI: 10.1111/j.1432-1033.1995.0460h.x

[79] Battista T, Colotti G, Ilari A, Fiorillo A. Targeting trypanothione reductase, a key enzyme in the redox trypanosomatid metabolism, to develop new drugs against Leishmaniasis and trypanosomiases. Molecules. 2020;**25**:1924. DOI: 10.3390/molecules25081924

[80] Fairlamb AH, Cerami A. Metabolism and functions of trypanothione in the kinetoplastida. Annual Review of Microbiology. 1992;**46**:695-729. DOI: 10.1146/annurev.mi.46.100192.003403

[81] Tovar J, Cunningham ML, Smith AC, Croft SL, Fairlamb AH. Down-regulation of *Leishmania donovani* trypanothione reductase by heterologous expression of a trans-dominant mutant homologue: Effect on parasite intracellular survival. Proceedings of the National Academy of Sciences of the United States of America. 1998;**95**:5311-5316. DOI: 10.1073/pnas.95.9.5311

[82] Khan MOF, Austin SE, Chan C, Yin H, Marks D, Vaghjiani SN, et al. Use of an additional hydrophobic binding site, the Z site, in the rational drug design of a new class of stronger trypanothione reductase inhibitor, quaternary alkylammonium phenothiazines. Journal of Medicinal Chemistry. 2000;**43**:3148-3156. DOI: 10.1021/jm000156+

[83] Parveen S, Khan MOF, Austin SE, Croft SL, Yardley V, Rock P, et al. Antitrypanosomal, antileishmanial, and antimalarial activities of quaternary arylalkylammonium 2-amino-4-chlorophenyl phenyl sulfides, a new class of trypanothione reductase inhibitor, and of N-acyl derivatives of 2-amino-4-chlorophenyl phenyl sulfide. Journal of Medicinal Chemistry. 2005;**48**:8087-8097. DOI: 10.1021/jm050819t

[84] Girault S, Davioud-Charvet E, Maes L, Dubremetz JF, Debreu MA, Landry V, et al. Potent and specific inhibitors of trypanothione reductase from Trypanosoma cruzi: bis(2-aminodiphenylsulfides) for fluorescent labeling studies. Bioorganic & Medicinal Chemistry. 2001;**9**:837-846. DOI: 10.1016/S0968-0896(00)00312-6

[85] Chibale K, Haupt H, Kendrick H, Yardley V, Saravanamuthu A, Fairlamb AH, et al. Antiprotozoal and cytotoxicity evaluation of sulfonamide and urea analogues of quinacrine. Bioorganic & Medicinal Chemistry Letters. 2001;**11**:2655-2657. DOI: 10.1016/S0960-894X(01)00528-5

[86] Galarreta BC, Sifuentes R, Carrillo AK, Sanchez L, Amado MRI, Marenda H. The use of natural product scaffolds as leads in the search for trypanothione reductase inhibitors. Bioorganic & Medicinal Chemistry. 2008;**16**:6689-6695. DOI: 10.1016/j.bmc.2008.05.074

[87] Blackie MAL, Saravanamuthu A, Fairlamb AH, Chibale K. Inhibition of trypanothione reductase and glutathione reductase by ferrocenic 4-aminoquinoline ureas. ARKIVOC. 2008;**VI**:52-60. DOI: 10.3998/ark.5550190.0009.605

[88] Holloway GA, Charman WN, Fairlamb AH, Brun R, Kaiser M, Kostewicz E, et al. Trypanothione reductase high-throughput screening campaign identifies novel classes of inhibitors with antiparasitic activity. Antimicrobial Agents and Chemotherapy. 2009;**53**:2824-2833. DOI: 10.1128/AAC.01568-08

[89] Baiocco P, Ilari A, Ceci P, Orsini S, Gramiccia M, di Muccio T, et al. Inhibitory effect of silver nanoparticles on trypanothione reductase activity and *Leishmania infantum* proliferation. ACS Medicinal Chemistry Letters. 2011;**2**:230-233. DOI: 10.1021/ml1002629

[90] Portas AS, Miguel DC, Yokoyama-Yasınaka JKU, Uliana SR, Esposito BP. Increasing the activity of copper(II) complexes against *Leishmania* through lipophilicity and pro-oxidant ability. Journal of Biological Inorganic Chemistry. 2012;**17**:107-112. DOI: 10.1007/s00775-011-0834-3

[91] Baiocco P, Poce G, Alfonso S, Cocozza M, Porretta GC, Colotti G, et al. Inhibition of *Leishmania infantum* trypanothione reductase by Azole-based compounds: A comparative analysis with its physiological substrate by X-ray crystallography. ChemMedChem. 2013;**8**:1175-1183. DOI: 10.1002/cmdc.201300176

[92] Chauhan SS, Pandey S, Shivahare R, Ramalingam K, Krishna S, Vishwakarma P, et al. Novel β-carboline–quinazolinone hybrid as an inhibitor of *Leishmania donovani* trypanothione reductase: Synthesis, molecular docking and bioevaluation. MedChemComm. 2015;**6**:351-356. DOI: 10.1039/C4MD00298A

[93] Marcu A, Schurigt U, Müller K, Moll H, Krauth-Siegel RL, Prinz H. Inhibitory effect of phenothiazine- and phenoxazine-derived chloroacetamides on *Leishmania major* growth and *Trypanosoma brucei* trypanothione reductase. European Journal of Medicinal Chemistry. 2016;**108**:436-443. DOI: 10.1016/j.ejmech.2015.11.023

[94] Baquedano Y, Alcolea V, Toro MA, Gutierrez KJ, Nguewa P, Font M, et al. Novel heteroaryl selenocyanates and diselenides as potent antileishmanial agents. Antimicrobial Agents and Chemotherapy. 2016;**60**:3802-3812. DOI: 10.1128/AAC.02529-15

[95] Garnica P, Etxebeste-Mitxeltorena M, Plano D, Moreno E, Espuelas S, Palop JA, et al. Pre-clinical evidences of the antileishmanial effects of diselenides and selenocyanates. Bioorganic & Medicinal Chemistry Letters. 2020;**30**:127371. DOI: 10.1016/j.bmcl.2020.127371

[96] Arndt A, Liria CW, Yokoyama-Yasunaka JKU, Machini MT, Uliana SRB, Esposito BP. New iminodibenzyl derivatives with anti-leishmanial activity. Journal of Inorganic Biochemistry. 2017;**172**:9-15. DOI: 10.1016/j.jinorgbio.2017.04.004

[97] Saccoliti F, Angiulli G, Pupo G, Pescatori L, Madia VN, Messore A, et al. Inhibition of *Leishmania infantum* trypanothione reductase by diaryl

sulfide derivatives. Journal of Enzyme Inhibition and Medicinal Chemistry. 2017;**32**:304-310. DOI: 10.1080/14756366.2016.1250755

[98] Vishwakarna P, Parmar N, Chandrakar P, Sharma T, Kathuria M, Agnihotri PK, et al. Ammonium trichloro [1,2-ethanediolato-*O,O′*]-tellurate cures experimental visceral leishmaniasis by redox modulation of *Leishmania donovani* trypanothione reductase and inhibiting host integrin linked PI3K/Akt pathway. Cellular and Molecular Life Sciences. 2018;**75**:563-588. DOI: 10.1007/s00018-017-2653-3

[99] Ruiz-Santaquiteria M, de Castro S, Toro MA, de Lucio H, Gutierrez KJ, Sanchez-Murcia PA, et al. Trypanothione reductase inhibition and anti-leishmanial activity of all-hydrocarbon stapled α-helical peptides with improved proteolytic stability. European Journal of Medicinal Chemistry. 2018;**149**:238-247. DOI: 10.1016/j.ejmech.2018.02.071

[100] Aziz H, Saeed A, Jabeen F, Florke U, Ui-Ain Q, Akhter N. Synthesis, crystal structure, cytotoxic, antileishmanial and docking evaluation of 3-(4-chloro-3-nitrophenyl)-1-phenylprop-2-en-1-one. Chinese Journal of Structural Chemistry. 2018;**37**:1250-1258. DOI: 10.14102/j.cnki.0254-5861.2011-1908

[101] Rodriguez F, Iniguez E, Contreras GP, Ahmed H, Costa TEMM, Skouta R, et al. Development of thiophene compounds as potent chemotherapies for the treatment of cutaneous Leishmaniasis caused by Leishmania major. Molecules. 2018;**23**:1626. DOI: 10.3390/molecules23071626

[102] Revuelto A, Ruiz-Santaquiteria M, de Lucio H, Gamo A, Carriles AA, Gutierrez KJ, et al. Pyrrolopyrimidine vs imidazole-phenyl-thiazole scaffolds in nonpeptidic dimerization inhibitors of *Leishmania infantum* trypanothione reductase. ACS Infectious Diseases. 2019;**5**:873-891. DOI: 10.1021/acsinfecdis.8b00355

[103] Harikandei KB, Salehi P, Ebrahimi SN, Bararjanian M, Kaiser M, Al-Harrasi A. Synthesis, *in-vitro* antiprotozoal activity and molecular docking study of isothiocyanate derivatives. Bioorganic & Medicinal Chemistry. 2020;**28**:115185. DOI: 10.1016/j.bmc.2019.115185

[104] Colotti G, Saccoliti F, Gramiccia M, di Muccio T, Prakash J, Yadav S, et al. Structure-guided approach to identify a novel class of anti-leishmaniasis diaryl sulfide compounds targeting the trypanothione metabolism. Amino Acids. 2020;**52**:247-259. DOI: 10.1007/s00726-019-02731-4

[105] Mukherjee D, Yousuf M, Dey S, Chakraborty S, Chaudhuri A, Kumar, et al. Targeting the trypanothione reductase of tissue-residing *Leishmania* in hosts' reticuloendothelial system: A flexible water-soluble ferrocenylquinoline-based preclinical drug candidate. Journal of Medicinal Chemistry. 2020;**63**:15621-15638. DOI: 10.1021/acs.jmedchem.0c00690

[106] Revuelto A, de Lucio H, Garcia-Soriano JC, Sanchez-Murcia PA, Gago F, Jimenz-Ruiz A, et al. Efficient dimerization disruption of *Leishmania infantum* trypanothione reductase by Triazole-phenyl-thiazoles. Journal of Medicinal Chemistry. 2021;**64**:6137-6160. DOI: 10.1021/acs.jmedchem.1c00206

[107] Kuldeep J, Karthik R, Kaur P, Goyal N, Siddiqi MI. Identification of potential anti-leishmanial agents using computational investigation and biological evaluation against trypanothione reductase. Journal of Biomolecular Structure and Dynamics. 2021;**39**:960-969. DOI: 10.1080/07391102.2020.1721330

[108] Tunes LG, Morato RE, Garcia A, Schmitz V, Steindel M, Correa-Junior JD, et al. Preclinical gold complexes as oral drug candidates to treat Leishmaniasis are potent trypanothione reductase inhibitors. ACS Infectious Diseases. 2020;**6**:1121-1139. DOI: 10.1021/acsinfecdis.9b00505

[109] Krstin S, Sobeh M, Braun MS, Wink M. *Tulbaghia violacea* and *Allium ursinum* extracts exhibit anti-parasitic and antimicrobial activities. Molecules. 2018;**23**:313. DOI: 10.3390/molecules23020313

[110] Pramanik PK, Chakraborti S, Bagchi A, Chakraborti T. Bioassay-based *Corchorus capsularis L.* leaf-derived β-sitosterol exerts antileishmanial effects against *Leishmania donovani* by targeting trypanothione reductase. Scientific Reports. 2020;**10**:20440. DOI: 10.1038/s41598-020-77066-2

[111] Fiorillo A, Colotti G, Boffi A, Baiocco P, Ilari A. The crystal structures of the tryparedoxin-tryparedoxin peroxidase couple unveil the structural determinants of Leishmania detoxification pathway. PLoS Neglected Tropical Diseases. 2012;**6**:e1781. DOI: 10.1371/journal.pntd.0001781

[112] Moore KJ, Matlashewski G. Intracellular infection by *Leishmania donovani* inhibits macrophage apoptosis. Journal of Immunology. 1994;**152**:2930-2937

[113] Heussler VT, Küenzi P, Rottenberg S. Inhibition of apoptosis by intracellular protozoan parasites. International Journal for Parasitology. 2001;**31**:1166-1176. DOI: 10.1016/S0020-7519(01)00271-5

[114] Fukao T, Tanabe M, Terauchi Y, Ota T, Matsuda S, Asano T, et al. PI3K-mediated negative feedback regulation of IL-12 production in DCs. Nature Immunology. 2002;**3**:875-881. DOI: 10.1038/ni825

[115] Ruhland A, Leal N, Kima PE. *Leishmania* promastigotes activate PI3K/Akt signalling to confer host cell resistance to apoptosis. Cellular Microbiology. 2007;**9**:84-96. DOI: 10.1111/j.1462-5822.2006.00769.x

[116] Cooke NG, Fernandes GDS, Furet P, Hebach C, Högenauer K, Hollingworth G, et al. Use of Inhibitors of the Activity or Function of PI3K. 2013. WO 2013/088404 A1

[117] Khadem F, Jia P, Mou Z, Barazandeh AF, Liu D, Keynan Y, et al. Pharmacological inhibition of p110δ subunit of PI3K confers protection against experimental leishmaniasis. Journal of Antimicrobial Chemotherapy. 2017;**72**:467-477. DOI: 10.1093/jac/dkw448

[118] Phan TN, KH BA, Lee N, Byun SY, Shum D, No JH. *In vitro* and *in vivo* activity of mTOR kinase and PI3K inhibitors against *Leishmania donovani* and *Trypanosoma brucei*. Molecules. 2020;**25**:1980. DOI: 10.3390/molecules25081980

[119] Bendjeddou LZ, Loaec N, Villiers B, Prina E, Spath GF, Galons H, et al. Exploration of the imidazo[1,2-b] pyridazine scaffold as a protein kinase inhibitor. European Journal of Medicinal Chemistry. 2017;**125**:696-709. DOI: 10.1016/j.ejmech.2016.09.064

[120] Sanchez-Fernandez EM, Garcia-Moreno MI, Arroba AI, Aguilar-Diosdado M, Padron JM, Garcia-Hernandez R, et al. Synthesis of polyfluoroalkyl sp2-iminosugar glycolipids and evaluationof their immunomodulatory properties towards anti-tumor, anti-leishmanial and anti-inflammatory therapies. European Journal of Medicinal Chemistry. 2019;**182**:111604. DOI: 10.1016/j.ejmech.2019.111604

[121] Grant KM, Dunion MH, Yardley V, Skaltsounis AL, Marko D,

Eisenbrand G, et al. Inhibitors of *Leishmania mexicana* CRK3 cyclin-dependent kinase: Chemical library screen and antileishmanial activity. Antimicrobial Agents and Chemotherapy. 2004;**48**:3033-3042. DOI: 10.1128/AAC.48.8.3033-3042.2004

[122] Das S, Banerjee A, Kamran M, Ejazi SA, Asad M, Ali N, et al. A chemical inhibitor of heat shock protein 78 (HSP78) from *Leishmania donovani* represents a potential antileishmanial drug candidate. The Journal of Biological Chemistry. 2020;**295**:9934-9947. DOI: 10.1074/jbc.RA120.014587

[123] Chakraborty AK, Majumder HK. An ATP-independent catenating enzyme from the kinetoplast hemoflagellate *Leishmania donovani*. Biochemical and Biophysical Research Communications. 1991;**180**:279-285

[124] Chakraborty AK, Gupta A, Majumder HK. A type 1 DNA topoisomerase from the kinetoplast hemoflagellate *Leishmania donovani*. Indian Journal of Biochemistry and Biophysics. 1993;**30**:257-263

[125] Jean-Moreno V, Rojas R, Goyeneche D, Coombs GH, Walker J. *Leishmania donovani*: Differential activities of classical topoisomerase inhibitors and antileishmanials against parasite and host cells at the level of DNA topoisomerase I and in cytotoxicity assays. Experimental Parasitology. 2006;**112**:21-30. DOI: 10.1016/j.exppara.2005.08.014

[126] Chakraborty AK, Majumder HK. Mode of action of pentavalent antimonials: Specific inhibition of type I DNA topoisomerase of *Leishmania donovani*. Biochemical and Biophysical Research Communications. 1988;**152**:605-611. DOI: 10.1016/S0006-291X(88)80081-0

[127] Werbovetz KA, Lehnert EK, Macdonald TL, Pearson RD. Cytotoxicity of acridine compounds for *Leishmania* promastigotes *in vitro*. Antimicrobial Agents and Chemotherapy. 1992;**36**: 495-497. DOI: 10.1128/AAC.36.2.495

[128] Carballeira NM, Morales-Guzman C, Alvarez-Benedicto E, Torres-Martinez Z, Delgado-Reyes Y, Griebenow KH, et al. First total synthesis of ω-phenyl Δ6 fatty acids and their Leishmanicidal and anticancer properties. Current Topics in Medicinal Chemistry. 2018;**18**:418-427. DOI: 10.2174/1568026618666180516125056

[129] Tejeria A, Perez-Pertejo Y, Reguera RM, Balana-Fouce R, Alonso C, Gonzalez M, et al. Substituted 1,5-naphthyridine derivatives as novel antileishmanial agents. Synthesis and biological evaluation. European Journal of Medicinal Chemistry. 2018;**152**:137-147. DOI: 10.1016/j.ejmech.2018.04.033

[130] Lee H, Baek KH, Phan TN, Park IS, Lee S, Kim JK, et al. Discovery of *Leishmania donovani* topoisomerase IB selective inhibitors by targeting protein-protein interactions between the large and small subunits. Biochemical and Biophysical Research Communications. 2021;**569**:193-198. DOI: 10.1016/j.bbrc.2021.07.019

[131] Yardley V, Snowdon D, Croft S, Hazra B. *In vitro* activity of diospyrin and derivatives against *Leishmania donovani*, *Trypanosoma cruzi* and *Trypanosoma brucei brucei*. Phytotherapy Research. 1996;**10**:559-562. DOI: 10.1002/(SICI)1099-1573(199611)10:7%3C559::AID-PTR891%3E3.0.CO;2-V

[132] Ray S, Hazra B, Mittra B, Das A, Majumder HK. Diospyrin, A bisnaphthoquinone: A novel inhibitor of type I DNA topoisomerase of *Leishmania donovani*. Molecular Pharmacology. 1998;**54**:994-999. DOI: 10.1124/mol.54.6.994

[133] Chowdhury AR, Mandal S, Goswami A, Ghosh M, Mandal L, Chakraborty D, et al. Dihydrobetulinic acid induces apoptosis in *Leishmania donovani* by targeting DNA topoisomerase I and II: Implications in antileishmanial therapy. Molecular Medicine. 2003;**9**:26-36

[134] Marquis JF, Drolet M, Olivier M. Consequence of Hoechst 33342-mediated Leishmania DNA topoisomerase-I inhibition on parasite replication. Parasitology. 2003;**126**:21-30. DOI: 10.1017/s0031182002002524

[135] Marquis JF, Makhey D, LaVoie EJ, Olivier M. Effects of topoisomerases inhibitors protoberberine on *Leishmania donovani* growth, macrophage function, and infection. J. Parasitol. 2003;**89**: 1048-1052. DOI: 10.1645/GE-3161

[136] Poorrajab F, Ardestani SK, Foroumadi A, Emami S, Kariminia A, Behrouzi-Fardmoghadam M, et al. Selective leishmanicidal effect of 1,3,4-thiadiazole derivatives and possible mechanism of action against *Leishmania* species. Experimental Parasitology. 2009;**121**:323-330. DOI: 10.1016/j.exppara.2008.12.004

[137] Carballeira NM, Cartagena MM, Prada CF, Rubio CF, Balana-Fouce R. Total synthesis and antileishmanial activity of the natural occurring acetylenic fatty acids 6-heptadecynoic acid and 6-icosynoic acid. Lipids. 2009;**44**:953-961. DOI: 10.1007/s11745-009-3345-z

[138] Carballeira NM, Cartagena MM, Sanabria D, Tasdemir D, Prada CF, Reguera RM, et al. 2-Alkynoic fatty acids inhibit topoisomerase IB from *Leishmania donovani*. Bioorganic & Medicinal Chemistry Letters. 2012;**22**:6185-6189. DOI: 10.1016/j.bmcl.2012.08.019

[139] Roy A, Chowdhury S, Sengupta S, Mandal M, Jaisankar P, D'Anessa I, et al. Development of derivatives of 3, 3'-diindolylmethane as potent *Leishmania donovani* bi-subunit topoisomerase IB poisons. PLoS One. 2011;**6**:e28493. DOI: 10.1371/journal.pone.0028493

[140] Sharma G, Chowdhury S, Sinha A, Majumder HK, Kumar SV. Antileishmanial activity evaluation of bis-lawsone analogs and DNA topoisomerase-I inhibition studies. Journal of Enzyme Inhibition and Medicinal Chemistry. 2014;**29**:185-189. DOI: 10.3109/14756366.2013.765413

[141] Saha S, Acharya C, Pal U, Chowdhury SR, Sarkar K, Maiti NC, et al. A novel spirooxindole derivative inhibits the growth of *Leishmania donovani* parasites both *in vitro* and *in vivo* by targeting type IB topoisomerase. Antimicrobial Agents and Chemotherapy. 2016;**60**:6281-6293. DOI: 10.1128/AAC.00352-16

[142] Tejeira A, Perez-Pertejo Y, Reguera RM, Balana-Fouce R, Alonso C, Fuertes M, et al. Antileishmanial effect of new indeno-1,5-naphthyridines, selective inhibitors of *Leishmania infantum* type IB DNA topoisomerase. European Journal of Medicinal Chemistry. 2016;**124**:740-749. DOI: 10.1016/j.ejmech.2016.09.017

[143] Yang G, Choi G, No JH. Antileishmanial mechanism of diamidines involves targeting kinetoplasts. Antimicrobial Agents and Chemotherapy. 2016;**60**:6828-6836. DOI: 10.1128/AAC.01129-16

[144] Singh MK, Bhaumik SK, Karmakar S, Paul J, Sawoo S, Majumder HK, et al. Copper salisylaldoxime (CuSAL) imparts protective efficacy against visceral leishmaniasis by targeting *Leishmania donovani* topoisomerase IB. Experimental Parasitology. 2017; **175**:8-20. DOI: 10.1016/j.exppara.2017.02.010

[145] Fyfe PK, Westrop GD, Ramos T, Müller S, Coombs GH, Hunter WN. Structure of *Leishmania major* cysteine synthase. Acta Crystallographica Section F. 2012;**F68**:738-743. DOI: 10.1107/S1744309112019124

[146] Luis JAS, Costa NAS, Luis CCS, Lira BF, Athayde-Filho PF, Lima TKS, et al. Synthesis of new cyclic imides derived from Safrole, structure- and ligand-based approaches to evaluate potential new multitarget agents against species of Leishmania. Medicinal Chemistry. 2020;**16**:39-51. DOI: 10.2174/1573406415666190430144950

[147] Swenerton RK, Zhang S, Sajid M, Medzihradszky KF, Craik CS, Kelly BL, et al. The oligopeptidase B of *Leishmania* regulates parasite enolase and immune evasion. The Journal of Biological Chemistry. 2011;**286**:429-440. DOI: 10.1074/jbc.M110.138313

[148] McLuskey K, Paterson NG, Bland ND, Isaacs NW, Mottram JC. Crystal structure of *Leishmania major* oligopeptidase B gives insight into the enzymatic properties of a trypanosomatid virulence factor. The Journal of Biological Chemistry. 2010;**285**:39249-39259. DOI: 10.1074/jbc.M110.156679

[149] Souza-Silva F, Bourguignon SC, Pereira BAS, Côrtes LMDC, de Oliveira LFG, Henriques-Pons A, et al. Epoxy-a-lapachone has in vitro and in vivo anti-*Leishmania (Leishmania) amazonensis* effects and inhibits serine proteinase activity in this parasite. Antimicrobial Agents and Chemotherapy. 2015;**59**:1910-1918. DOI: 10.1128/AAC.04742-14

[150] Silva-Lopez RE, Morgado-Diaz JA, Chavez MA, Giovanni-De-Simone S. Effects of serine protease inhibitors on viability and morphology of *Leishmania (Leishmania) amazonensis* promastigotes. Parasitology Research. 2007;**101**:1627-1635. DOI: 10.1007/s00436-007-0706-5

[151] Meshnick SR, Eaton JW. Leishmanial superoxide dismutase: A possible target for chemotherapy. Biochemical and Biophysical Research Communications. 1981;**102**:970-976. DOI: 10.1016/0006-291X(81)91633-8

[152] Paramchuk WJ, Ismail SO, Bhatia A, Gedamu L. Cloning, characterization and overexpression of two ironsuperoxide dismutase cDNAs fromLeishmania chagasi:role in pathogenesis. Molecular and Biochemical Parasitology. 1997;**90**:203-221. DOI: 10.1016/S0166-6851(97)00141-2

[153] Phan IQH, Davies DR, Moretti NS, Shanmugam D, Cestari I, Anupama A, et al. Iron superoxide dismutases in eukaryotic pathogens: New insights from Apicomplexa and *Trypanosoma* structures. Acta Cryst. 2015;**F71**:615-621. DOI: 10.1107/S2053230X15004185

[154] Sanchez-Moreno M, Gomez-Contreras F, Navarro P, Marin C, Ramirez-Macias I, Rosales MJ, et al. Imidazole-containing phthalazine derivatives inhibit Fe-SOD performance in *Leishmania* species and are active *in vitro* against visceral and mucosal leishmaniasis. Parasitology. 2015;**142**:1115-1129. DOI: 10.1017/S0031182015000219

[155] Martin-Montes A, Santivanez-Veliz M, Moreno-Viguri E, Martin-Escolano R, Jimenez-Montes C, Lopez-Gonzalez C, et al. *In vitro* antileishmanial activity and iron superoxide dismutase inhibition of arylamine Mannich base derivatives. Parasitology. 2017;**144**:1783-1790. DOI: 10.1017/S0031182017001123

[156] Brito CCB, da Silva HVC, Brondani DJ, de Faria AR, Ximenes RM, da Silva IM, et al. Synthesis and biological evaluation of thiazole

derivatives as *Lb*SOD inhibitors. Journal of Enzyme Inhibition and Medicinal Chemistry. 2019;**34**:333-342. DOI: 10.1080/14756366.2018.1550752

[157] Marin C, Clares MP, Ramirez-Macias I, Blasco S, Olmo F, Soriano C, et al. *In vitro* activity of scorpiand-like azamacrocycle derivatives in promastigotes and intracellular amastigotes of Leishmania infantum and *Leishmania braziliensis*. European Journal of Medicinal Chemistry. 2013;**62**:466-477. DOI: 10.1016/j.ejmech.2013.01.001

[158] Marin C, Inclan M, Ramirez-Macias I, Albelda MT, Canas R, Clares MP, et al. *In vitro* antileishmanial activity of aza-scorpiand macrocycles. Inhibition of the antioxidant enzyme iron superoxide dismutase. RSC Advances. 2016;**6**:17446-17455. DOI: 10.1039/C5RA21262F

[159] Navarro P, Sanchez-Moreno M, Marin C, Garcia-Espana E, Ramirez-Macias I, Olmo F, et al. *In vitro* leishmanicidal activity of pyrazole-containing polyamine macrocycles which inhibit the Fe-SOD enzyme of *Leishmania infantum* and *Leishmania braziliensis* species. Parasitology. 2014;**141**:1031-1043. DOI: 10.1017/S0031182014000201

[160] Gupta S, Raychaudhuri B, Banerjee S, Das B, Mukhopadhaya S, Datta SC. Momordicatin purified from fruits of *Momordica charantia* is effective to act as a potent antileishmania agent. Parasitology International. 2010;**59**:192-197. DOI: 10.1016/j.parint.2010.01.004

[161] Sanchez-Moreno M, Gomez-Contreras F, Navarro P, Marin C, Ramirez-Macias I, Olmo F, et al. *In vitro* leishmanicidal activity of imidazole- or pyrazole-based benzo[g] phthalazine derivatives against *Leishmania infantum* and *Leishmania braziliensis* species. The Journal of Antimicrobial Chemotherapy. 2012;**67**:387-397. DOI: 10.1093/jac/dkr480

[162] Raychaudhury B, Banerjee S, Gupta S, Singh RV, Datta SC. Antiparasitic activity of a triphenyl tin complex against *Leishmania donovani*. Acta Tropica. 2005;**95**:1-8. DOI: 10.1016/j.actatropica.2005.03.008

[163] Martin-Montes A, Plano D, Martin-Escolano R, Alcolea V, Diaz M, Perez-Silanes S, et al. Library of seleno-compounds as novel agents against *Leishmania* species. Antimicrobial Agents and Chemotherapy. 2017;**61**:e02546-e02516. DOI: 10.1128/AAC.02546-16

[164] Fandzloch M, Arriaga JMM, Sanchez-Moreno M, Wojtczak A, Jezierska J, Sitkowski J, et al. Strategies for overcoming tropical disease by ruthenium complexes with purine analog: Application against *Leishmania spp*. and *Trypanosoma cruzi*. Journal of Inorganic Biochemistry. 2017;**176**:144-155. DOI: 10.1016/j.jinorgbio.2017.08.018

[165] Reviriego F, Olmo F, Navarro P, Marin C, Ramirez-Macias I, Garcia-Espana E, et al. Simple dialkyl pyrazole-3,5-dicarboxylates show *in vitro* and *in vivo* activity against disease-causing trypanosomatids. Parasitology. 2017;**144**:1133-1143. DOI: 10.1017/S0031182017000415

[166] Wilkinson SR, Taylor MC, Horn D, Kelly JM, Cheeseman. A mechanism for cross-resistance to nifurtimox and benznidazole in trypanosomes. PNAS. 2008;**105**:5022-5027. DOI: 10.1073/pnas.0711014105

[167] Voak AA, Gobalakrishnapillai V, Seifert K, Balczo E, Hu L, Hall BS, et al. An essential type I nitroreductase from *Leishmania major* can be used to activate Leishmanicidal prodrugs. Journal of Biological Chemistry. 2013;**288**:28466-28476. DOI: 10.1074/jbc.M113.494781

[168] Voak AA, Seifert K, Helsby NA, Wilkinson SR. Evaluating aziridinyl nitrobenzamide compounds as leishmanicidal prodrugs. Antimicrobial Agents and Chemotherapy. 2014;**58**:370-377. DOI: 10.1128/AAC.01459-13

[169] Pedron J, Boudot C, Hutter S, Bourgeade-Delmas S, Stigliani JL, Sournia-Saquet A, et al. Novel 8-nitroquinolin-2(1H)-ones as NTR-bioactivated antikinetoplastid molecules: Synthesis, electrochemical and SAR study. European Journal of Medicinal Chemistry. 2018;**155**:135-152. DOI: 10.1016/j.ejmech.2018.06.001

[170] Fersing C, Boudot C, Pedron J, Hutter S, Primas N, Castera-Ducros C, et al. 8-Aryl-6-chloro-3-nitro-2-(phenylsulfonylmethyl)imidazo[1,2-a] pyridines as potent antitrypanosomatid molecules bioactivated by type 1 nitroreductases. European Journal of Medicinal Chemistry. 2018;**157**:115-126. DOI: 10.1016/j.ejmech.2018.07.064

[171] Pacheco JS, Costa DS, Cunha-Junior EF, Andrade-Neto VV, Fairlamb AH, Wyllie S, et al. Monocyclic nitro-heteroaryl nitrones with dual mechanism of activation: Synthesis and antileishmanial activity. ACS Medicinal Chemistry Letters. 2021;**12**(9):1405-1412. DOI: 10.1021/acsmedchemlett.1c00193

[172] Koszalka GW, Krenitsky TA, Nucleosidases from Leishmania donovani. Pyrimidine ribonucleosidase, purine ribonucleosidase, and a novel purine 2′-deoxyribonucleosidase. Journal of Biological Chemistry. 1979;**254**:8185-8193. DOI: 10.1016/S0021-9258(19)86874-6

[173] Goeminne A, Berg M, McNaughton M, Bal G, Surpeteanu G, der Veken PV, et al. N-Arylmethyl substituted iminoribitol derivatives as inhibitors of a purine specific nucleoside hydrolase. Bioorganic & Medicinal Chemistry. 2008;**16**:6752-6763. DOI: 10.1016/j.bmc.2008.05.056

[174] Berg M, Kohl L, der Veken PV, Joosens J, Al-Salabi MI, Castagna V, et al. Evaluation of nucleoside hydrolase inhibitors for treatment of African trypanosomiasis. Antimicrobial Agents and Chemotherapy. 2010;**54**:1900-1908. DOI: 10.1128/AAC.01787-09

[175] Freitas EO, Nico D, Guan R, Meyer-Fernandes JR, Clinch K, Evans GB, et al. Immucillins impair *Leishmania (L.) infantum chagasi* and *Leishmania (L.) amazonensis* multiplication *in vitro*. PLoS One. 2015;**10**:e0124183. DOI: 10.1371/ journal.pone.0124183

[176] Alves MA, Nirma C, Moreira MM, Soares RO, Pascutti PG, Noel F, et al. Non-competitive inhibitor of nucleoside hydrolase from *Leishmania donovani* identified by fragment-based drug discovery. RSC Advances. 2016;**90**:87738-87744. DOI: 10.1039/C6RA15143D

[177] Nirma C, Rangel GT, Alves MA, Casanova LM, Moreira MM, Rodrigues LM, et al. New *Leishmania donovani* nucleoside hydrolase inhibitors from Brazilian flora. RSC Advances. 2019;**9**:18663-18669. DOI: 10.1039/C9RA02382H

[178] Palatnik-e-Sousa CB, Nico D. The delay in the licensing of protozoal vaccines: A comparative history. Frontiers in Immunology. 2020;**11**:204. DOI: 10.3389/fimmu.2020.00204

[179] Sakanari JA, Nadler SA, Chan VJ, Engel JC, Leptak C, Bouvier J. *Leishmania major*: Comparison of the cathepsin L- and B-like cysteine protease genes with those of other trypanosomatids. Experimental Parasitology. 1997;**85**:63-76. DOI: 10.1006/expr.1996.4116

[180] Schuright U, Schad C, Glowa C, Baum U, Thomale K, Schnitzer JK, et al. Aziridine-2,3-dicarboxylate-based cysteine cathepsin inhibitors induce cell

death in *Leishmania major* associated with accumulation of debris in autophagy-related lysosome-like vacuole. Antimicrobial Agents and Chemotherapy. 2010;**54**:5028-5041. DOI: 10.1128/AAC.00327-10

[181] de Sousa LRF, Wu H, Nebo L, Fernandes JB, da Silva MFGF, Kiefer W, et al. Natural products as inhibitors of recombinant cathepsin L of *Leishmania Mexicana*. Experimental Parasitology. 2015;**156**:42-48. DOI: 10.1016/j.exppara.2015.05.016

[182] Schad C, Baum U, Frank B, Dietzel U, Mattern F, Gomes C, et al. Development of a new antileishmanial aziridine-2,3-dicarboxylate-based inhibitor with high selectivity for parasite cysteine proteases. Antimicrobial Agents and Chemotherapy. 2016;**60**:797-805. DOI: 10.1128/AAC.00426-15

[183] Pimentel IAS, Paladi CS, Katz S, WAdS J, RLOR C, et al. *In vitro* and *in vivo* activity of an organic tellurium compound on *Leishmania (Leishmania) chagasi*. PLoS One. 2012;7(11):e48780. DOI: 10.1371/journal.pone.0048780

[184] Paladi CS, Pimentel IAS, Katz S, Cunha RLOR, Judice WAS, et al. *In vitro* and *in vivo* activity of a palladacycle complex on *Leishmania (Leishmania) amazonensis*. PLoS Neglected Tropical Diseases. 2012;**6**(5):e1626. DOI: 10.1371/journal.pntd.0001626

[185] dos Santos IB, da Silva DAM, Paz FACR, Garcia DM, Carmona AK, Teixeira D, et al. Leishmanicidal and immunomodulatory activities of the palladacycle complex DPPE 1.1, a potential candidate for treatment of cutaneous leishmaniasis. Frontiers in Microbiology. 2018;**9**:1427. DOI: 10.3389/fmicb.2018.01427

[186] Royo S, Shirmeister T, Kaiser M, Jung S, Rodriguez S, Bautita JM, et al. Antiprotozoal and cysteine proteases inhibitory activity of dipeptidyl enoates. Bioorganic & Medicinal Chemistry. 2018;**26**:4624-4634. DOI: 10.1016/j.bmc.2018.07.015

[187] Hannaert V, Blaauw M, Kohl L, Allert S, Opperdoes FR, Michels PAM. Molecular analysis of the cytosolic and glycosomal glyceraldehyde- 3-phosphate dehydrogenase in Leishmania Mexicana. Molecular and Biochemical Parasitology. 1992;**55**:115-126. DOI: 10.1016/0166-6851(92)90132-4

[188] Suresh S, Bressi JC, Kennedy KJ, Verlinde CLMJ, Gelb MH, Hol WGJ. Conformational changes in *Leishmania mexicana* glyceraldehyde-3-phosphate dehydrogenase induced by designed inhibitors. Journal of Molecular Biology. 2001;**309**:423-435. DOI: 10.1006/jmbi.2001.4588

[189] Cordeiro AT, Felicisno PR, Nonato MC. Crystallization and preliminary X-ray diffraction analysis of *Leishmania major* dihydroorotate dehydrogenase. Acta Cryst. 2006;**F62**:1049-1051. DOI: 10.1107/S1744309106038966

[190] Chibli LA, Rosa AL, Nonato MC, da Costa FB. Untargeted LC–MS metabolomic studies of Asteraceae species to discover inhibitors of *Leishmania major* dihydroorotate dehydrogenase. Metabolomics. 2019;**15**:59. DOI: 10.1007/s11306-019-1520-7

[191] Larson ET, Kim JE, Zucker FH, Kelley A, Mueller N, Napuli AJ, et al. Structure of *Leishmania major* methionyl-tRNA synthetase in complex with intermediate products methionyladenylate and pyrophosphate. Biochimie. 2011;**93**:570-582. DOI: 10.1016/j.biochi.2010.11.015

[192] Torrie LS, Brand S, Robinson DA, Ko EJ, Stojanovski L, Simeons FRC, et al. Chemical validation of methionyl-tRNA synthetase as a druggable target in

Leishmania donovani. ACS Infectious Diseases. 2017;**3**:718-727. DOI: 10.1021/acsinfecdis.7b00047

[193] Torrie LS, Robinson DA, Thomas MG, Hobrath JV, Shepherd SM, Post JM, et al. Discovery of an allosteric binding site in kinetoplastid methionyl-tRNA synthetase. ACS Infectious Diseases. 2020;**6**:1044-1057. DOI: 10.1021/acsinfecdis.9b00453

[194] Walter RD, Buse E, Ebert F. Effect of cyclic AMP on transformation and proliferation of leishmania cells. Tropenmedizin und Parasitologie. 1978;**29**:439-442

[195] Wang H, Yan Z, Geng J, Kunz S, Seebeck T, Ke H. Crystal structure of the *Leishmania major* phosphodiesterase LmjPDEB1 and insight into the design of the parasite-selective inhibitors. Molecular Microbiology. 2007;**66**: 1029-1038. DOI: 10.1111/j.1365-2958.2007.05976.x

[196] Piaz VD, Rascon A, Dubra ME, Giovannoi MP, Vergelli C, Castallena MC. Isoxazolo[3,4-d]pyridazinones and analogues as *Leishmania mexicana* PDE inhibitors. Il Farmaco. 2002;**57**:89-96. DOI: 10.1016/S0014-827X(01)01188-0

[197] Ebastián-Pérez V, Hendrickx S, Munday JC, Kalejaiye T, Martínez A, Campillo NE, et al. Cyclic nucleotide-specific phosphodiesterases as potential drug targets for anti-Leishmania therapy. Antimicrobial Agents and Chemotherapy. 2018;**62**:e00603-e00618. DOI: 10.1128/AAC.00603-18

[198] Bhargava P, Kumar K, Chaudhaery SS, Saxena AK, Roy U. Cloning, overexpression and characterization of *Leishmania donovani* squalene synthase. FEMS Microbiology Letters. 2010;**311**:82-92. DOI: 10.1111/j.1574-6968.2010.02071.x

[199] Urbina JA, Concepcion JL, Rangel S, Visbal G, Lira R. Squalene synthase as a chemotherapeutic target in *Trypanosoma cruzi* and *Leishmania Mexicana*. Molecular and Biochemical Parasitology. 2002;**125**:35-45. DOI: 10.1016/S0166-6851(02)00206-2

[200] Lorente SO, Gomez R, Jimenez C, Cammerer S, Yardley V, de Luca-Fradley K, et al. Biphenylquinuclidines as inhibitors of squalene synthase and growth of parasitic protozoa. Bioorganic & Medicinal Chemistry. 2005;**13**:3519-3529. DOI: 10.1016/j.bmc.2005.02.060

[201] Rodrigues JCF, Concepcion JL, Rodrigues C, Caldera A, Urbina JA, de Souza W. *In vitro* activities of ER-119884 and E5700, two potent squalene synthase inhibitors, against *Leishmania amazonensis*: Antiproliferative, biochemical, and ultrastructural effects. Antimicrobial Agents and Chemotherapy. 2008;**52**:4098-4114. DOI: 10.1128/AAC.01616-07

[202] Lamerz AC, Haselhorst T, Bergfeld AK, von Itzstein M, Gerardy-Schahn R. Molecular cloning of the *Leishmania major* UDP-glucose pyrophosphorylase, functional characterization, and ligand binding analyses using NMR spectroscopy. Journal of Biological Chemistry. 2006;**281**:16314-16322. DOI: 10.1074/jbc.M600076200

[203] Steiner T, Lamerz AC, Hess P, Breithaupt C, Krapp S, Bourenkov G, et al. Open and closed structures of the UDP-glucose pyrophosphorylase from *Leishmania major*. Journal of Biological Chemistry. 2007;**282**:13003-13010. DOI: 10.1074/jbc.M609984200

[204] Camacho A, Arrebola R, Pena-Diaz J, Ruiz-Perez LM, Gonzalez-Paanowska D. Description of a novel eukaryotic deoxyuridine 5′-triphosphate nucleotidohydrolase in *Leishmania major*. The Biochemical Journal. 1997;**325**:441-447. DOI: 10.1042/bj3250441

[205] Camacho A, Hidalgo-Zarco F, Bernier-Villamor V, Ruiz-Perez LM, Gonzalez-Pacanowska D. Properties of *Leishmania major* dUTP nucleotidohydrolase, a distinct nucleotide-hydrolysing enzyme in kinetoplastids. The Biochemical Journal. 2000;**346**:163-168. DOI: 10.1042/bj3460163

[206] Hemsworth GR, Moroz OV, Fogg MJ, Scott B, Bosch-Navarrete C, Gonzalez-Pacanowska D, et al. The crystal structure of the *Leishmania major* deoxyuridine triphosphate nucleotidohydrolase in complex with nucleotide analogues, dUMP, and deoxyuridine. Journal of Biological Chemistry. 2011;**286**:16470-16481. DOI: 10.1074/jbc.M111.224873

[207] Nguyen C, Kasinathan G, Leal-Cortijo I, Musso-Buendia A, Kaiser M, Brun R, et al. Deoxyuridine triphosphate nucleotidohydrolase as a potential antiparasitic drug target. Journal of Medicinal Chemistry. 2005;**48**:5942-5954. DOI: 10.1021/jm050111e

[208] Agnihotri P, Singh SP, Shakya AK, Pratap JV. Biochemical and biophysical characterization of *Leishmania donovani* gamma-glutamylcysteine synthetase. Biochemistry and Biophysics Reports. 2016;**8**:127-138. DOI: 10.1016/j.bbrep.2016.08.016

[209] Agnihotri P, Mishra AK, Mishra S, Sirohi VK, Sahasrabuddhe AA, Pratap JV. Identification of novel inhibitors of *Leishmania donovani* γ-glutamylcysteine synthetase using structure-based virtual screening, docking, molecular dynamics simulation, and *in vitro* studies. Journal of Chemical Information and Modeling. 2017;**57**:815-825. DOI: 10.1021/acs.jcim.6b00642

[210] Venugopal V, Datt AK, Bhattacharyya D, Dasgupta D, Banerjee R. Structure of cyclophilin from *Leishmania donovani* bound to cyclosporin at 2.6 A resolution: Correlation between structure and thermodynamic data. Acta Crystallographica. Section D, Biological Crystallography. 2009;**65**:1187-1195. DOI: 10.1107/S0907444909034234

[211] Zheng ZW, Li J, Vhen H, He JL, Chen QW, Zhang JH, et al. Evaluation of *in vitro* antileishmanial efficacy of cyclosporin A and its non-immunosuppressive derivative, dihydrocyclosporin A. Parasites & Vectors. 2020;**13**:94. DOI: 10.1186/s13071-020-3958-x

Chapter 10

microRNAs: Are They Important in the Development of Resistance in Leishmaniasis?

Sandra Alves de Araújo, Tatiane Aranha da Penha-Silva, Jaqueline Diniz Pinho, Marcelo de Souza Andrade and Ana Lucia Abreu-Silva

Abstract

Leishmaniasis is an infectious and parasitic disease of great importance in public health. Numerous studies indicate that biochemical and molecular mechanisms are factors that contribute to the emergence of antileishmanial drug resistance. Currently, miRNAs have been identified as targets for the invasion of pathogens to control the immune response and imply resistance to treatments. Considering the alarming growth in drug resistance, new possibilities for controlling leishmaniasis have been emerging. Natural compounds originating from medicinal plants are being increasingly explored as promising antileishmanial alternatives. The chapter aims to provide a brief review on mechanisms of action associated with traditional agents used to treat leishmaniasis, focusing mainly on molecular bases associated with the resistance of *Leishmania* spp. to current drugs and identifying the possible miRNAs involved in this process. In addition, we seek to describe some of the promising plant molecules that can be used as potential antileishmanial agents and their possible mechanisms of action.

Keywords: Leishmaniasis, drug resistance, miRNAs, mechanisms of action, natural products

1. Introduction

Leishmaniasis is an infectious and parasitic disease of major importance to public health worldwide due to its difficult control, mainly because the commonly used antileishmanial drugs have contributed to the increasing increase in parasite resistance [1, 2].

Biochemical, molecular and/or genetic mechanisms are factors that contribute to the emergence of resistance [3–5]. Among these mechanisms, we highlight microRNAs (miRNAs), small non-coding RNAs functionally involved in various biological processes of an organism [6–8]. Currently, these structures have been identified as the main targets for invasion by pathogens, including *Leishmania* spp., aiming to control the immune response and possibly implying resistance to treatments [9, 10].

Due to the alarming increase in drug resistance, the search for new drugs or natural compounds to control leishmaniasis has grown [11, 12]. Natural compounds originating from plants are increasingly being explored as promising antileishmanial alternatives, since, when compared to currently available drugs, these products can selectively act on the parasite besides that the most of them present low cytotoxicity and low market value [13, 14].

Although, researches demonstrate the importance of natural products for the treatment of leishmaniasis, little is known about the influence of miRNAs on the mechanisms of action of natural products. However, recent evidence suggests that some phytochemical substances regulate the expression of several pathological miRNAs [15, 16]. For example, in breast cancer, phytochemical substances extracted from plant foods have acted directly on the regulation of miRNA expression and these are pointed out as promising alternative chemopreventive and chemotherapeutic agents [17].

In this context, to understand the mechanisms of action of natural compounds and the emergence of resistance by parasites, this review was developed based on the following question: Is it possible that certain natural compounds also act by inhibiting or activating miRNAs that interfere with the parasitic action against *Leishmania*? The chapter aims to provide a brief review on mechanisms of action associated with traditional agents used to treat leishmaniasis, focusing mainly on molecular basis associated with resistance in *Leishmania* spp. to current drugs and identifying the possible miRNAs involved in this process. In addition, we seek to describe some of the promising plant molecules that can be used as potential antileishmanial agents and their possible mechanisms of action.

2. Traditional therapeutic agents and mechanisms of action

Leishmaniasis presents different clinical manifestations, ranging from skin lesions to severe visceral forms, depending on the species of the parasite of the genus *Leishmania* [4].

Chemotherapy is the only effective alternative to treat all forms of the disease. Therapeutic approaches to control leishmaniasis comprise five main drugs: pentavalent antimony, amphotericin B, miltefosine, paromomycin and pentamidine, however, these drugs are associated with serious problems, such as toxicity and especially with the emergence of resistant strains, making treatment difficult [18].

Although, current antileishmanial drugs have been used for decades, their mechanisms of action remain obscure, however, some assumptions are accepted. Pentavalent antimonials, for example, eliminate parasites through the process of apoptosis and also inhibit trypanothione reductase, an important enzyme for the survival of the parasite in the host [19]. Miltefosine, in turn, also induces cell death by apoptosis, in addition to inducing various immunological and inflammatory effects on macrophages [20]. The mechanism of action of amphotericin B may involve interaction with membrane sterols, resulting in membrane disorganization, increased permeability and cell damage in the parasite [21, 22]. Paromomycin inhibits protein synthesis and modifies the fluidity and permeability of the membrane and also decreases mitochondrial potential [3, 23]. While pentamidine acts as a DNA-binding drug, causing the parasite mitochondrial membrane potential collapse and induction of kinetoplast DNA destruction [24, 25].

The prolonged use of these drugs has contributed to the acceleration of leishmaniasis resistance; however, little is known about the cellular and molecular mechanisms, especially about the importance of miRNAs involved in the emergence of this resistance (**Figure 1**).

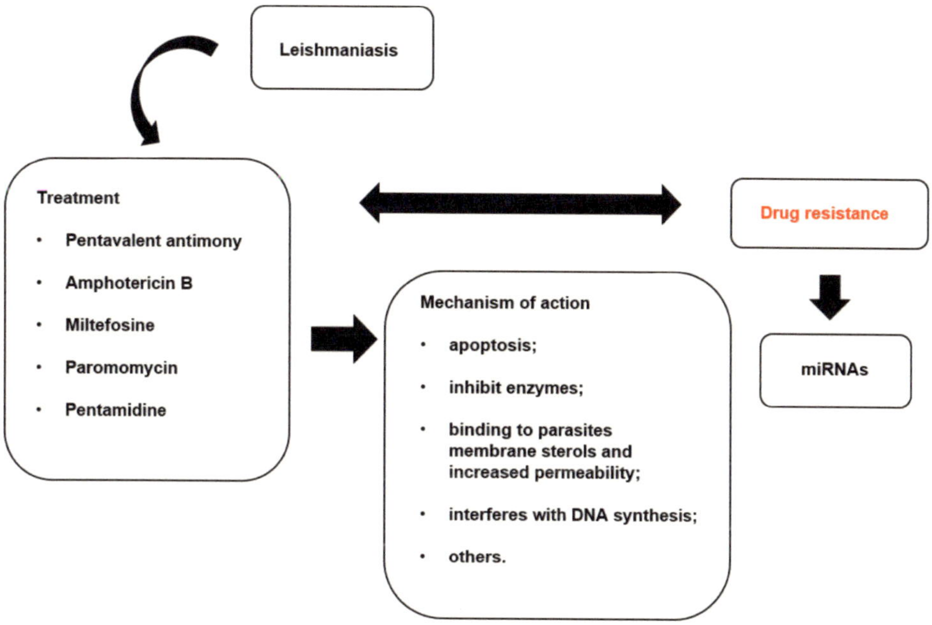

Figure 1.
Antileishmanial drugs and mechanism of action. The pentavalent antimony, amphotericin B, miltefosine, paromomycin and pentamidine drugs act mainly by inducing apoptosis; inhibiting important enzymes; binding to the parasite's membrane sterols, increasing permeability and interfering with DNA synthesis. The prolonged use of these drugs and consequently the increase in parasite resistance has been explained by molecular mechanisms, for example, the expression of miRNAs.

3. miRNAs and drug resistance

MicroRNAs (miRNAs) are a small class of non-coding RNAs composed of 18–24 nucleotides, present in a variety of organisms, including parasites, plants, animals and humans [7, 8, 26, 27]. The first description of these structures occurred after studies with the nematode parasite *Caenorhabditis elegans* [28].

The canonical biosynthesis of a miRNA starts with a primary miRNA (pri-miRNA) that is transcribed and recognized by a microprocessor complex. This process includes the double-stranded RNA-specific endoribonuclease enzymes (DROSHA) and the DiGeorge syndrome critical region gene 8 (DGCR8), which are cleaved to form a miRNA precursor (pre-miRNA). The pre-miRNAs are then exported to the cytoplasm for further processing by the DICER enzyme and cofactors such as protein kinase R activator (PACT) or transactivation response RNA binding protein (TRBP) [29].

The mature duplex miRNA is finally loaded into an RNA-induced silencing complex (RISC) that is multiprotein and a corrected miRNA strand (–5p or -3p) that binds to the Argonaute protein (AGO) guiding the complex to its mRNA target [30]. Both biogenesis and maturation of miRNAs are tightly regulated processes. The first level of adjustment is represented by single nucleotide polymorphisms (SNPs) and epigenetic control of transcription through mechanisms of acetylation, DNA methylation and histones. The biosynthesis and maturation of miRNAs can also be influenced by RNA binding proteins (RBPs), which can interact with key enzyme processes such as DROSHA, DGCR8, DICER and the complex RISC [31].

In addition to impacting the actions of miRNAs on their targets, editing pri and pre-miRNAs is also an important mechanism that modulates the biosynthesis and maturation of specific miRNAs. Degradation of the miRNA strand (–5p or -3p strand) or incorporation into the RISC complex (lead strand) determines the pool of target mRNAs. The complementarity between the miRNA response elements (MRE) in the mRNA and the seed sequence in the miRNA strand determines the specificity of the action of the RISC complex for mRNAs. Furthermore, the degree of complementarity between the MRE and the seed sequences generally dictates whether the mRNA is degraded or its translation is blocked [32]. The mechanism of biogenesis and maturation of miRNA is described in **Figure 2**.

miRNAs are involved in important biological processes in organisms, including the control of gene and pathological expression, cell and organ development, differentiation and homeostasis, tumor suppression and stem cell regulation [26]. miRNAs are also known to be involved in the development of human parasitic diseases. For example, in *Schistosoma mansoni*, the causative agent of schistosomiasis, it was shown that miRNAs can control the development of the parasite and also of liver pathology [33]. While in Chagas disease, caused by *Trypanosoma cruzi*, there are reports of the involvement of miRNAs in cardiovascular disorders caused by illness [34–36].

In toxoplasmosis, a disease caused by the agent *Toxoplasma gondii*, some miRNAs may be related to the degree of virulence, inhibition of apoptosis and immune response [37, 38]. While in malaria (*Plasmodium* spp.), evidence has shown that the agent manipulates the host miRNA expression, supporting its growth and survival, and also regulates important genes for the host immune response [39–41].

In leishmaniasis, miRNAs play an important role in the biology of infection, pathogenicity, recognition and activation of the immune response by macrophages and dendritic cells, host–parasite interaction and drugs resistance [42–44].

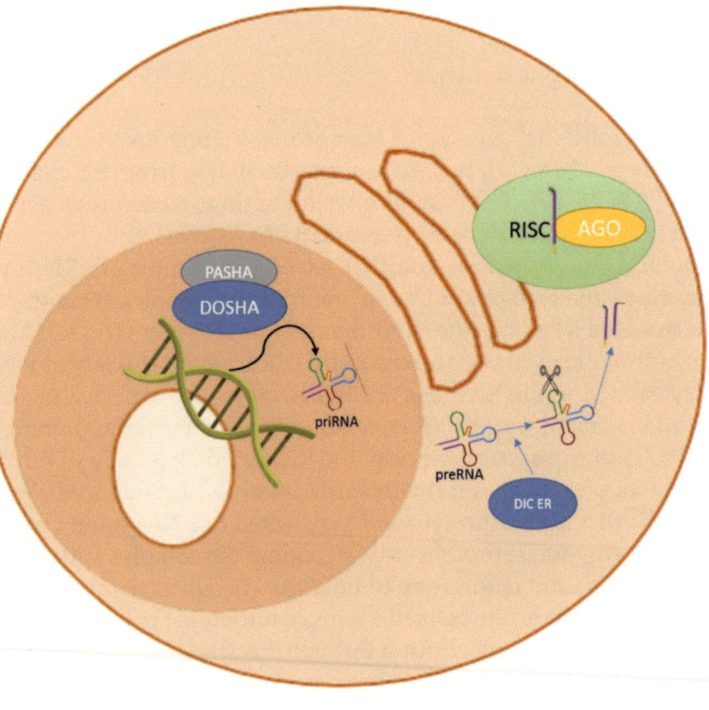

Figure 2.
Biogenesis or generation of miRNAs and the mechanisms of protein synthesis inhibition. A primary miRNA (pri-miRNA) is transcribed or produced in the nucleus. It is processed or modified by the Drosha enzyme and exported to the cytoplasm. In the cytoplasm, now called pre-miRNA, it is again processed by another enzyme, Dicer, finally forming the mature miRNA. Mature miRNA associates with a complex or set of enzymes called RISC and represses or inhibits protein synthesis by cleaving (breaking) messenger RNAs (mRNA) or may impede mRNA reading (prevent translation) by inhibiting protein production.

Although, research emphasizes the importance of studying miRNAs during infection or pathogenesis by different parasites, the role of these structures in the development of antiparasitic resistance remains unclear. Drug resistance is a growing problem worldwide. Resisting a drug means saying that there was a reduction in the drug effectiveness in the total elimination of the pathogen responsible for the disease [45]. miRNAs have been identified as targets for pathogen invasion and immune response control, in addition to resistance to chemotherapy in a variety of organisms and diseases (**Figure 3**) [6, 10].

In recent years, studies have shown that miRNAs are involved in tumor cell resistance to chemotherapy [46–48]. According to the studies, miRNAs regulate different target genes, especially genes that affect the cell response to chemotherapy drugs. In insects, some miRNAs are involved in resistance to the insecticide diamide in the control of *Plutella xylostella*, mainly miR-7a and miR-8519 [49]. Other studies have reported the importance of miR-2, miR-13, miR-7, miR-92a and miR-13,664 expression in the *Culex pipiens* insect resistance to the drug deltamethrin [50–52].

The resistance of some parasites is also related to miRNAs. In the nematode *C. elegans*, miR-1 down-regulates the expression of two nicotinic acetylcholine receptor subunits (nAChR), unc-29 and unc-63 [53]. According to the authors, when the expression of these subunits is increased, it corresponds to a decrease in muscle sensitivity to acetylcholine by levamisole, that is, the drug action is decreased. In *Toxocara* spp., the causative agent of toxocariasis in humans and other animals, computational studies predict that some miRNAs function as targets associated with drug resistance, such as Tc-miR-2861, Tc-miR-2881 and Tc-miR -5126 [54]. Additionally, miR-9551 is regulated in *Teladorsagia circumcincta*, the most prevalent parasite in United Kingdom animals with proven multiple drug resistance [55]. Recently, miR-9551 expression was also correlated with an anthelmintic resistance phenotype of *Haemonchus contortus* to the drug ivermectin [9].

The role of miRNAs in drug resistance is clear for a wide variety of organisms, for protozoan parasites, mainly *Leishmania* spp. it's still not well elucidated. However, the expression of miRNAs in leishmaniasis can be used as a strategy to escape the host immune system [13, 14]. For example, the pentavalent

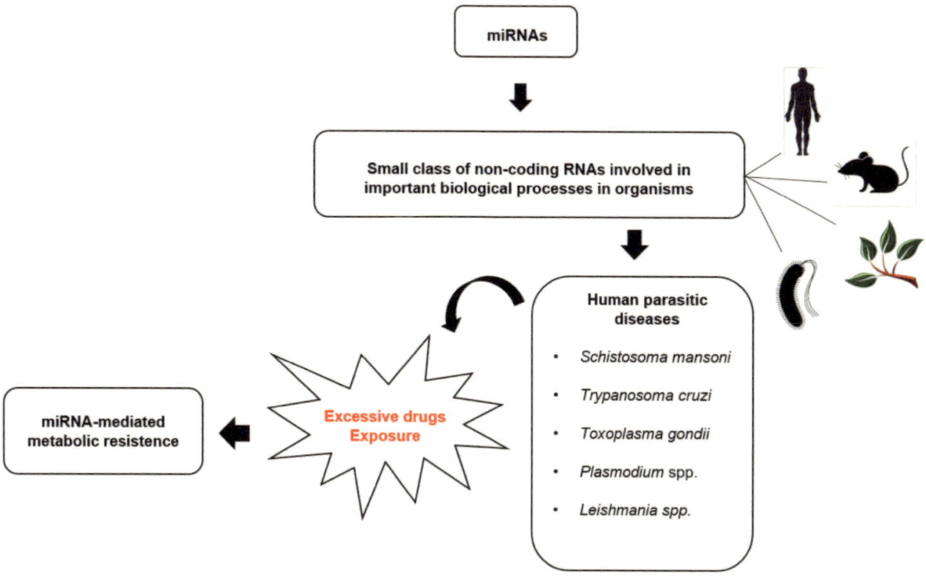

Figure 3.
miRNAs and human parasitic diseases.

antimony-resistant *Leishmania donovani* species exploits miR-466i to regulate levels of inflammatory cytokines produced by macrophages during infection, and in other cases, it decreases miR-122 expression by hepatocytes to facilitate infection, ensuring its differentiation and intracellular multiplication [56, 57].

For years, pentavalent antimony was the main treatment against leishmaniasis and with this, the parasites acquired resistance and the drug lost its effectiveness [58]. The resistance mechanism of *Leishmania donovani* to pentavalent antimonals can be explained by the increased production of IL-10 and TGF-β inducing the upregulation of the multiresistant protein-1 (MDR1) and causing the expulsion of the drug by macrophages [58]. Also, according to the authors, during infection by the resistant parasite, miRNAs control the expression of pro and anti-inflammatory cytokines in macrophages internally regulated by the proteins Ago2, PP2A and HuR. HuR positively inhibits PP2A expression by activating the modulatory function of HuR and PP2A antagonist miRNAs and acting as a balancing factor for immune responses in macrophages to interrupt or prevent infection by pentavalent antimonal resistant *L. donovani* [59].

Tiwari et al. [10] pointed out that *Leishmania* parasites possibly induce macrophages to express miRNA regulatory proteins that help expel drugs from cells. This drug resistance has been associated with the downregulation of miRNA-763, −1264, and -3473f by parasitized macrophages that induced upregulation of ABC transporters [10]. Recent studies have revealed that miRNA deficiency can also influence the emergence of host resistance to leishmaniasis. According to Varikuti et al. [60], miR-21 is positively expressed in dendritic cells and macrophages and in organs such as the spleen and liver infected by *L. donovani*. During infection, the lack of miR-21 increases IL-12 production and the Th1 immune response and consequently increases host resistance. miR-21 plays an essential role in the pathogenesis of the disease and is considered a potential target in the treatment of leishmaniasis. miRNAs alter transporters, receptors and ion channels drug, reducing sensitivity and consequently developing resistance [61, 62]. The change in the miR profile may be a strategy of infection or drug resistance of parasites.

Thus, these studies highlight the importance of these structures in the development of leishmaniasis resistance to currently available drugs and indicate that the identification of miRNAs can provide strategies for controlling leishmaniasis.

To contain the acceleration of resistance by parasites, the search for new treatments has emerged. The discovery of new drugs with fewer side effects and more advantageous cost-benefits than current treatments has gained strength, in this sense, the use of natural products in the treatment of leishmaniasis has become an excellent alternative.

4. Natural products as an anti-*Leishmania* source

Natural products originating from plants are being increasingly explored as promising therapeutic alternatives, and the action of these products is mainly attributed to existing bioactive phytochemicals [63, 64].

The concentration of these compounds depends on the nature of the chemical used as a solvent during the extraction and handling process, as well as the storage conditions [65]. Terpenoids, phenolic compounds, alkaloids and flavonoids are the most important phytochemical groups. Terpenoids from essential oils are extracted by hydrodistillation and mechanical pressing techniques, while phenolic compounds, alkaloids and flavonoids are extracted using organic solvents, mainly dichloromethane, methanol, ethanol, ethyl acetate, n-butanol, chloroform, ether and benzene [65–67].

After extraction, the phytochemical analysis to identify the main classes of compounds is performed using chromatographic and colorimetric techniques [68]. Approximately 10,000 phytochemicals have been identified so far and their numerous medicinal properties are being investigated. Leaves, seeds, fruits and flowers are the plant organs richest in phytochemicals [69, 70].

Currently, these groups of phytochemicals have anti-*Leishmania* properties and mechanisms of action already described. Terpenoids, aromatic and lipophilic substances, possibly can cross the plasma membrane, interfering with cell composition, inducing mitochondrial rupture and chromatin condensation and causing parasite death by apoptosis [71, 72]. The glycyrrhizic acid, a triterpene extracted from the root of *Glycyrrhiza glabra*, was found to be responsible for the change in the host immune system, inducing an increase in the release of inflammatory cytokines in macrophages infected by *Leishmania*, facilitating a more efficient response against the parasite [73].

Phenolic compounds primarily function as antioxidants and free radical scavengers [74]. Its action on *Leishmania* is attributed to its ability to induce cell death through apoptosis and inhibition of cell replication through iron chelation [75–77]. Recently, Antwi et al. [78] also suggested that rosmarinic acid exerts an antileishmanial effect through iron chelation, however, its mechanism of action results in morphological alterations and interruption of the parasite cell cycle.

Alkaloids are alkaline compounds and can be classified based on the presence and activity of specific amino acids [79]. Many alkaloids have been described as having biological activities against *Leishmania* spp., however, the mechanism of action of these compounds is not fully understood. According to Fournet et al. [80] alkaloids can inhibit an essential antioxidant enzyme in the parasite, trypanothione reductase. Additionally, a study showed that different synthetic quinoline alkaloids caused ultrastructural changes in *Leishmania*, such as loss of cell membrane integrity in the parasites, in addition to inducing apoptosis [81].

Flavonoids, in turn, are a class of natural compounds with several known biological activities, including anti-*Leishmania*. Flavonoids subdivide into classes such as chalcones, flavones, isoflavones, flavonols and anthocyanidins [82]. Quercetin, a flavonol extracted from *Kalanchoe pinnata*, showed activity against *Leishmania amazonensis* promastigotes [83]. According to the authors, the compound increased the levels of reactive oxygen species, causing mitochondrial damage and leading to parasite death. Recently, Araújo et al. [84] demonstrated that flavonoids isolated from *Solanum paludosum* had an antiproliferative effect on *Leishmania* parasites inducing cell cycle blockage and autophagy.

In general, plants contain biomolecules with high active potential against leishmaniasis. However, the process of discovering these molecules is considered complex and time-consuming, since it involves phases such as isolation, identification, optimization of their properties and selection of safe and effective compounds for drug development [64, 70].

Studies have identified that the expression of miRNAs in different types of cancer is specifically regulated by phytochemicals [15]. In the treatment of breast cancer, several phytochemicals have been identified as tumor suppressors, directly controlling the expression of miRNAs [15–17]. According to Baselga-Escudero et al. [85] polyphenols can bind directly to miRNAs and that the chemical structure of these compounds influences the expression of miRNAs. Recently, through *in vitro* and *in vivo* studies, quercetin was able to modulate miRNAs and, consequently, suppress oncogenes or stimulate tumor suppressor genes by altering the expression of miRNAs [86].

These studies show the importance of natural compounds in the regulation of miRNAs and the possible influence of these in their action on diseases. However, it remains unclear whether miRNAs can interact with phytochemicals so that they are not absorbed and/or metabolized by the parasites and thus contribute to the resistance mechanism of leishmaniasis (**Figure 3**).

5. Conclusions

In conclusion, miRNAs have a wide range of important biological functions for parasites, including leishmaniasis. Although, the role of these structures in the development of antiparasitic resistance remains unclear, this work provides suggestive information about the strong contribution of miRNAs in this process. Furthermore, natural compounds with anti-*Leishmania* activity may play an important role in the regulation of miRNAs, influencing their action on the parasite. Therefore, the identification and characterization of specific miRNAs, as well as the clarification of their interaction with natural compounds are crucial for understanding the resistance mechanism of leishmaniasis.

Acknowledgements

The authors would like to thank CAPES (the Brazilian Federal Agency for support and evaluation of graduate education) for the scholarship to S.A. Araujo.

Conflict of interest

The authors declare no conflict of interest.

Author details

Sandra Alves de Araújo[1,2,3], Tatiane Aranha da Penha-Silva[4*], Jaqueline Diniz Pinho[2], Marcelo de Souza Andrade[1,3*] and Ana Lucia Abreu-Silva[1,2]

1 Postgraduate Program in Biotechnology, RENORBIO, São Luís, Brazil

2 State University of Maranhão, São Luís, Brazil

3 Federal University of Maranhão, São Luís, Brazil

4 Faculdade Pitágoras de São Luis, Brazil

*Address all correspondence to: tatianearanha@hotmail.com and marcelo.andrade@ufma.br

References

[1] Ponte-Sucre A, Gamarro F, Dujardin JC, Barrett MP, López-Vélez R, García-Hernández R, et al. Drug resistance and treatment failure in leishmaniasis: A 21st century challenge. PLoS Neglected Tropical Diseases. 2017;**11**(12):e0006052. DOI: 10.1371/journal.pntd.0006052

[2] Sundar S, Chakravarty J, Meena LP. Leishmaniasis: Treatment, drug resistance and emerging therapies. Expert Opinion on Orphan Drugs. 2019;**7**(1):1-10. DOI: 10.1080/21678707.2019.1552853

[3] Maltezou HC. Drug resistance in visceral leishmaniasis. Journal of Biomedicine & Biotechnology. 2010;**2010**:617521. DOI: 10.1155/2010/617521

[4] Ouellette M, Drummelsmith J, El-Fadili A, Kündig C, Richard D, Roy G. Pterin transport and metabolism in Leishmania and related trypanosomatid parasites. International Journal for Parasitology. 2002;**32**(4):385-398. DOI: 10.1016/s0020-7519(01)00346-0

[5] Capela R, Moreira R, Lopes F. An overview of drug resistance in protozoal diseases. International Journal of Molecular Sciences. 2019;**20**(22):5748. DOI: 10.3390/ijms20225748

[6] Britton C, Winter AD, Gillan V, Devaney E. microRNAs of parasitic helminths - Identification, characterization and potential as drug targets. International Journal for Parasitology: Drugs and Drug Resistance. 2014;**4**(2):85-94. DOI: 10.1016/j.ijpddr.2014.03.001

[7] Judice CC, Bourgard C, Kayano AC, Albrecht L, Costa FT. MicroRNAs in the Host-Apicomplexan Parasites Interactions: A review of immunopathological aspects. Frontiers in Cellular and Infection Microbiology. 2016;**6**:5. DOI: 10.3389/fcimb.2016.00005

[8] Acuña SM, Floeter-Winter LM, Muxel SM. MicroRNAs: Biological regulators in pathogen-host interactions. Cell. 2020;**9**(1):113. DOI: 10.3390/cells9010113

[9] Gillan V, Maitland K, Laing R, Gu H, Marks ND, Winter AD, et al. Increased expression of a MicroRNA correlates with anthelmintic resistance in parasitic nematodes. Frontiers in Cellular and Infection Microbiology. 2017;**7**:452. DOI: 10.3389/fcimb.2017.00452

[10] Tiwari N, Kumar V, Gedda MR, Singh AK, Singh VK, Gannavaram S, et al. Identification and characterization of miRNAs in response to leishmania donovani infection: Delineation of their roles in macrophage dysfunction. Frontiers in Microbiology. 2017;**8**:314. DOI: 10.3389/fmicb.2017.00314

[11] Hefnawy A, Berg M, Dujardin JC, De Muylder G. Exploiting knowledge on leishmania drug resistance to support the quest for new drugs. Trends in Parasitology. 2017;**33**(3):162-174. DOI: 10.1016/j.pt.2016.11.003

[12] Raj S, Sasidharan S, Balaji S, Dubey VK, Saudagar P. Review on natural products as an alternative to contemporary anti-leishmanial therapeutics. Journal of Proteins and Proteomics. 2020;**11**:135-158. DOI: 10.1007/s42485-020-00035-w

[13] Geraci NS, Tan JC, McDowell MA. Characterization of microRNA expression profiles in Leishmania-infected human phagocytes. Parasite Immunology. 2015;**37**(1):43-51. DOI: 10.1111/pim.12156

[14] Bayer-Santos E, Marini MM, da Silveira JF. Non-coding RNAs in

host-pathogen interactions: Subversion of mammalian cell functions by protozoan parasites. Frontiers in Microbiology. 2017;**8**:474. DOI: 10.3389/fmicb.2017.00474

[15] Kang H. MicroRNA-mediated health-promoting effects of phytochemicals. International Journal of Molecular Sciences. 2019;**20**(10): 2535. DOI: 10.3390/ijms20102535

[16] Ganapathy A, Ezekiel U. Phytochemical modulation of MiRNAs in colorectal cancer. Medicines (Basel). 2019;**6**(2):48. DOI: 10.3390/medicines6020048

[17] Abbasi BA, Iqbal J, Mahmood T, Khalil AT, Ali B, Kanwal S, et al. Role of dietary phytochemicals in modulation of miRNA expression: Natural swords combating breast cancer. Asian Pacific Journal of Tropical Medicine. 2018;**11**(9):501. DOI: 10.4103/1995-7645.242314

[18] Tiwari N, Gedda MR, Tiwari VK, Singh SP, Singh RK. Limitations of current therapeutic options, possible drug targets and scope of natural products in control of leishmaniasis. Mini Reviews in Medicinal Chemistry. 2018;**18**(1):26-41. DOI: 10.2174/1389557517666170425105129

[19] Singh N. Drug resistance mechanisms in clinical isolates of Leishmania donovani. The Indian Journal of Medical Research. 2006; **123**(3):411-422

[20] Pérez-Victoria FJ, Sánchez-Cañete MP, Seifert K, Croft SL, Sundar S, Castanys S, et al. Mechanisms of experimental resistance of Leishmania to miltefosine: Implications for clinical use. Drug Resistance Updates. 2006;**9**(1-2):26-39. DOI: 10.1016/j.drup.2006.04.001

[21] Mohapatra S. Drug resistance in leishmaniasis: Newer developments. Trop Parasitol. 2014;**4**(1):4-9. DOI: 10.4103/2229-5070.129142

[22] Légaré D, Ouellette M. Drug resistance in leishmania. In: Gotte MB, Matlashewski A, Wainberg G, Mark A, Donald S, editors. Handbook of Antimicrobial Resistance. New York, NY: Springer; 2017. pp. 313-341. DOI: 10.1007/978-1-4939-0694-9_17

[23] Jhingran A, Chawla B, Saxena S, Barrett MP, Madhubala R. Paromomycin: uptake and resistance in Leishmania donovani. Molecular and Biochemical Parasitology. 2009;**164**(2):111-117. DOI: 10.1016/j.molbiopara.2008.12.007

[24] Thomas JA, Baker N, Hutchinson S, Dominicus C, Trenaman A, Glover L, et al. Insights into antitrypanosomal drug mode-of-action from cytology-based profiling. PLoS Neglected Tropical Diseases. 2018;**12**(11):e0006980. DOI: 10.1371/journal.pntd.0006980

[25] Baker CH, Welburn SC. The long wait for a new drug for human African trypanosomiasis. Trends in Parasitology. 2018;**34**(10):818-827. DOI: 10.1016/j.pt.2018.08.006

[26] Bartel DP. MicroRNAs: Genomics, biogenesis, mechanism, and function. Cell. 2004;**116**(2):281-297. DOI: 10.1016/s0092-8674(04)00045-5

[27] Kim YK, Kim VN. Processing of intronic microRNAs. The EMBO Journal. 2007;**26**(3):775-783. DOI: 10.1038/sj.emboj.7601512

[28] Lee RC, Ambros V. An extensive class of small RNAs in Caenorhabditis elegans. Science. 2001;**294**(5543):862-864. DOI: 10.1126/science.1065329

[29] Sousa MC, Gjorgjieva M, Dolicka D, Sobolewski C, Foti M. Deciphering miRNAs' Action through miRNA

Editing Int. J. Mol. Sci. 2019;**20**:6249. DOI: 10.3390/ijms20246249

[30] Van den Berg A, Mols J, Han J. RISC-target interaction: Cleavage and translational suppression. Biochimica et Biophysica Acta. 2008;**1779**:668-677. DOI: 10.1016/j.bbagrm.2008.07.005

[31] Ota H, Sakurai M, Gupta R, Valente L, Wul BE, Ariyoshi K, et al. ADAR1 forms a complex with Dicer to promote microRNA processing and RNA-induced gene silencing. Cell. 2013;**153**:575-589. DOI: 10.1016/j.cell.2013.03.024

[32] Sobolewski C, Calo N, Portius D, Foti M. MicroRNAs in fatty liver disease. Seminars in Liver Disease. 2015;**35**:12-25. DOI: 10.1055/s-0034-1397345

[33] Zhu L, Liu J, Cheng G. Role of microRNAs in schistosomes and schistosomiasis. Frontiers in Cellular and Infection Microbiology. 2014;**4**:165. DOI: 10.3389/fcimb.2014.00165

[34] Ferreira LRP, Frade AF, Santos RHB, Teixeira PC, Baron MA, Navarro IC, et al. MicroRNAs miR-1, miR-133a, miR-133b, miR-208a and miR-208b are dysregulated in Chronic Chagas disease Cardiomyopathy. International Journal of Cardiology. 2014;**175**(3):409-417. DOI: 10.1016/j.ijcard.2014.05.019

[35] Linhares-Lacerda L, Palu CC, Ribeiro-Alves M, Paredes BD, Morrot A, Garcia-Silva MR, et al. Differential expression of microRNAs in thymic epithelial cells from trypanosoma cruzi acutely infected mice: Putative role in thymic atrophy. Frontiers in Immunology. 2015;**6**:428. DOI: 10.3389/fimmu.2015.00428

[36] Navarro IC, Ferreira FM, Nakaya HI, Baron MA, Vilar-Pereira G, Pereira IR, et al. MicroRNA transcriptome profiling in heart of trypanosoma cruzi-infected mice: Parasitological and cardiological outcomes. PLoS Neglected Tropical Diseases. 2015;**9**(6):e0003828

[37] Braun L, Cannella D, Ortet P, Barakat M, Sautel CF, Kieffer S, et al. A complex small RNA repertoire is generated by a plant/fungal-like machinery and effected by a metazoan-like Argonaute in the single-cell human parasite Toxoplasma gondii. PLoS Pathogens. 2010;**6**(5):e1000920. DOI: 10.1371/journal.ppat.1000920

[38] Cai Y, Chen H, Jin L, You Y, Shen J. STAT3-dependent transactivation of miRNA genes following Toxoplasma gondii infection in macrophage. Parasites & Vectors. 2013;**6**:356. DOI: 10.1186/1756-3305-6-356

[39] Rathjen T, Nicol C, McConkey G, Dalmay T. Analysis of short RNAs in the malaria parasite and its red blood cell host. FEBS Letters. 2006;**580**(22):5185-5188. DOI: 10.1016/j.febslet.2006.08.063

[40] Taganov KD, Boldin MP, Chang KJ, Baltimore D. NF-kappaB-dependent induction of microRNA miR-146, an inhibitor targeted to signaling proteins of innate immune responses. Proceedings of the National Academy of Sciences of the United States of America. 2006;**103**(33):12481-12486. DOI: 10.1073/pnas.0605298103

[41] Hakimi MA, Ménard R. Do apicomplexan parasites hijack the host cell microRNA pathway for their intracellular development? F1000 Biol Rep. 2010;**2**:42. DOI: 10.3410/B2-42

[42] Frank B, Marcu A, de Oliveira Almeida Petersen AL, Weber H, Stigloher C, Mottram JC, et al. Autophagic digestion of Leishmania major by host macrophages is associated with differential expression of BNIP3, CTSE, and the miRNAs miR-101c, miR-129, and miR-210. Parasites & Vectors. 2015;**8**:404. DOI: 10.1186/s13071-015-0974-3

[43] Muxel SM, Laranjeira-Silva MF, Zampieri RA, Floeter-Winter LM. Leishmania (Leishmania) amazonensis induces macrophage miR-294 and miR-721 expression and modulates infection by targeting NOS2 and L-arginine metabolism. Scientific Reports. 2017;7:44141. DOI: 10.1038/srep44141

[44] Bragato JP, Melo LM, Venturin GL, Rebech GT, Garcia LE, Lopes FL, et al. Relationship of peripheral blood mononuclear cells miRNA expression and parasitic load in canine visceral leishmaniasis. PLoS One. 2018;**13**(12): e0206876. DOI: 10.1371/journal.pone.0206876

[45] Loke MF, Hanafi A. Molecular Mechanisms Responsible for Drug Resistance. In: Ranganathan S, Gribskov M, Nakai K, Schönbach C, editors. Encyclopedia of Bioinformatics and Computational Biology, Academic Press, 2019;**3**:926-931. DOI: 10.1016/B978-0-12-809633-8.20467-6

[46] Hu S, Yuan Y, Song Z, Yan D, Kong X. Expression profiles of microRNAs in drug-resistant non-small cell lung cancer cell lines using microRNA sequencing. Cellular Physiology and Biochemistry. 2018;**51**(6):2509-2522. DOI: 10.1159/000495921

[47] Si W, Shen J, Zheng H, Fan W. The role and mechanisms of action of microRNAs in cancer drug resistance. Clinical Epigenetics. 2019;**11**(1):25. DOI: 10.1186/s13148-018-0587-8

[48] Duan L, Yang W, Feng W, Cao L, Wang X, Niu L, et al. Molecular mechanisms and clinical implications of miRNAs in drug resistance of colorectal cancer. Ther Adv Med Oncol. 2020;**12**: 1758835920947342. DOI: 10.1177/1758835920947342

[49] Li X, Guo L, Zhou X, Gao X, Liang P. miRNAs regulated overexpression of ryanodine receptor is involved in chlorantraniliprole resistance in Plutella xylostella (L.). Scientific Reports. 2015;**5**(1):1-9. DOI: 10.1038/srep14095

[50] Guo Q, Huang Y, Zou F, Liu B, Tian M, Ye W, et al. The role of miR-2~13~71 cluster in resistance to deltamethrin in Culex pipiens pallens. Insect Biochemistry and Molecular Biology. 2017;**84**:15-22. DOI: 10.1016/j.ibmb.2017.03.006

[51] Ma K, Li X, Hu H, Zhou D, Sun Y, Ma L, et al. Pyrethroid-resistance is modulated by miR-92a by targeting CpCPR4 in Culex pipiens pallens. Comparative Biochemistry and Physiology. Part B, Biochemistry & Molecular Biology. 2017;**203**:20-24. DOI: 10.1016/j.cbpb.2016.09.002

[52] Sun XH, Xu N, Xu Y, Zhou D, Sun Y, Wang WJ, et al. A novel miRNA, miR-13664, targets CpCYP314A1 to regulate deltamethrin resistance in Culex pipiens pallens. Parasitology. 2019;**146**(2):197-205. DOI: 10.1017/S0031182018001002

[53] Simon DJ, Madison JM, Conery AL, Thompson-Peer KL, Soskis M, Ruvkun GB, et al. The microRNA miR-1 regulates a MEF-2-dependent retrograde signal at neuromuscular junctions. Cell. 2008;**133**(5):903-915. DOI: 10.1016/j.cell.2008.04.035

[54] Ma G, Luo Y, Zhu H, Korhonen PK, Young ND, Gasser RB, et al. MicroRNAs of Toxocara canis and their predicted functional roles. Parasites & Vectors. 2016;**9**:229. DOI: 10.1186/s13071-016-1508-3

[55] Sargison ND, Jackson F, Bartley DJ, Wilson DJ, Stenhouse LJ, Penny CD. Observations on the emergence of multiple anthelmintic resistance in sheep flocks in the south-east of Scotland. Veterinary Parasitology. 2007;**145**(1-2):65-76. DOI: 10.1016/j.vetpar.2006.10.024

[56] Ghosh J, Bose M, Roy S, Bhattacharyya SN. Leishmania donovani targets Dicer1 to downregulate miR-122, lower serum cholesterol, and facilitate murine liver infection. Cell Host & Microbe. 2013;**13**(3):277-288. DOI: 10.1016/j.chom.2013.02.005

[57] Mukherjee B, Paul J, Mukherjee S, Mukhopadhyay R, Das S, Naskar K, et al. Antimony-resistant leishmania donovani exploits miR-466i to deactivate host MyD88 for regulating IL-10/IL-12 levels during early hours of infection. Journal of Immunology. 2015;**195**(6):2731-2742. DOI: 10.4049/jimmunol.1402585

[58] Mukherjee B, Mukherjee K, Nanda P, Mukhopadhayay R, Ravichandiran V, Bhattacharyya SN, et al. Probing the molecular mechanism of aggressive infection by antimony resistant *Leishmania donovani*. Cytokine. 2021;**145**:155245. DOI: 10.1016/j.cyto.2020.155245

[59] Goswami A, Mukherjee K, Mazumder A, Ganguly S, Mukherjee I, Chakrabarti S, et al. MicroRNA exporter HuR clears the internalized pathogens by promoting pro-inflammatory response in infected macrophages. EMBO Molecular Medicine. 2020;**12**(3):e11011. DOI: 10.15252/emmm.201911011

[60] Varikuti S, Verma C, Holcomb E, Jha BK, Viana A, Maryala R, et al. MicroRNA-21 Deficiency Promotes the Early Th1 Immune Response and Resistance toward Visceral Leishmaniasis. Journal of Immunology. 2021;**207**(5):1322-1332. DOI: 10.4049/jimmunol.2001099

[61] Ren N, Gao G, Sun Y, Zhang L, Wang H, Hua W, et al. MicroRNA signatures from multidrug-resistant Mycobacterium tuberculosis. Molecular Medicine Reports. 2015;**12**(5):6561-6567. DOI: 10.3892/mmr.2015.4262

[62] Nawaz M, Malik MI, Hameed M, Zhou J. Research progress on the composition and function of parasite-derived exosomes. Acta Tropica. 2019;**196**:30-36. DOI: 10.1016/j.actatropica.2019.05.004

[63] Carter NS, Stamper BD, Elbarbry F, Nguyen V, Lopez S, Kawasaki Y, et al. Natural products that target the arginase in. Microorganisms. 2021;**9**(2):267. DOI: 10.3390/microorganisms9020267

[64] Oliveira RM, Melo SA, Penha-Silva TA, Almeida-Souza F, Abreu-Silva AL. Alternative treatment for leishmaniasis. In: Afrin F, Hemeg H, editors. Leishmaniases as Re-emerging Diseases. Rijeka: IntechOpen; 2018. DOI: 10.5772/intechopen.75895

[65] Martins N, Barros L, Henriques M, Silva S, Ferreira IC. In vivo anti-candida activity of phenolic extracts and compounds: Future perspectives focusing on effective clinical interventions. BioMed Research International. 2015;**2015**:247382. DOI: 10.1155/2015/247382

[66] Santos HLLR, Souza N, Macedo NR, Ramos JPS, Dias AF, Nascimento A. Phytochemical analysis of extracts from the atlantic forest wood species. Floresta e Ambiente. 2019;**26**. DOI: 10.1590/2179-8087.038118

[67] Wilkin PJ, Al-Yozbaki M, George A, Gupta GK, Wilson CM. The Undiscovered Potential of Essential Oils for Treating SARS-CoV-2 (COVID-19). Current Pharmaceutical Design. 2020;**26**(41):5261-5277. DOI: 10.2174/1381612826666201015154611

[68] Acquavia MA, Pascale R, Foti L, Carlucci G, Scrano L, Martelli G, et al. Analytical methods for extraction and identification of primary and secondary metabolites of apple (Malus domestica) fruits: A review. Separations. 2021;**8**(7):91. DOI: 10.3390/separations8070091

[69] Reddy MV, Reddy MK, Gunasekar D, Caux C, Bodo B. A flavanone and a dihydrodibenzoxepin from Bauhinia variegata. Phytochemistry. 2003;**64**(4):879-882. DOI: 10.1016/s0031-9422(03)00416-3

[70] Altemimi A, Lakhssassi N, Baharlouei A, Watson DG, Lightfoot DA. Phytochemicals: Extraction, isolation, and identification of bioactive compounds from plant extracts. Plants (Basel). 2017;**6**(4):42. DOI: 10.3390/plants6040042

[71] Corpas-López V, Merino-Espinosa G, Díaz-Sáez V, Morillas-Márquez F, Navarro-Moll MC, Martín-Sánchez J. The sesquiterpene (−)-α-bisabolol is active against the causative agents of Old World cutaneous leishmaniasis through the induction of mitochondrial-dependent apoptosis. Apoptosis. 2016;**21**(10):1071-1081. DOI: 10.1007/s10495-016-1282-x

[72] Hajaji S, Sifaoui I, López-Arencibia A, Reyes-Batlle M, Jiménez IA, Bazzocchi IL, et al. Leishmanicidal activity of α-bisabolol from Tunisian chamomile essential oil. Parasitology Research. 2018;**117**(9): 2855-2867. DOI: 10.1007/s00436-018-5975-7

[73] Bhattacharjee S, Bhattacharjee A, Majumder S, Majumdar SB, Majumdar S. Glycyrrhizic acid suppresses Cox-2-mediated anti-inflammatory responses during Leishmania donovani infection. The Journal of Antimicrobial Chemotherapy. 2012;**67**(8):1905-1914. DOI: 10.1093/jac/dks159

[74] Verruck S, Prudencio ES, da Silveira SM. Compostos bioativos com capacidade antioxidante e antimicrobiana em frutas. Revista do Congresso Sul Brasileiro de Engenharia de Alimentos; 2018;**4**(1):111. DOI: 10.5965/24473650412018111.

[75] Montrieux E, Perera WH, García M, Maes L, Cos P, Monzote L. In vitro and in vivo activity of major constituents from Pluchea carolinensis against Leishmania amazonensis. Parasitology Research. 2014;**113**(8):2925-2932. DOI: 10.1007/s00436-014-3954-1

[76] Fonseca-Silva F, Canto-Cavalheiro MM, Menna-Barreto RF, Almeida-Amaral EE. Effect of apigenin on leishmania amazonensis is associated with reactive oxygen species production followed by mitochondrial dysfunction. Journal of Natural Products. 2015;**78**(4): 880-884. DOI: 10.1021/acs.jnatprod.5b00011

[77] Belkhelfa-Slimani R, Djerdjouri B. Caffeic acid combined with autoclaved Leishmania major boosted the protection of infected BALB/c mice by enhancing IgG2 production, IFN-γ/TGF-β and iNO synthase/arginase1 ratios, and the death of infected phagocytes. Inflammopharmacology. 2018;**26**(2):621-634. DOI: 10.1007/s10787-017-0399-z

[78] Antwi CA, Amisigo CM, Adjimani JP, Gwira TM. In vitro activity and mode of action of phenolic compounds on Leishmania donovani. PLoS Neglected Tropical Diseases. 2019;**13**(2):e0007206. DOI: 10.1371/journal.pntd.0007206

[79] Gervazoni LFO, Barcellos GB, Ferreira-Paes T, Almeida-Amaral EE. Use of natural products in leishmaniasis chemotherapy: An overview. Frontiers in Chemistry. 2020;**8**:579891. DOI: 10.3389/fchem.2020.579891

[80] Fournet A, Rojas de Arias A, Ferreira ME, Nakayama H, Torres de Ortiz S, Schinini A, et al. Efficacy of the bisbenzylisoquinoline alkaloids in acute and chronic Trypanosoma cruzi murine model. International Journal of Antimicrobial Agents. 2000;**13**(3):189-195. DOI: 10.1016/s0924-8579(99)00117-x

[81] Torres Suarez E, Granados-Falla DS, Robledo SM, Murillo J, Upegui Y, Delgado G. Antileishmanial activity of synthetic analogs of the naturally occurring quinolone alkaloid N-methyl-8-methoxyflindersin. PLoS One. 2020;**15**(12):e0243392. DOI: 10.1371/journal.pone.0243392

[82] Seleem D, Pardi V, Murata RM. Review of flavonoids: A diverse group of natural compounds with anti-Candida albicans activity in vitro. Archives of Oral Biology. 2017;**76**:76-83. DOI: 10.1016/j.archoralbio.2016.08.030

[83] Fonseca-Silva F, Inacio JD, Canto-Cavalheiro MM, Almeida-Amaral EE. Reactive oxygen species production by quercetin causes the death of Leishmania amazonensis intracellular amastigotes. Journal of Natural Products. 2013;**76**(8):1505-1508. DOI: 10.1021/np400193m

[84] Araújo MV, Queiroz AC, Silva JFM, Silva AE, Silva JKS, Silva GR, et al. Flavonoids induce cell death in Leishmania amazonensis: in vitro characterization by flow cytometry and Raman spectroscopy. The Analyst. 2019;**144**(17):5232-5244. DOI: 10.1039/c9an00948e

[85] Baselga-Escudero L, Blade C, Ribas-Latre A, Casanova E, Suárez M, Torres JL, et al. Resveratrol and EGCG bind directly and distinctively to miR-33a and miR-122 and modulate divergently their levels in hepatic cells. Nucleic Acids Research. 2014;**42**(2):882-892. DOI: 10.1093/nar/gkt1011

[86] Ramos YAL, Souza OF, Novo MCT, Guimarães CFC, Popi AF. Quercetin shortened survival of radio-resistant B-1 cells. Oncotarget. 2021;**12**(4):355-365. DOI: 10.18632/oncotarget.27883

Chapter 11

Molecular Informatics of Trypanothione Reductase of *Leishmania major* Reveals Novel Chromen-2-One Analogues as Potential Leishmanicides

Samuel K. Kwofie, Gabriel B. Kwarko, Emmanuel Broni, Michael B. Adinortey and Michael D. Wilson

Abstract

Trypanothione reductase (TR), a flavoprotein oxidoreductase is an important therapeutic target for leishmaniasis. Ligand-based pharmacophore modelling and molecular docking were used to predict selective inhibitors against TR. Homology modelling was employed to generate a three-dimensional structure of *Leishmania major* trypanothione reductase (*Lm*TR). A pharmacophore model used to screen a natural compound library generated 42 hits, which were docked against the *Lm*TR protein. Compounds with lower binding energies were evaluated via *in silico* pharmacological profiling and bioactivity. Four compounds emerged as potential leads comprising Karatavicinol (7-[(2E,6E,10S)-10,11-dihydroxy-3,7,11-trimethyldodeca-2,6-dienoxy]chromen-2-one), Marmin (7-[(E,6R)-6,7-dihydroxy-3,7-dimethyloct-2-enoxy]chromen-2-one), Colladonin (7-[[(4*a*S)-6-hydroxy-5,5,8*a*-trimethyl-2-methylidene-3,4,4*a*,6,7,8-hexahydro-1*H*-naphthalen-1-yl]methoxy]chromen-2-one), and Pectachol (7-[(6-hydroxy-5,5,8*a*-trimethyl-2-methylidene-3,4,4*a*,6,7,8-hexahydro-1*H*-naphthalen-1-yl)methoxy]-6,8-dimethoxychromen-2-one) with good binding energies of −9.4, −9.3, 8.8, and −8.5 kcal/mol, respectively. These compounds bound effectively to the FAD domain of the protein with some critical residues including Asp35, Thr51, Lys61, Tyr198, and Asp327. Furthermore, molecular dynamics simulations and molecular mechanics Poisson-Boltzmann surface area (MMPBSA) computations corroborated their strong binding. The compounds were also predicted to possess anti-leishmanial activity. The molecules serves as templates for the design of potential drug candidates and can be evaluated *in vitro* with optimistic results in producing plausible attenuating infectivity in macrophages.

Keywords: *Leishmania*, trypanothione reductase, oxidative stress, natural product, pharmacophore modeling, virtual screening, molecular dynamics

1. Introduction

Leishmaniasis is a disease caused by a single-cell eukaryotic parasite of the *Leishmania* species. This protozoan parasite causes a substantial level of morbidity and mortality. *Leishmania* has a digenetic life cycle [1]. In mammals, the parasite colonizes macrophages, transforming into intracellular amastigotes. The parasite has an adaptive way to life conditions. The amastigotes tolerate low pH and are hydrolase resistant [2].

Trypanothione is a major product of the trypanothione biosynthesis pathway in trypanosomes which is crucial in maintaining cellular redox potential and is essential for the parasite's survival. This molecule is catalyzed by so many enzymes for which *Leishmania major* trypanothione reductase (*Lm*TR, E.C. 1.6.4.8) plays a critical role in the biosynthetic pathway. TR reduces trypanothione ($T[S]_2$) to dithiol ($T[SH]_2$). They catalyze the transfer of electrons from NADPH to their specific substrate via an FAD prosthetic group [3]. The reduced form is critical in regulating oxidative stress by reacting with reactive oxygen species (ROS) that are produced by the macrophage. $T[SH]_2$ is not only needed for detoxification of peroxides but also required for the synthesis of DNA precursors, homeostasis of ascorbate, sequestration and export of thiol conjugate [4].

Trypanothione reductase is a member of the disulphide oxidoreductase family of enzymes. It has an analogue in the human body, glutathione reductase (GR) which also carries out oxidoreductive reactions. But *Lm*TR does not process GSSG and host GR does not reduce $T[S]_2$ [5, 6]. The ascribed reasons for targeting *Lm*TR include the following: (i) trypanothione reductase is a key enzyme in regulating a reducing environment aiding in disease pathogenesis, (ii) this parasite does not depend on the host for reduced trypanothione, (iii) it has a less close known homologous protein in humans; (iv) the availability of template homologs for modeling purpose; and (v) moreover, *in vitro* trials have proven *Lm*TR to be a good therapeutic target [7].

Several inhibitors have been screened against this enzyme causing a reduction of infectivity and decreased capacity of the parasite to survive within intracellular macrophages. Potent compounds, such as 7-chloro-4-nitro-5-quinazolin-4-ylsulfanyl-2,1,3-benzothiadia-zole (CNQB) and 4-phenyl-5-(4-nitro-cinnamoyl)-1,3,4-thiadiazolium-2-phenylamine-chloride (PNTPC) with IC_{50} values 0.58 and 1.63 μM, respectively have already been tested in an *in vitro* assay against trypanothione reductase of trypanosomatids [8, 9].

Computer-aided drug designing is an *in-silico* approach for drug discovery that combines computational and pharmaceutical research [10]. This application helps in spanning the drug discovery pipeline and helps to speed up and rationalize the drug design process while reducing costs [11]. Ehrlich in 1909 first defined the term pharmacophore as 'a molecular framework that carries (*phoros*) the essential features responsible for a drug's (*pharmacon*) biological activity [12]. These features are essential functional groups of atoms in a three-dimensional position that interact with a receptor. Ligand-based drug design can be performed in association with molecular docking. These methods can be combined to identify a number of new hit compounds with potent inhibitory activity and to understand the main interactions at the binding sites. Appropriate use of these methods can improve the ability to identify and optimize hits and confirm their potential to serve as scaffolds for producing new therapeutic agents [13].

Drugs currently used for the treatment of human leishmaniasis are toxic, having severe adverse reactions which limit their use. Aside this includes, increase in resistance by the parasite, high cost of available drugs, lack of efficacy against VL \HIV co-infections with standard chemotherapy, and the development of a single drug or formulation for all forms of leishmaniasis [14–17]. Therefore, the development of novel, effective drugs with reduced side effects, is still a major priority for health researchers, in spite of many compelling research reports published on antileishmanial agents in the last 10 years [18]. In this study, *in silico* method of identifying leads was used incorporating the knowledge of pharmacophore and virtual screening to arrive at lead molecules. The overall goal of the study was to predict with high degree potent selective inhibitors of *Lm*TR from the African Natural Product Database (AfroDb) and North African Natural Product Database (NANPDB).

2. Materials and methods

2.1 Protein homology modeling

The protein sequence of trypanothione reductase of *Leishmania major* was retrieved from the NCBI database with the accession number XP_001687512.1, having 491 amino acids [19]. Using the Basic Local Alignment Search Tool (BLAST), the query sequence was compared to known structures which generated structures similar to *Lm*TR. Modeller 9.20 [20] was used for modeling the structure of *Lm*TR.

2.2 Active site prediction and quality assessment

To predict the active site, the protein was submitted to CASTp 3.0 [21, 22]. The predicted active site was corroborated via a blind docking process using AutoDock Vina within PyRx version 0.9.7 [23, 24]. The active region was confirmed by the 'Toggle selection of Spheres' function which highlighted predicted residues from CASTp 3.0. Binding pocket was also viewed with PyMOL v2.0.0 [25]. The quality of the modeled protein was assessed by some quality measure tools. This included PROSA which determines the quality of experimentally solved structures and theoretical models in protein engineering by comparing these to that of experimentally solved protein structures in the PDB database [26]. Verify3D was used to validate the three-dimensional structure of the model [27]. PROCHECK, a quality assessment tool was also used to check the stereochemical properties of the model by generating a Ramachandran plot [28]. ProQ was also used to carry out further validation. ProQ predicted protein quality based on the LGscore and MaxSub scores [29].

2.3 Energy minimization of protein target

The modeled *Lm*TR was energy minimized using GROMACS 5.1.1 [30, 31]. Simulations were performed with the force field, GROMOS96 43a1. The system was solvated using an equilibrated SPCE216 water model. The charged protein had a net charge of −9 which was neutralized with an equal amount of Na^+ ions. Energy minimization of the protein was then carried out.

2.4 Pharmacophore modeling and screening

2.4.1 Pharmacophore generation

Pharmacophore model, virtual screening, and molecular docking studies were performed to find novel *Lm*TR inhibitors. The ligand-based structural design incorporates the absence of the macromolecular structure by generating pharmacophore models from a set of ligands. This method takes advantage of the conformational flexibility of the ligands [32]. The active compounds, CNQB and PNTPC were retrieved with IDs CID1323435 and CHEMBL242165 from PubChem (https://pubchem.ncbi.nlm.nih.gov)and CHEMBL (https://www.ebi.ac.uk/chembl) [33, 34], respectively and were used to generate the pharmacophore. These ligands served as a training set for pharmacophore generation. All customized settings were kept in default.

2.4.2 Library preparation and pharmacophore validation

LigandScout 4.3 was used for screening a total of 5813 compounds including 885 AfroDb entries found in ZINC database [35] and 4928 NANPDB compounds [36]. The two actives were converted to SMILES format and submitted to the Directory of useful decoys and enhanced (DUD-E) database to generate decoys for the screening [37]. A total of 100 decoys were generated and used as a decoy library. The libraries were then converted into a .ldb file format. The reliability of the pharmacophore model was validated by the area under the receiver operating characteristic (ROC) curve (AUC) [38] using two descriptors, selectivity and sensitivity.

2.4.3 Screening with pharmacophore

LigandScout 4.3 allows *in-silico* screening of compound libraries using pharmacophore models as filter criteria. Database of active ligands was selected and marked in green with decoys marked in red. The screening process was initiated to generate hits corresponding to the pharmacophore model. These compounds were saved in an “sdf” file format to be used in the docking process.

2.5 Molecular docking

2.5.1 Docking of LmTR

The generated hit compounds were uploaded into PyRx (Version 0.9.6) [23]. The energy of the ligands was minimized using Universal Force Field (UFF) option in Open Babel incorporated in PyRx prior to docking. This was done to obtain 3D ligand structures which constitute atomic elements that have proper bond lengths between their atoms [39]. Ligands were converted to PDBQT format using AutoDock Vina embedded in the PyRx. Predicted active site residues were selected within a grid box of dimensions X: 42.39 Å, Y: 35.47 Å, and Z: 31.05.14 Å; and centre X: 28.58 Å, Y: 57.09 Å, and Z: −2.24 Å within the AutoDock Vina environment of PyRx for docking process.

2.5.2 Docking validation with AUC

Validation of the algorithm used for the docking process was carried out by generating an AUC plot. Decoys of five known inhibitors in complex with *Leishmania* trypanothione reductase of several species of *Leishmania* which included 2,3,4,6-tetra-*O*-acetyl-1-thio-beta-beta-D-glucopyranose (Auranofin); 4-[[1-(4-ethylphenyl)-2-methyl-5-(4-methylsulfonylphenyl)pyrrol-3-yl]methyl] thiomorpholine (CHEMBL1277380); 6-sec-butoxy-2-[(3-chlorophenyl)sulfanyl]-4-pyramidinamine (RDS); 2-(diethylamino)ethyl4-((3-(4-nitrophenyl)-3-oxopropyl) amino)benzoate (ZINC8782981); {N}-(4-azanylbutyl)- ~ {N}-(2-azanyl-2-oxidanylidene-ethyl)-7-(3-azanyl-3-oxidanylidene-propyl)-4-(dimethylamino)-2-(2-naphthal en-2-ylethylamino)pyrrolo[2,3-d]pyrimidine-6-carboxamide (H6H) were retrieved from DUD-E to generate an AUC curve. The result was correlated and plotted using their respective binding energies as the only variable via easyROC (Ver. 1.3) [40].

2.5.3 Docking validation via superimposition and alignment

Superimposition of the crystallographic ligand and re-docking poses was used as a means of validating docking. The five crystallographic ligands in complex with *Leishmania* trypanothione reductase were removed from the co-crystallized complex and re-docked. The pdb files of the re-docked complex were uploaded into PyMOL together with the solved complex from the Protein Data Bank. LigAlign [41] was then used to calculate the root mean square deviation between the superimposed re-docked and co-crystalized ligands. Superimposition also allowed the identification of critical overlapping residues via LigPlot$^+$. The FAD molecule from the template selected for modeling (PDB ID: 2JK6) was also extracted and docked in *Lm*TR. A comparative study of the original FAD-2JK6 complex and FAD-*Lm*TR complex was done using LigPlot$^+$.

2.6 Identification of lead compounds

To identify lead compounds the binding energy, molecular bond interactions, pharmacological, and physiochemical properties were considered. This step helped to filter generalized hit compounds. These compounds in SMILES format were submitted to SwissADME [42], which calculates the corresponding ADME (absorption, distribution, metabolism, and excretion) properties of the compounds. Hydrogen bond interactions of the ligand–protein complexes were studied using LigPlot$^+$ and PyMOL.

The hit compounds were physiochemically profiled to identify their drug-likeness and solubility in water. Lipinski's rule of 5 was used as a metric to narrow down druggable compounds [43]. Pharmacokinetic properties of predicted compounds were determined *in silico*. This included cytochrome inhibition, P-glycoprotein (P-gp) substrates, gastrointestinal (GI) absorption, and the blood–brain barrier (BBB) permeant.

2.7 Prediction of activity spectra for substances (PASS) for leads

PASS assesses the probability that a compound has a suspected biological activity [44]. It has been well known that each substance has a wide spectrum of biological activities as evident from some new uses of many old drugs. The SMILES format of the leads were submitted to Way2Drug.com [45] to predict possible biological activity.

2.8 Molecular dynamics simulation and MM-PBSA calculation of protein–ligand complexes

By employing GROMACS 2018 [31], the chain A of *Lm*TR and the *Lm*TR–ligand complexes were subjected to molecular dynamics simulations. Ligand topologies were generated via PRODRG which were converted to .gro files. Solvation of each of the protein–ligand complexes in a dodecahedron box was followed by neutralization of the output with sodium and chlorine ions. Each complex was minimized using the steepest descent algorithm coupled with the GROMOS43A force field. Equilibration protocol was carried out to restrain and relax protein–ligand positions. The MD production run was carried out for 100 ns. The output file was used in downstream processes to generate root mean-square deviation (RMSD), root mean-square fluctuation (RMSF) and radius of gyration (Rg) plots with Xmgrace (https://plasma-gate.weizmann.ac.il/Grace/). Molecular mechanics Poisson–Boltzmann surface area (MM-PBSA) was employed in calculating the free energies of the complexes. MM-PBSA was carried out using g_mmpbsa, which calculates binding energy components and the per-residue energy decomposition [46]. Graphs were generated using R-programming showing energy interactions.

3. Results and discussion

3.1 Homology modeling

L. major trypanothione reductase was modeled with an appreciable degree of accuracy and validated via several bioinformatics tools (**Figure 1A**). The protein sequence of *L. major* with the accession number XP_001687512.1, having 491 amino acids when searched amongst protein homologs in NCBI resulted in a list of similar structures with PDB codes 2JK6, 2X50, 6ER5, 1FEA from *Leishmania infantum* with their respective percentage identity of 95.72, 95.71, 95.70, and 78.78%, respectively. The similarity of structure and sequence between *Lm*TR protein sequence and the template 2JK6 was 95.72%. This favored its selection for the modeling process. The best model selection was based on the least discrete optimization potential energy (DOPE) score which informs about the energy of the protein.

3.2 Active site prediction

In predicting the active site of the protein, results obtained showed 73 binding pockets. Several pockets were identified but the pocket with the largest volume and surface area of 595.278 Å^3 and 924.887 Å^2, respectively was selected. Larger pockets favor conformational rotation during virtual screening. A total of 80 amino acid active site residues were predicted from CASTp 3.0 (**Table A1**). The predicted binding site was visualized using PyMOL (**Figure 1B**).

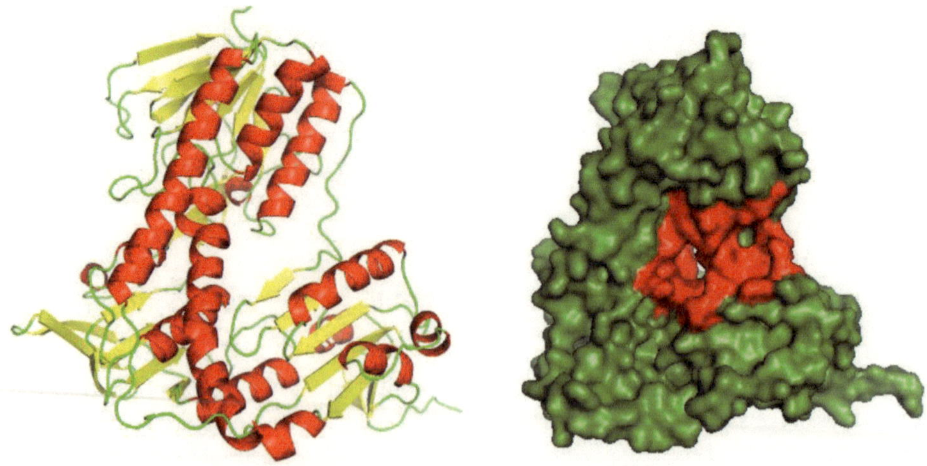

(a) (b)

Figure 1.
(a) 3D structure of modeled protein in cartoon representation. A monomer of LmTR *with alpha helices represented in red, the beta sheets in yellow and the loops in green. (b) Surface representation of the* LmTR. *Active site (in red) is the FAD binding region.*

The predicted active site was finally confirmed to be FAD binding site. TR has been studied to be a homodimer protein constituting FAD-binding, NADPH-binding, central, and interface domains [5]. The predicted site was concluded to be an FAD site in *Lm*TR by comparative studies between the FAD-2JK6 and FAD-*Lm*TR complexes (**Figure A1-A**). The study showed common hydrogen bonding residues including Ser14, Gly15, Arg287, and Thr335 interacting with FAD. These residues correlate with that which was predicted by CASTp 3.0 including other several common residues participating in hydrophobic interactions such as Gly13, Asp35, Ala46, Gly50, Thr51, and Cys52 (**Figure A1-A**).

3.3 Structural validation and quality prediction

PROSA was used to determine the quality of the structure by comparing it to protein structures that are experimentally solved in the PDB database. It validated the model based on the "quality score or *z*-score" with a value of −11.68. The *z*-score shows whether the predicted model is of X-ray or NMR quality with regards to the amino acid residues length. This *z*-score value showed that the modeled protein fell in the range of proteins solved experimentally by X-ray crystallography (**Figure A2-A**). Verify3D validated the 3D structure of the model. A good 3D structure is expected to have at least 80% of its amino acids to have scored greater than or equal to 0.2 in a 3D/1D profile. This model passed with an appreciable result of 91.65% of residues having a score greater or equal to 0.2 (**Figure A2-B**). Further validation with PROCHECK resulted in the generation of a Ramachandran plot (**Figure A3**). The plot described the rotations of the polypeptide backbone around the bonds between N-Cα (Phi, φ) and Cα-C (Psi, ψ). The plot allowed the viewing of the distribution of these torsional angles taking into consideration the allowed rotations and rotations that are unfavored which can result in a collision or steric hindrance. A protein with 90% of its residues in the most favorable region is considered a good model. ProQ predicted the quality of protein based on the MaxSub and LGscore scores [29]. The predicted LG score was 6.447 and MaxSub score was 0.520. LGscore >4 implied that the model was extremely good. Also, a MaxSub score > 0.5 implied that the model was very good [47].

3.4 Pharmacophore modeling

The active ligands used as training sets to develop a pharmacophore allowed features similar to the two compounds to be identified and combined into a single geometric function as the basis for the generation of the pharmacophore (**Figure 2**). Pharmacophore generated utilized features that contributed regions of hydrophobicity and hydrogen bond acceptors incorporated in the model for selective screening. The oxygen from nitrogen dioxide contributed to hydrogen bond acceptors with aromatic and alkene groups contributing to the hydrophobic region (**Figure A4**). A number of 10 hypotheses were developed for the model. The best hypothesis with a similarity of 58.12% had a score of 0.8537 and was selected based on the AUC score of 0.99 generated by LigandScout (**Figure A5-A**). The AUC score was used as a metric to validate how best the pharmacophore model created could distinguish rightly between active compounds and decoys. This intends to reduce false positives and negatives during the screening process.

The screening process was successfully completed with the model which identified 42 compounds that matched the pharmacophore model with a pharmacophore fit score ranging from 55.32 to 57.98 (**Table A2**).

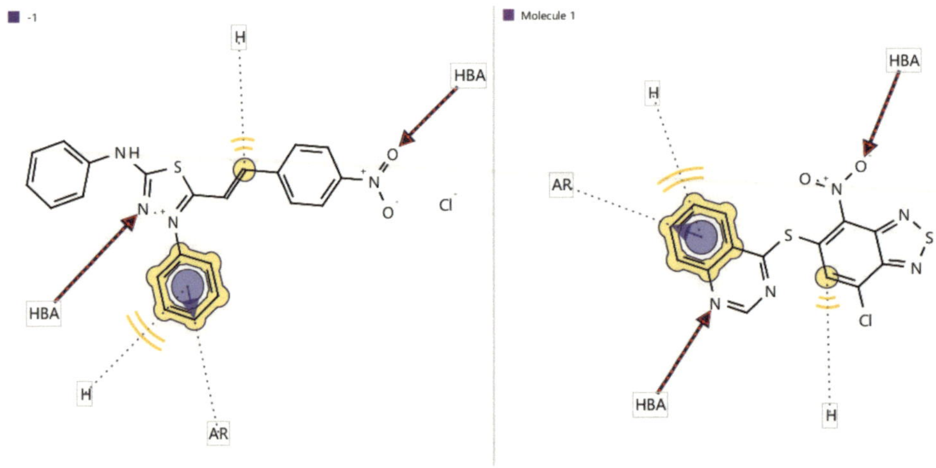

Figure 2.
2D structure of PNTPC (left) and CNQB (right) showing shared features. PNTPC and CNQB showed two hydrogen bond acceptors. Both compounds had an aromatic ring as a common feature. These served as active ligand for the training set.

3.5 Docking validation

The docking system was validated using the five inhibitors and 250 decoys generated with DUD-E and further used their binding energies to plot an AUC with a value of 0.702 (**Figure A5-B**). AUC value of 1.0 verifies that the prediction of hits obtained from the hypothesis is perfect whereas values of 0.5 and less than 0.70 imply average and moderate random selection respectively [48].

Furthermore, the validation of the molecular docking was also undertaken by aligning the re-docked ligands with their respective co-crystallized complexes taken from PDB. The RMSD values of the alignment between the re-docked ligands and the co-crystalized ligands in complexes of 2YAU, 4APN, 5EBK, 6ER5, 6I7N were 1.483, 3.020, 1.920, 2.712, and 2.465 Å, respectively. Only two of the RMSD values (5EBK and 2YAU) of the alignments were below 2.0 Å, which is considered the threshold for good alignment.

Superimposition also validated the accuracy of docking at the predicted active site. The FAD molecule from the template selected for modeling, 2JK6 when extracted and docked in *Lm*TR, showed similar surrounding residues in the pocket of FAD-2JK6 and FAD-*Lm*TR complex. Ligand alignment of these two complexes gave an RMSD of 3.291 Å which is above the expected threshold. Nonetheless, the FAD-*Lm*TR docking simulated a pose that showed common residues such as Ser14, Gly15, Arg287, and Thr335 taking part in hydrogen bonding in these complexes (**Figure A1**). All these verified that the docking system performed very well in docking ligands to the active site.

3.6 Virtual screening of pharmacophore hits

When docking validation was verified, molecular docking was carried out. Molecular docking predicted various conformations of each ligand in the binding site of the *Lm*TR. Compounds were selected based on their binding energies. The binding energies gave a theoretical value that relates the affinity of the ligand to the protein model. The results of the respective pharmacophore fit scores and binding energies are well documented (**Table A2**). The 42 compounds obtained were narrowed down to 11 by considering their binding energies and pharmacophore fit scores (**Table 1**). With respect to these studies to find inhibitors of the FAD binding site for which FAD is a prosthetic group that already binds tightly to the catalytic site, it was reasonable to select the compounds with binding energies below −9.0 kcal/mol or relatively closer to −9.0 kcal/mol which can provide a plausible binding advantage when acting as inhibitors at the site. The compound ZINC95486081 had the lowest binding energy of −9.8 kcal/mol and the highest was observed from evoxine as −6.2 kcal/mol (**Table A2**).

Predicted ligands	Pharmacophore fit score	Binding energy/ (kcal/mol)	Hydrogen bond Residues and length (Å)	Hydrophobic bond interacting residues
ZINC95486081	55.95	−9.8	Lys60 (2.92) Ser178 (2.87)	Gly13, Gly15, Asp32, Ala46, Thr51, Cys52, Val55, Gly56, Ala159, Thr160, Tyr198, Arg287, Asp327, Met333, Leu334, Thr335
MTPA	56.37	−9.4	Thr51 (3.12) Thr293 (2.89) Asp327 (3.13) Ser14 (3.17)	Gly11, Gly13, Gly15, Asp32, Val36, Ala46, Gly50, Cys52, Val55, Gly56, Ala159, Thr160, Tyr198, Arg287, Met333, Leu334, Thr335
Karatavicinol	56.5	−9.4	Thr51 (3.28) Arg287 (3.00) Thr293 (3.01, 2.97) Asp327 (2.82)	Ser14, Gly11, Gly13, Val34, Asp35, Val36, Gly50, Cys52, Ala46, Phe126, Gly127, Ala159, Thr160, Gly161, Tyr198, Arg290, Met333, Ala338
Taccalin	56.42	−9.4	Ser14 (3.21) Ala365 (3.25)	Gly13, Thr51, Cys52 Gly56, Cys57, Lys60, Gly161, Ile199, Thr198, Gly326, Met333, Leu334, Thr335, Ala338
Marmin	56.18	−9.3	Val34 (3.17) Thr51 (2.99, 3.04) Thr160 (2.83) Thr335 (2.87)	Leu10, Gly11, Gly13, Ser14, Asp35, Ala46 Gly50, Cys52, Gly127, Ala159, Gly161, Arg290, Leu294, Ala327, Leu334, Ala338
13-Hydroxyfeselol	55.62	−9.1	Val362 (2.79) Thr374 (2.85) Gly376 (3.20, 3.26)	Lys60, Thr198, Gly229, Phe230, Gly326, Leu334, Cys364, Ala365
Betaxanthin	57.51	−8.9	Ser14 (2.85) Cys52 (3.03) Gly127 (3.03, 3.22, 3.30) Thr335	Gly11, Gly13, Val34, Asp35, Val36, Gly50, Cys52, Ala46, Phe126, Ala159, Thr160, Gly161, Tyr198, Arg290, Asp327 Met333, Ala338
Colladonin	55.90	−8.8	Asn330 (2.85)	Lys60, Gly197, Tyr198, Tyr221, Arg287, Phe230, Leu334, Ala365
Feselol	55.63	−8.8	Asn330 (2.87)	Lys60, Gly197, Tyr198, Tyr221, Arg287, Phe230, Leu334, Ala365

Predicted ligands	Pharmacophore fit score	Binding energy/ (kcal/mol)	Hydrogen bond Residues and length (Å)	Hydrophobic bond interacting residues
ZINC38658035	55.95	−8.7	Tyr198 (3.31) Val362 (2.92) Tyr374 (3.30) Gly376 (2.86, 3.05)	Ile199, Phe230, Gly286 Arg287, Met333, Leu334, Cys364, Cys375
Pectachol	57.18	−8.5	Lys60 (2.93) Gly376 (3.11)	Tyr198, Gly229, Phe230, Val332, Met333, Leu334, Ala365, Val362, Cys364, Val366, Phe367
FAD molecule and inhibitors from 6ER5 and 4APN				
ZINC8782981	_	−7.2	Lys60 (3.12) Arg287 (3.08)	Cys52, Cys57, Tyr198, Gly229, Phe230, Val332, Met333, Leu334, Ala365, Val362, Cys364
CHEMBL1277380	_	−8.2	Lys60 (2.89)	Tyr198, Gly229, Phe230, Val332, Met333, Leu334, Ala365, Val362, Gly376
FAD	_	−9.0	Ser14 (3.11) Gly15 (2.96) Ala159 (2.97) Tyr198 (2.87) Arg287 (2.75) Met333 (2.78) Thr335 (2.88, 3.31)	Gly13, Gly50, Thr51, Cys52, Ser162, Gly197, Gly229, Phe230, Asp327, Leu334, Ala338

Table 1.
The table shows parameters involved in the selection of lead compounds. This included pharmacophore fit score, the binding energy and the number of hydrogen and hydrophobic bond interacting residues.

3.7 Protein–ligand interaction

Molecular interaction studies are important for understanding the mechanism of biological regulation at the molecular level and as such also provides a theoretical basis for drug design and discovery [49, 50]. Hydrogen and hydrophobic interactions are key players in stabilizing energetically favored ligands, in an open conformational environment of protein structures [29]. The intermolecular interaction and bond lengths of these 11 compounds were observed. The compound which showed the highest binding affinity, ZINC95486081 formed two hydrogen bonds with residues Lys60 and Ser178 with respective bond lengths of 2.92 Å and 2.87 Å. Five compounds including MTPA, Karatavicinol, Marmin, Betaxanthin and ZINC38658035 had four residues as the highest number of residues partaking in hydrogen bonding. MTPA formed hydrogen bonds with residues Thr51, Thr293, Asp327, and Ser14. Karatavicinol on the other hand formed hydrogen bonds with Thr51, Arg287, Thr293, and Asp327 (**Figure A6-A**). Marmin formed hydrogen bonds with Val34, Thr51, Thr160, and Thr335 (**Figure A6-B**). Betaxanthin also bonded with Ser14, Cys52, Gly127, and Thr335. Finally, ZINC38658035 formed hydrogen bonds with Tyr198, Val362, Tyr374, and Gly376. The compound 13-hydroxyfeselol was the only hit that formed three hydrogen bonds with Val362, Thr374, and Gly376. Taccalin and Pectachol formed only two hydrogen bonds with Ser14 and Ala365. On the other hand, Colladonin and Feselol formed the least hydrogen bond residues with Asn330. The shortest bond length of 2.83 Å was exhibited by Marmin with Thr160. Betaxanthin showed the highest pharmacophore fit score of 57.51 followed by Pectachol (57.18). 13-Hydroxyfeselol showed the lowest fit score of 55.62.

3.8 Pharmacological profiling

To identify lead compounds, the binding energy, molecular bond interactions, pharmacological, and physiochemical properties were considered. This step helped to filter generalized hit compounds. The top 11 compounds were profiled *in silico* to characterize compounds with drug-likeness and good water solubility. Lipinski's rule of 5 was used as a metric to narrow down druggable compounds. The rule factors in the compound's molecular weight which should not exceed 500 g/mol, hydrogen bond donors must not be more than 5, log-p value must be less than or equal to 5 and hydrogen bond acceptors must not be more than 10. All the 11 top hits passed Lipinski's rule of 5 with a good bioavailability score of 0.55 (**Table A3**).

3.9 Pharmacokinetic properties

Further filtering analysis subjected all 11 pharmacophore hits to pharmacokinetics profiling taking into consideration parameters such as gastrointestinal (GI) absorption, blood–brain barrier (BBB) permeation, the permeability of glycoprotein (Pgp), and cytochrome P450 (CYP). Physical parameters such as drug solubility may affect oral bioavailability but in most cases, the major determining factors are likely to be metabolism by CYP and absorption at the intestinal level [51]. CYP3A4 has been known to be responsible for the metabolism of about 50% of all drugs [52] and therefore inhibition of cytochrome can affect oxidation of substrates in cells. Absorption of drugs in the intestine if found high favors the efficacy of the compound as a drug. Multi-drug resistance transporters, such as P-glycoproteins, are essential for many cellular processes that require the transport of substrates across cell membranes [53]. Compounds that are P-gp substrates may face continual efflux which can affect the efficacy of drugs. The blood–brain barrier (BBB) prevents the brain uptake of most pharmaceuticals [54]. This is a disadvantage to neurological diseases but would be of merit since the disease of study is not related to the brain. Compounds that cross the blood–brain barrier may elucidate unwanted biological activities that could be dangerous to health. Therefore, the negative inference would be good for the compound. ZINC95486081 was predicted to show inhibition to three CYP isoenzymes. Karatavicinol, ZINC38658035, and Marmin excelled with an appreciable result (**Table A4**). For the purpose of narrowing down leads with potential for further computational analysis, compounds with low gastrointestinal absorption were side-lined. This included Taccalin and Betaxanthin.

3.10 Prediction activity spectra for substance (PASS)

The biological activity of the selected drug-like candidates was then evaluated using PASS. It is well known that each substance has a wide spectrum of biological activities as evident from some new uses of many old drugs. This allows the tool to utilize this information to predict biological activities based on their probable activity (Pa) and probable inactivity (Pi). When Pa is greater than Pi (Pa > Pi), the compound is likely to possess the predicted biological activity [55, 56]. PASS predicted Karatavicinol, Marmin, Colladonin and Pectachol to be potential antileishmanial agents (**Table A5**). Colladonin showed the highest Pa of 0.768 and Pi of 0.006 followed by Taccalin (Pa of 0.711 and Pi of 0.009) and

Pectachol with a Pa of 0.694 and Pi of 0.009. Betaxanthin had no prediction as an antileishmanial agent.

3.11 Selection of lead compounds for MD and MM-PBSA analysis

The various lead compounds were considered for selection based on the criteria above. ZINC95486081 and MTPA compound although had high binding energy trailed in pharmacokinetic properties and showed Pa less than 0.500. We eliminated Taccalin and Betaxanthin because of their low GI absorption and low Pa values (**Tables A3** and **A4**). Compounds predicted with good probable activity for antileishmanial activities included Karatavicinol, Taccalin, Marmin, 13-hydroxyfeselol, Colladonin, Feselol and Pectachol. A literature search revealed Feselol to have antiprotozoal activity against *Trypanosoma brucei* (IC_{50} 8.1 μM), *Trypanosoma cruzi* (IC_{50} 8.6 μM), and *Leishmania infantum* (IC_{50} 6.8 μM). Similarly, 10′*R*-karatavacinol has presented activity against *T. brucei* (IC_{50} 32.4 μM), *T. cruzi* (IC_{50} 9.4 μM), and *L. infantum* (IC_{50} 32.4 μM) [57]. That of Feselol and hydroxyfeselol was eliminated because it had been worked on experimentally and also extracts from *Ferula genus* which is known to exhibit antiviral, antibacterial, and antileishmanial properties [58]. Marmin and Pectachol presented optimistic potential to look into. The high number of hydrogen bonds and binding energy allowed for the inclusion of Karatavicinol in the MM-PBSA to observe their stabilization with this protein target. Also, the high prediction of Colladonin as a compound with probable activity also increased the chance of this compound for MM-PBSA analysis. Therefore, Marmin Pectachol, Karatavicinol, and Colladonin were considered for further analysis in molecular dynamics.

3.12 Molecular dynamic simulation of protein–ligand complex

Molecular dynamics simulation allowed the early view of proteins as relatively rigid structures to be replaced by a dynamic model in which the internal motions and resulting conformational changes play an essential role in its function [59]. An RMSD plot generated after molecular dynamics simulation showed a deviation of about 0.25 Å (**Figure A7**). Further scrutinized with molecular dynamics simulations gave the protein a dynamic dimension to its 3D structural form producing a realistic environment for the ligand interactions that were carried out in the docking process.

Molecular dynamics simulations can also capture a wide variety of important biomolecular processes, including conformational change, ligand binding, and protein folding [60]. The stability of docked protein–ligand complexes was determined by their (RMSD) plots generated from the MD simulation output file. The backbones of the four complexes were observed to be stable over time (**Figure 3**). The fluctuations of the protein–ligand complexes were analyzed within the system to check for movement and structural stability during the course of the simulation. These movements and stability are significant for the complex functioning inside living systems. The backbone of the *Lm*TR-ZINC8782981 complex showed the greatest stability with an average RMSD of 0.25 nm amongst all the complexes. The *Lm*TR-CHEMBL1277380 complex was fairly stable with RMSD of 0.4 nm. Amongst the four leads, Pectachol was found with the lowest RMSD of 0.3 nm. In terms of stability, the compound Marmin and Colladonin proved to be very much stable around 0.73 nm over the production time of 100 ns. The RMSD of Karatavicinol was observed to show stability from 0 to 60 ns and increased its RMSD to 0.5 nm from 60 to 100 ns.

The flexibility of residues contribution by the *Lm*TR was assessed by the root mean square fluctuation (RMSF). RMSF indicates the flexibility of different regions of a protein, which can be related to crystallographic B factors [61]. The results of

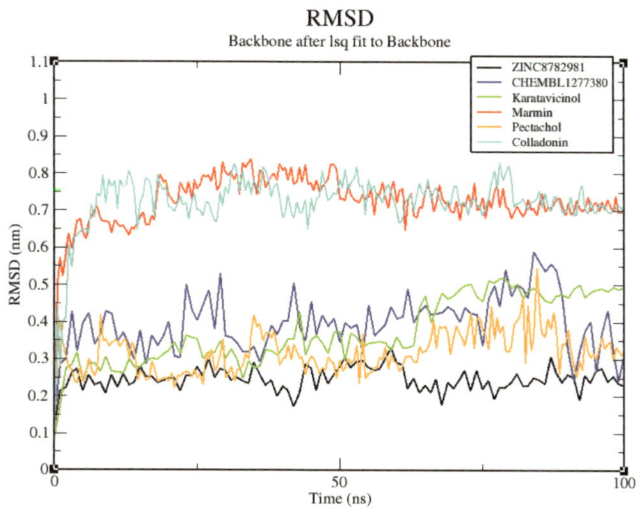

Figure 3.
RMSD values of the LmTR*-ligand complexes of the four leads (Karatavicinol, Marmin, Pectachol, and Colladonin) and the two known inhibitors after 100 ns. The complexes in the graph are color coded.*

the RMSF plots showed consistency for the docked complexes (**Figure A8**). The highest fluctuations exhibited was observed around residue numbers 70–90, with Karatavicinol and CHEMBL1277380 showing higher fluctuation levels followed by ZINC8782981 and Marmin complexes. Other regions where good fluctuations were observed include residues between 395 and 410 and 465–480. Overall, Marmin showed more fluctuations around most residues with a distinct difference at residue numbers 260 and 310.

The compactness of the complexes over simulation time is determined by the Rg. If a protein is folded well, it will likely maintain a relatively steady value of Rg, whereas its value will change over time if the protein unfolds [62]. Rg values of all complexes indicated stable complexes over 100 ns (**Figure A9**). The Rg graph showed most compounds experienced a fairly stable Rg. Marmin experienced the lowest Rg value around 2.33 nm compared to other complexes. This was followed by Colladonin, Pectachol and Karatavicinol with Rg values of 2.37, 2.42, and 2.45 nm, respectively. Between the known inhibitors, CHEMBL1277380 was observed to have an average Rg value of 2.46 nm whilst ZINC8782981 showed the average highest value of around 2.5 nm. Inferring from the Rg graph, the compactness of the *Lm*TR–Marmin, –Colladonin and –Pectachol complexes were maintained after complex formation.

3.13 Evaluation of leads using MM-PBSA

MM-PBSA was employed to calculate free binding energies by per-residue decomposition of the protein complexes. At a quantitative level, simulation-based methods provide substantially more accurate estimates of ligand binding affinities (free energies) than other computational approaches such as docking [63]. Residues contributing binding free energy greater than 5 kJ/mol or less than −5 kJ/mol are considered critical for binding of a ligand to a protein [64]. MM-PBSA results showed only Asp327 amongst the hydrogen bonding residues of Karatavicinol to contribute a per residue decomposition energy of 13.65 kJ/mol. Amino acid residue Asp35 (21.89 kJ/mol) was observed with such greater contribution (**Figure A10**). The complex of *Lm*TR–Marmin also showed surrounding hydrophobic residues Asp35 (−8.62 kJ/mol), Ala46 (−7.65 kJ/mol), Arg290 (8.83 kJ/mol), and Glu141

(−5.12 kJ/mol) with their energy decomposition to be greater than 5 kJ/mol and less than −5 kJ/mol. The only hydrogen bonding residue that showed a relevant contribution of energy decomposition was Thr51 (−16.36 kJ/mol) (**Figure 4**). Hydrophobic amino acid residues Lys61 (−5.16 kJ/mol), Tyr198 (−11.29 kJ/mol), Asp327 (5.56 kJ/mol), and Arg331 (6.38 kJ/mol) showed relevant contribution to the total binding energy of the *Lm*TR–Colladonin complex (**Figure A11**). Moreover, only hydrogen bonding residue Lys60 (13.32 kJ/mol) in *Lm*TR–Pectachol complex showed to be a critical residue in binding. Other surrounding residues contributed substantially to the per residue energy decomposition in the *Lm*TR–Pectachol complex. This included Lys61 (−10.97 kJ/mol), Arg287 (−6.91 kJ/mol), Asp327 (9.30 kJ/mol), Met333 (−6.72 kJ/mol), Leu334 (−8.91 kJ/mol), Lys361 (6.46 kJ/mol), and Cys364 (−6.07 kJ/mol) (**Figure A12**). Deducing from the substantial contribution of energy per decomposition of residues, we propose Asp35, Thr51, Lys61, Tyr198, and Asp327 to be critical in intermolecular bonding and stabilization of ligands at the FAD active site.

3.14 Other energy terms

Van der Waals forces, electrostatic and polar solvation energies, and SASA are relevant energy terms contributing to the overall free binding energy of the complex. The van der Waals energy refers to the weak attraction existing between the intermolecular forces. The van der Waals energy observed in our study showed Karatavicinol and CHEMBL1277380 to have the lowest and highest energy of −228.565 and − 171.823 kJ/mol, respectively. Colladonin, Marmin, and Pectachol also showed relatively low van der Waals energy of −189.289, −189.229, and − 209.538 kJ/mol, respectively as compared with ZINC8782981 with −222.123 kJ/mol. Electrostatic energy refers to the potential energy of a system consisting of different electric charges [65–67]. The lowest electrostatic energy was exhibited by Marmin (−386.401 kJ/mol) followed by Pectachol (−286.260 kJ/mol), and Colladonin (−249.067 kJ/mol). Karatavicinol and the other two inhibitors were observed with high electrostatic energy (**Table 2**). Some studies have observed that

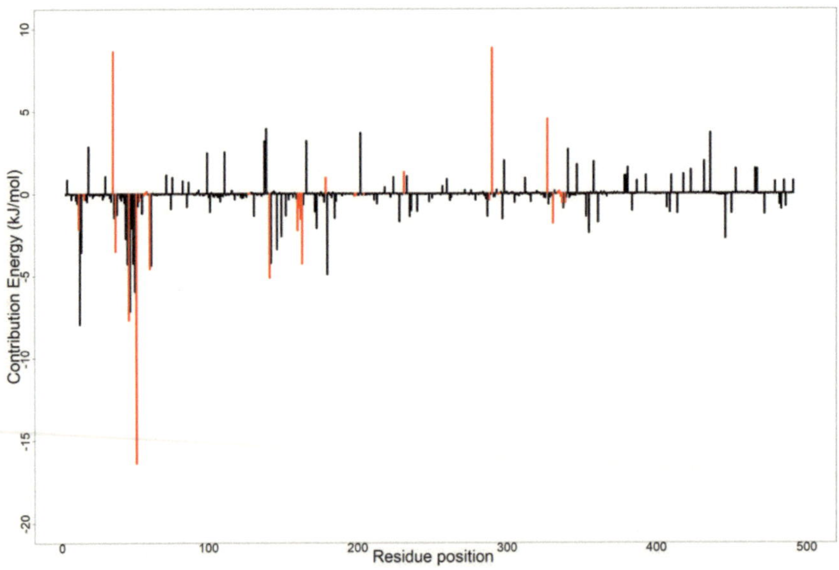

Figure 4.
MM-PBSA plot of the binding free energy decomposition contribution per residue of Lm*TR–Marmin complex. Coded red lines represent surrounding active site amino acid residues.*

van der Waals and electrostatic forces contribute favorably to the energetics of binding along with simulations that favor the binding of complexes [66, 68].

Polar solvation energy on the other hand refers to the electrostatic interaction that exists between the solute and the continuum solvent [69]. The highest polar solvation energy amongst the leads was exhibited by Marmin (484.074 kJ/mol) and the lowest by Karatavicinol (227.483 kJ/mol). Solvent accessible surface area (SASA) energy was calculated after MD. This represents the non-polar solvation energy [69]. This energy measures the interactions that exist between the complex and the solvents. Amongst the leads, Karatavicinol obtained the lowest SASA energy followed by Pectachol, Colladonin, and Marmin (**Table 2**). Relative to these were the low SASA energies of the inhibitors ZINC8782981 and CHEMBL1277380.

The total contribution of these energies enabled the final estimation of the free binding energies in the complexes (**Table 2**). The lowest free binding energy contributing to more stability of the protein–ligand complex was observed by Marmin (−109.114 kJ/mol). Next amongst the four complexes was Pectachol (−63.487), followed by Karatavicinol (−57.644 kJ/mol), and Colladonin (−48.936 kJ/mol). The low binding energy of Marmin was much closer to that of CHEMBL1277380 (−111.732 kJ/mol) with that of Pectachol higher than ZINC8782981 (−54.399 kJ/mol). These energies address the potential of Marmin and Pectachol to bind most effectively at the active site of *Lm*TR. *Lm*TR–Marmin's free binding energy correlated with the low binding energy (−9.3 kcal/mol) from docking. That of Pectachol showed a good free binding energy than that obtained from docking. This was better than that of Karatavicinol and Colladonin (**Table 1**).

3.15 Exploring possible implications and structure similarities of predicted leads

Karatavicinol and Marmin had lower binding energies of −9.4 and − 9.3 kcal/mol, respectively, as compared to Colladonin (−8.5 kcal/mol) and Pectachol (−8.5 kcal/mol). These binding energies are closer to that of FAD (−9.0 kcal/mol) for which can possibly compete in binding at the FAD domain. These compounds were concluded to have drug-likeness by satisfying Lipinski's rule of 5. They also do not pass the blood–brain barrier which is good. Also, Marmin and Karatavicinol checked false for p-glycoprotein substrate. This gives the compounds an advantage to maintain their concentrations in cellular level to maximize efficacy. Pectachol and Colladonin however were implicated as P-gp substrates. These predicted preferable properties can favor their lead likeness and chances of going a long way in experimental studies. The four lead compounds were predicted as antileishmanial compounds. The four leads are confirmed not to be already existing antileishmanial drugs by structural similarity searches in www.DrugBank.ca but rather observed to be analogues of chrome 2-one. In regard to this, studies over the years have however shown some novel compounds such as 7-{[(2R*)-3,3-dimethyloxiran-2-yl]methoxy}-8-[(2R*,3R*)-3-isopropenyloxiran-2-yl]-2H-chromen-2-one and 7-methoxy-8-(4-methyl-3-furyl)-2H-chromen-2-one against *Leishmania donovani* with EC_{50} of 9.9 and 10.5 μg/mL, respectively [70]. These tested compounds with antileishmanial effect tend to be analogues of chromen-2-one. We emphasize that Karatavicinol is not a unique lead compound since it has already been experimented on other *Leishmania* species excluding *L. major* [57]. But the study identified it via these computational processes and therefore would report it as a potential compound against *L. major*. This augments the fact that the computational drug discovery pipeline has an optimistic potential of yielding good candidates for experimental work. Colladonin on the other hand is an enantiomer of Feselol for which Feselol is experimented as an antileishmanial agent [57]. Marmin also holds a very good potential of being an anti-ulcerative agent [71]. This favors it being a good

Compound	Van der Waals energy (kJ/mol)	Electrostatic energy (kJ/mol)	Polar solvation energy (kJ/mol)	SASA energy (kJ/mol)	Binding energy (kJ/mol)
ZINC8782981	−222.123 ± 14.568	−52.495 ± 17.662	245.049 ± 33.654	−24.829 ± 0.962	−54.399 ± 20.084
CHEMBL1277380	−171.823 ± 14.173	−2.926 ± 5.485	82.884 ± 16.706	−19.869 ± 1.202	−111.732 ± 16.514
Karatavicinol	−228.565 ± 12.673	−32.345 ± 21.415	227.483 ± 27.305	−24.217 ± 1.100	−57.644 ± 24.019
Marmin	−189.289 ± 16.726	−386.401 ± 30.540	484.074 ± 28.991	−17.498 ± 1.050	−109.114 ± 23.461
Pectachol	−189.229 ± 18.203	−286.260 ± 49.152	430.604 ± 71.136	−18.602 ± 1.308	−63.487 ± 33.289`
Colladonin	−209.538 ± 18.908	−249.067 ± 40.851	427.216 ± 49.348	−17.548 ± 1.122	−48.936 ± 24.773

The energy values are presented as mean ± standard deviation kJ/mol.

Table 2.
The energy terms obtained after MM-PBSA analysis of the protein–ligand complexes.

compound for the treatment of cutaneous leishmaniasis. These compounds classified are coumarins and more other studies have reported good antileishmanial activities from this class of compounds [72, 73]. This work supports the fact that Karatavicinol, Marmin, Pectachol and Colladonin may possibly exhibit good antileishmanial activity if tested *in vitro* (**Table A6**).

Further in this study, the interaction of the active site residues with all four lead compounds showed hydrogen bonding with Val34, Thr51, Lys60, Thr160, Ala159, Arg287, Thr293, Asp327, Asn330, Thr335, and Gly376 (**Table 1**). Superimposition of the docked 2JK6 and co-crystallized revealed common residues such as Ser14, Gly15, Arg287, and Thr335 (**Figure A1**). These residues can be observed to be unique to the FAD domain of *Lm*TR in anchoring the FAD molecule. Comparing these residues to the hydrogen bonding residues from the four leads shows that possible interruption of any of these residues can cause conformational changes which might not favor the selective binding of FAD at its domain. Baiocco et al. in 2009 identified Thr335 of trypanothione reductase at the FAD catalytic site of *L. infantum* [74]. They proposed that the FAD molecule binds tightly to the protein and orients itself towards the hydride transfer region of the active site by hydrogen bonding with specific residues Lys60, Thr335, and His461. Having observed this, interrupting one of these residues can potentially inhibit the reduction of $T[S]_2$ by interfering with the hydride transfer. These compounds can potentially covey a competitive mode for binding to Thr355 which can affect the hydride transfer reaction in the active site preventing direct inactivation of trypanothione reductase. Other studies with quinone derivatives also have identified Thr355 and Ser14 as unique to the FAD domain of TR [75, 76].

4. Conclusion

Trypanothione reductase has been a well-investigated target essential for trypanosomatids. Its function in controlling oxidative stress in the parasite provided an opportunity to target the trypanothione biosynthesis pathway. A total of 11 hit compounds identified by pharmacophore modeling and virtual screening were filtered to four potential leads by considering their ADME with their molecular interactions in *Lm*TR. MM-PBSA enabled the individual computation of active site residues that contributed significantly to binding. Efficient selective blockade of *Lm*TR with these four coumarin compounds: Karatavicinol (7-[(2E,6E,10S)-10,11-dihydroxy-3,7,11-trimethyldodeca-2,6-dienoxy]chromen-2-one), Marmin (7-[(E,6R)-6,7-dihydroxy-3,7-dimethyloct-2-enoxy]chromen-2-one), Pectachol (7-[(6-hydroxy-5,5,8a-trimethyl-2-methylidene-3,4,4a,6,7,8-hexahydro-1*H*-naphthalen-1-yl)methoxy]-6,8-dimethoxychromen-2-one), and Colladonin (7-[[(4*aS*)-6-hydroxy-5,5,8*a*-trimethyl-2-methylidene-3,4,4*a*,6,7,8-hexahydro-1*H*-naphthalen-1-yl]methoxy]chromen-2-one) hold the potential to compromise the redox defenses of the parasites by inhibiting the FAD binding region and correspondingly increasing their sensitivity to redox-damage when carried out in *in vitro* and *in vivo* studies. Residues such as Asp35, Thr51, Lys61, Tyr198, and Asp327 are suspected to have critical role in the anchoring of FAD which contributes to the formation of reduced $T[SH]_2$ in the reducing environment of amastigotes.

Acknowledgements

The authors are grateful to the West African Centre for Cell Biology of Infectious Pathogens (WACCBIP) at the University of Ghana for making Zuputo, a Dell EMC high-performance computing cluster, available for this study.

Conflict of interest

The authors declare no conflict of interest.

A. Appendices and nomenclature

Leu10, Gly11, Gly13, Ser14, Gly15, Gly16, Val34, Asp35, Val36, Phe44, Ala46, Ala47, Gly50, Thr51, Cys52, Val55, Gly56, Cys57, Lys60, Lys61, Gly125, Phe126, Gly127, Ala128, Arg138, Ser140, Glu141, Pro143, Ala159, Thr160, Gly161, Ser162, Trp163, Pro164, Thr165, Thr177, Ser178, Asn179, Phe182, Tyr198, Ile199, Glu202, Phe203, Met282, Leu283, Ala284, Ile285, Gly286, Arg287, Arg290, Thr293, Leu294, Gln295, Ile325, Gly326, Asp327, Val332, Met333, Leu334, Thr335, Pro336, Val337, Ala338, Ile339, Asn340, Arg355, Thr357, Asp358, His359, Thr360, Lys361,Val362, Ala363, Cys364, Ala365, Phe367, Pro435, Glu436, Ile438, Gln439, Gly442, Ile443, Lys446

Table A1.
Predicted amino acid residues.

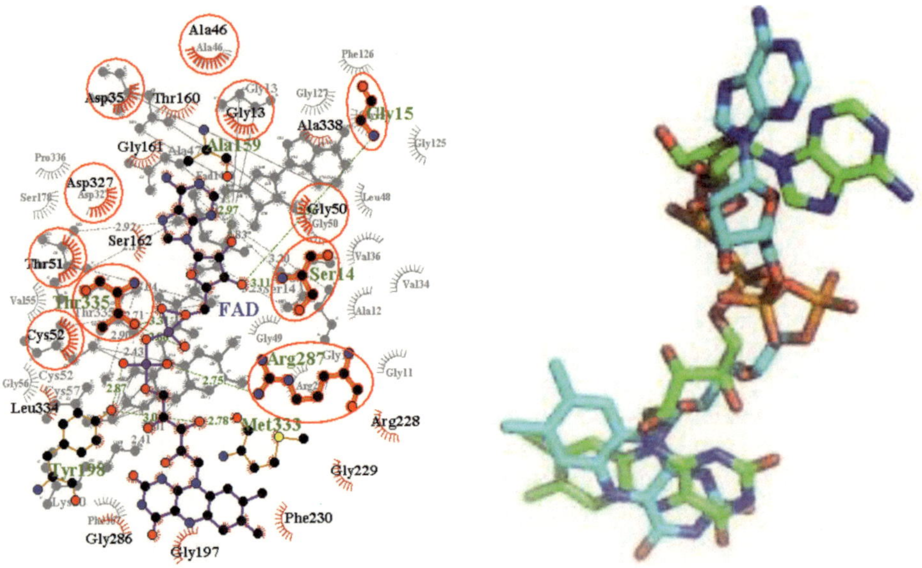

(a) (b)

Figure A1.
(a) The Z-score of the modeled LmTR *(represented in dot) estimated to be −11.68 which is within the range of experimentally determined proteins by X ray method. (b) Verify 3D plot of the modeled protein structure,* LmTR*. This shows 91.65% of its amino acid residues with an average 3D-1D score greater than or equal to 0.2, which is a positive inference to the expected 80% of amino acids with 3D-1D score above or equal to 0.2.*

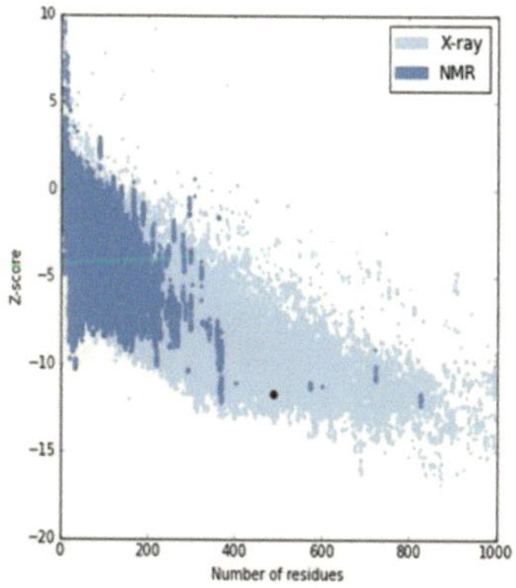

(a)

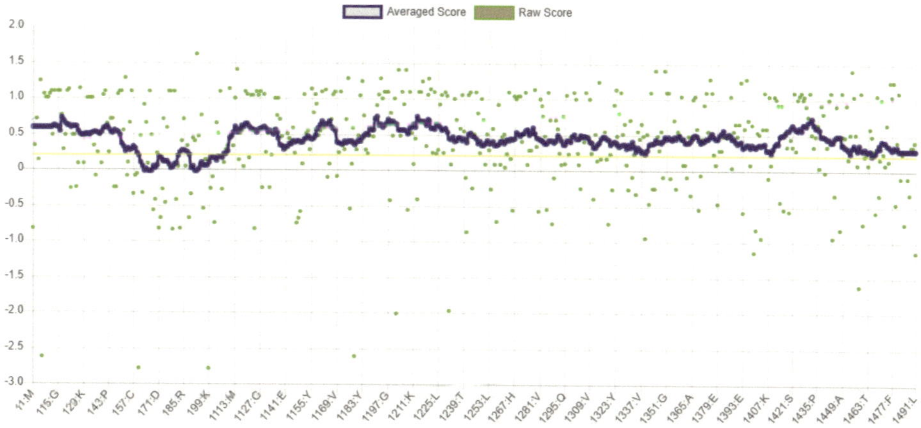

(b)

Figure A2.
Ramachandran plot of the modeled LmTR *protein structure. The percentage of residues in the most favored region (red) was 93.6% which is favorable for the protein's stereochemistry. The percentage of residues in the allowed region (yellow) was 6%. Only 0.2% of protein residues (Phe45) showed probable stereochemical hindrance or collision.*

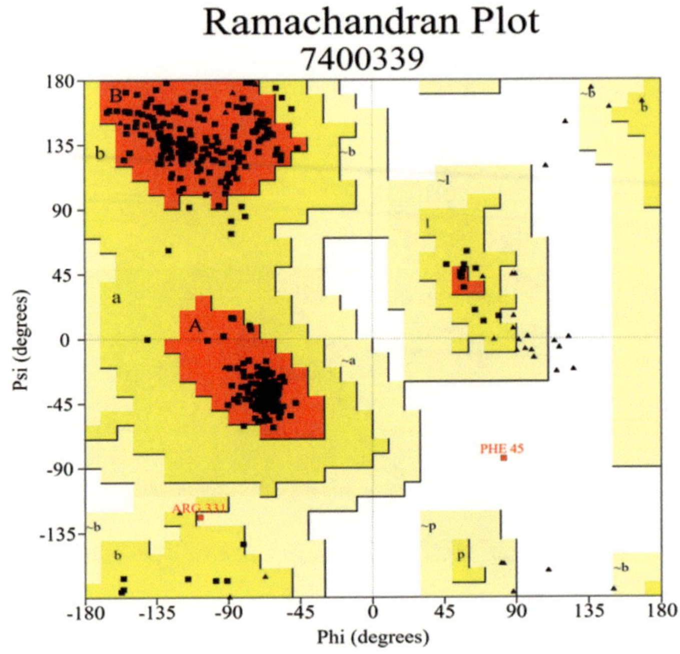

Figure A3.
A 3D geometry of the generated pharmacophore. The nitrogen on the bicyclic ring of CNQB with the oxygen from the nitro group on its purine ring derivative contributed a hydrogen bond acceptor HBA (red sphere). The oxygen from the nitrogen dioxide group on the conjugated benzene in addition to the nitrogen on the five-member ring of PNTPC also contributed to HBA. Both had an aromatic ring (blue ring) as a common feature (blue ring in yellow 3D sphere) which contributed to hydrophobic interactions and the alkene feature shared amongst them generated the same hydrophobicity.

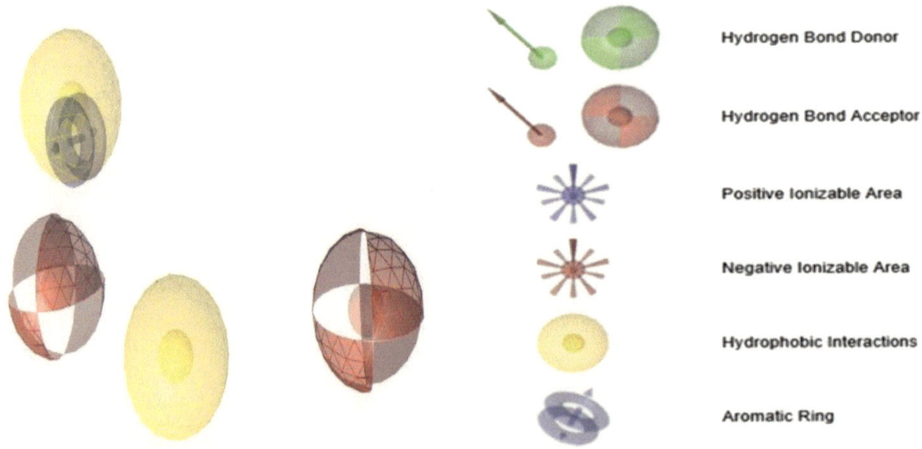

Figure A4.
*(A) AUC score of 0.99 for the pharmacophore model. Determined at 1, 5, 10, and 100% of the selected database were the AUC and EF values as shown. The median is shown by dotted lines. If the curve is closer to the median it would suggest poor model. (B) AUC score of 0.702 generated for validating the docking system used. It verified the correlation between virtual screening performance and binding site descriptors of protein targets model (*LmTR*).*

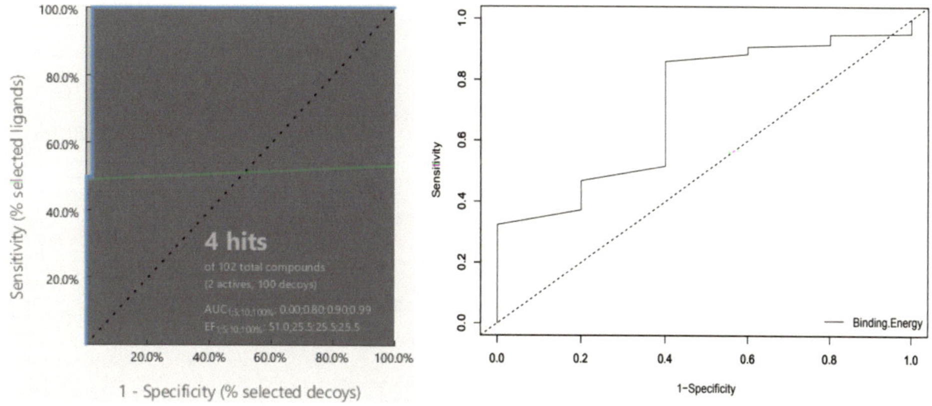

(A) **(B)**

Figure A5.
(a) 2D schematic diagram of co-crystallized FAD (PDB ID: 2JK6) and FAD docked in LmTR *superimposed together. Similar hydrogen bonding residues include Ser14, Gly15, Arg287, and Thr335. Similar hydrophobic residues in addition confirm the predicted active site. (b) Ligand alignment of co-crystalized FAD and FAD docked in* LmTR*.*

Name	P-fit score	Binding energy (kcal/mol)	Active/ decoy	Source database
ZINC95486081	55.95	−9.8	Active	AfroDB
(S)-alpha-methoxy-alpha-trifluoromethyl-alpha-phenylacetate (MTPA)	56.37	−9.4	Active	NANPDB
Karatavicinol	56.5	−9.4	Active	NANPDB
Taccalin	56.42	−9.4	Active	NANPDB
Marmin	56.18	−9.3	Active	NANPDB
3-Hydroxyfeselol	55.62	−9.1	Active	NANPDB
ZINC95486257	55.9	−9.0	Active	AfroDB
Betaxanthin	56.97	−8.9	Active	NANPDB
Coladonin	56.58	−8.8	Active	NANPDB
Feselol	56.41	−8.8	Active	NANPDB
ZINC38658035	55.9	−8.7	Active	AfroDB
Pectachol	57.18	−8.5	Active	NANPDB
ZINC85967928	55.85	−8.4	Active	AfroDB
Polyanthin	56.39	−8.4	Active	NANPDB
ZINC95486047	57.98	−8.3	Active	AfroDB
4′-Methyl gossypetin	56.17	−8.2	Active	NANPDB
2-(nonan-8-one)-4-methoxy-quinoline	56.41	−8.2	Active	NANPDB
Orientin	55.53	−8.1	Active	NANPDB
Kaempferol-3,6-dimethylether-7-glucoside	57.15	−7.8	Active	NANPDB
ZINC95486129	56.43	−7.8	Active	AfroDB
Ethuliaconyzophenone	56.9	−7.7	Active	NANPDB
ZINC95486209	56.55	−7.5	Active	AfroDB
(+)-1,2-bis-(4-hydroxy-3-methoxyphenyl)-propane-1,3-diol [erythro form]	55.9	−7.4	Active	NANPDB
4-Hydroxy-2′,4′-dimethoxy-dihydrochalcone	55.58	−7.4	Active	NANPDB
Drimartol A	56.31	−7.4	Active	NANPDB
Isoarnottinin-4′-*O*-beta-D-glucoside	55.71	−7.4	Active	NANPDB
4-Beta-hydroxy-6alpha-(4-hydroxy-3-methoxybenzoyl)-7-daucen-9-one	55.93	−7.4	Active	NANPDB
ZINC14686464	56.55	−7.4	Active	AfroDB
6-(3′,4′-dimethoxybenzoyl)-jaeschkeanadiol	57.17	−7.3	Active	NANPDB
ZINC14887523	56.88	−7.3	Active	AfroDB
Orientin-7-methoxide	56.26	−7.2	Active	NANPDB
ZINC14444870	56.35	−7.2	Active	AfroDB
ZINC14689062	56.5	−7.2	Active	AfroDB
1-Dehydrogingerdione	56.05	−7.1	Active	NANPDB
Onopordin	56.27	−7.1	Active	NANPDB
ZINC95486194	56.79	−7.1	Active	AfroDB
Methyl5-(3-4-dihydroxyphenyl)-3-hydroxypenta-2,4-dienoate	55.32	−7	Active	NANPDB

Name	P-fit score	Binding energy (kcal/mol)	Active/ decoy	Source database
Corniculatusin	56.23	−7	Active	NANPDB
3-(10-acetoxygeranyl)-4-acetoxy-*p*-coumaric acid	56.14	−7	Active	NANPDB
ZINC00035526	56.66	−7	Active	AfroDB
ZINC00608186	57.08	−6.8	Active	AfroDB
Evoxine	57.32	−6.2	Active	NANPDB

Table A2.
The 42 hits obtained from pharmacophore screening with their respective pharmacophore fit score, binding energies, and data sources.

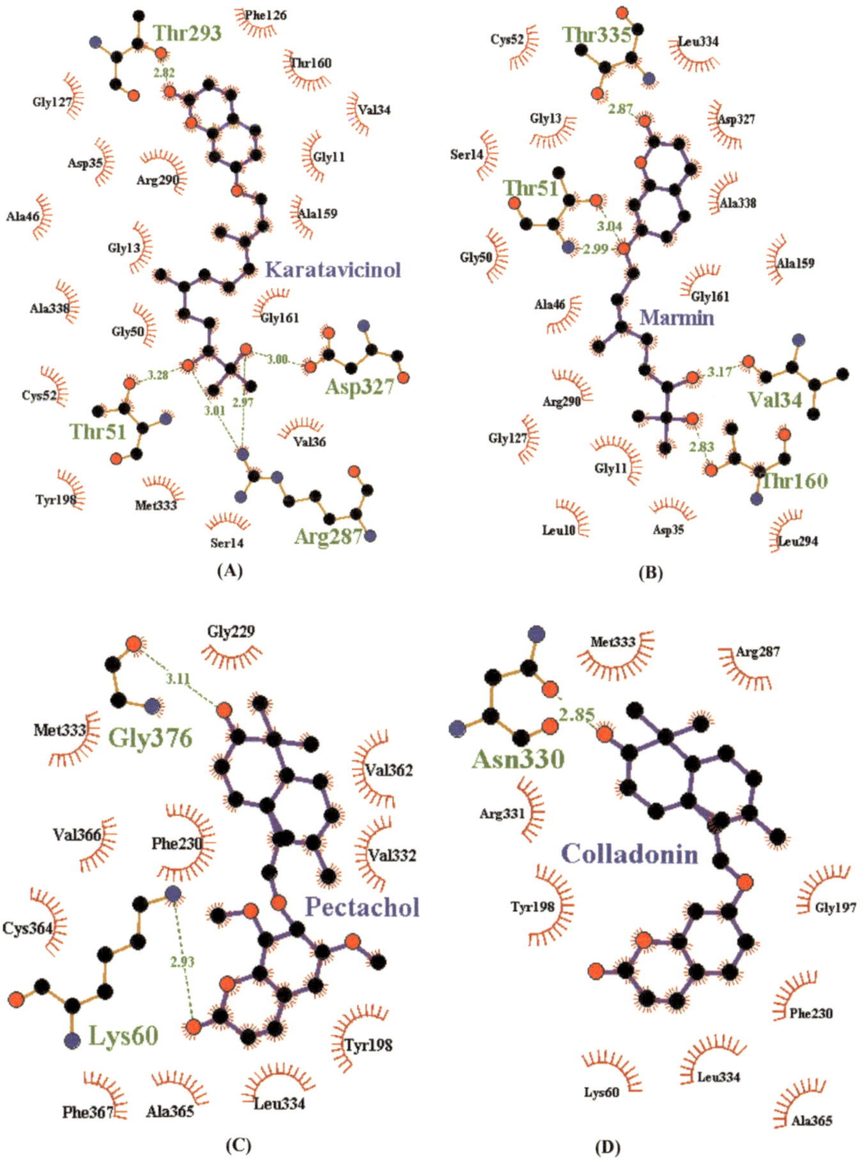

Figure A6.
2D schematic diagram showing protein-ligands interaction of some leads at the active site of Lm*TR. (A)* Lm*TR–Karatavicinol interaction profile, (B)* Lm*TR–Marmin interaction profile, (C)* Lm*TR–Pectachol interaction profile, and (D)* Lm*TR–Colladonin interaction profile.*

Compound ZINC ID/name	Number of Lipinski's rules violated	MW (g/mol)	No. HA	No. HD	xLogP	Water solubility (mg/mL)	Log S	Bio. Sc
ZINC95486081	0	382.45	5	2	4.52	Moderately soluble	−5.84	0.55
MTPA	0	470.52	8	0	6.35	Moderately soluble	−6.00	0.55
Karatavicinol	0	400.51	5	2	4.66	Moderately soluble	−4.85	0.55
Taccalin	0	418.48	9	6	−1.45	Moderately soluble	1.66	0.55
Marmin	0	332.39	5	2	2.81	Soluble	−3.52	0.55
13-Hydroxyfeselol	0	400.51	5	2	1.45	Moderately soluble	−5.93	0.55
Betaxanthin	0	370.44	8	7	−1.17	Moderately soluble	−2.11	0.55
Colladonin	0	384.51	4	1	5.76	Poorly soluble	−6.50	0.55
Feselol	0	384.51	4	1	5.76	Poorly soluble	−6.5	0.55
ZINC38658035	0	464.63	6	3	−4.47	Soluble	−3.28	0.55
Pectachol	0	444.56	6	1	5.70	Poorly soluble	−6.70	0.55

All the hits showed good druglikeness. MW, molecular weight; No. HD, number of H-bond donors; Bio Sc, bioavailability score, No. HA, number of H-bond acceptors.

Table A3.
Physicochemical profiling of the 11 hit compounds.

Compound ZINC ID	GI absorption	BBB permeant	P-gp substrate	CYP1A2 inhibitor	CYP2C19 inhibitor	CYP2C9 inhibitor	CYP2D6 inhibitor	CYP3A4 inhibitor
ZINC95486081	High	Yes	Yes	No	No	Yes	Yes	Yes
MTPA	High	No	No	No	No	No	Yes	Yes
Karatavicinol	High	No	No	No	No	No	No	Yes
Taccalin	Low	No	Yes	No	No	No	No	No
Marmin	High	No	No	No	No	No	No	No
13-Hydroxyfeselol	High	No	Yes	No	No	No	Yes	Yes
Betaxanthin	Low	No	No	No	No	No	No	No
Colladonin	High	Yes	No	No	No	No	Yes	No
Feselol	High	Yes	No	No	No	No	Yes	No
ZINC38658035	High	No	Yes	No	No	No	No	No
Pectachol	High	No	Yes	No	No	No	Yes	No

Four compounds out of the 11 showed an appreciable pharmacological property. This included Karatavicinol, Marmin, Colladonin, and Pectachol.

Table A4.
Pharmacological profiling of top 11 compounds characterized by gastrointestinal (GI) absorption, blood brain barrier (BBB) permeant, p-gp substrates, and cytochrome P450 inhibitors.

Lead compounds	Antileishmanial predicted activity	
	Pa	Pi
ZINC95486081	0.224	0.168
MTPA	0.263	0.130
Karatavicinol	0.513	0.021
Taccalin	0.711	0.009
Marmin	0.557	0.024
13-Hydroxyfeselol	0.658	0.030
Betaxanthin	—	—
Colladonin	0.768	0.006
Feselol	0.768	0.006
ZINC38658035	0.345	0.074
Pectachol	0.694	0.009

Karatavicinol, Taccalin, Marmin, 13-Hydroxyfeselol, Colladonin, Feselol, and Pectachol had a greater positive prediction above 0.5. If 0.5 < Pa < 0.7, the substance is likely to exhibit activity in experiment, but the probability of being a known pharmaceutical agent is less.

Table A5.
This table shows the 10 top hit compounds and their predicted antileishmanial activity.

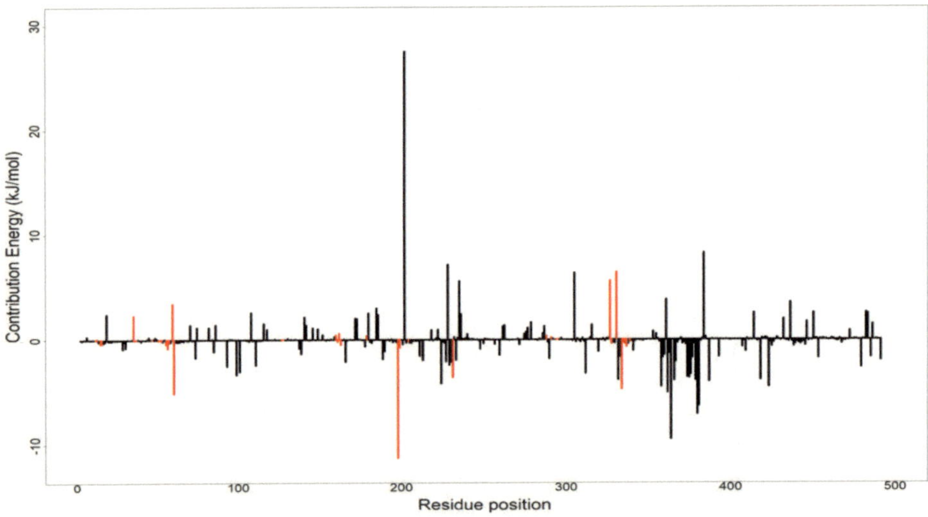

Figure A7.
Root mean square fluctuations of six complexes. The complexes are color coded in the graph. Karatavicinol and CHEMBL1277380 experienced the highest fluctuation at around residue number 80. Remaining complexes had similar patterns of fluctuations.

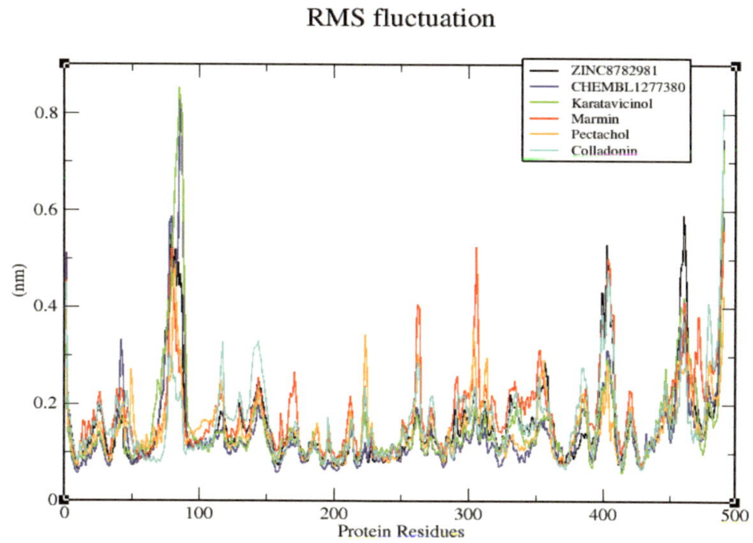

Figure A8.
The radius of gyration (Rg) plots of seven complexes within 100 ns simulation time. The complexes are represented in color code in the graph. Marmin showed the most preferentially well folded protein complex with Rg value of 2.33 nm.

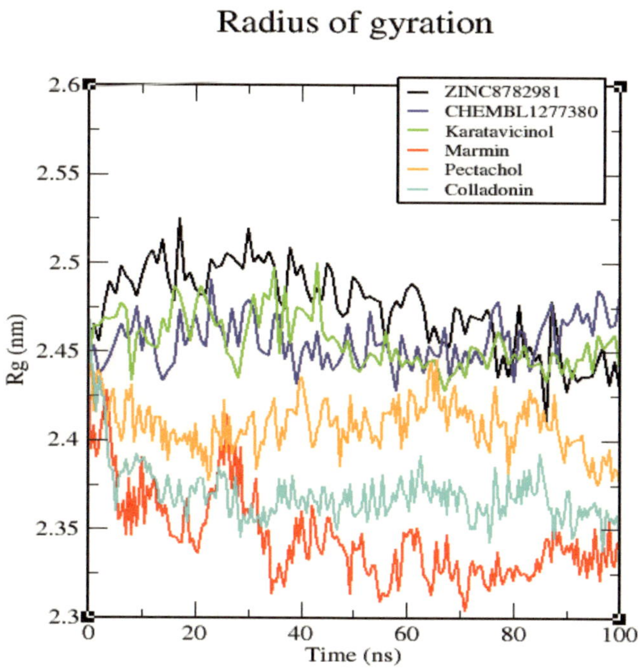

Figure A9.
MM-PBSA plot of the binding free energy decomposition contribution per residue of Lm*TR–Karatavicinol complex. Coded red lines represent surrounding active site amino acid residues.*

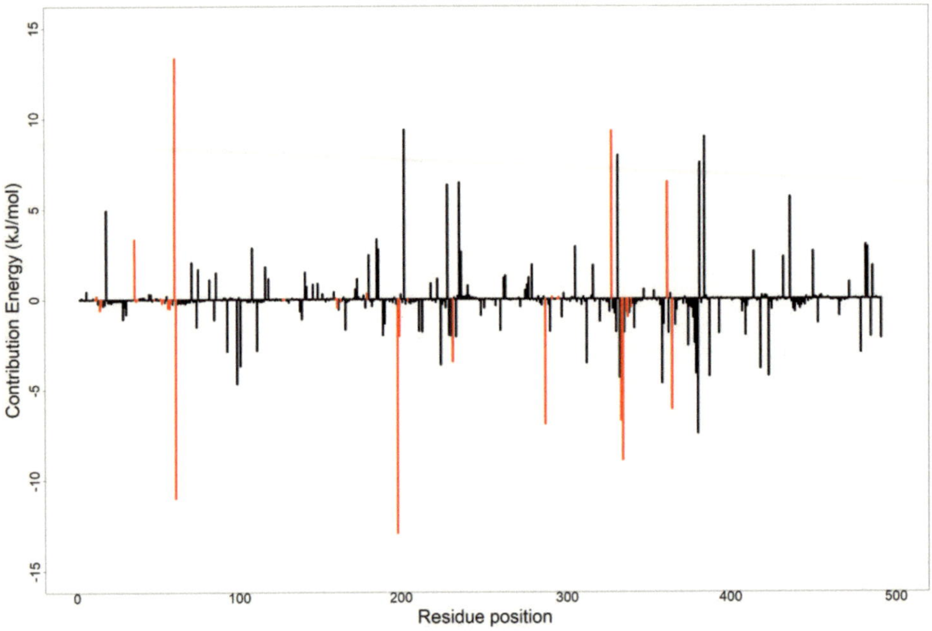

Figure A10.
MM-PBSA plot of the binding free energy decomposition contribution per residue of LmTR–Pectachol complex. Coded red lines represent surrounding active site amino acid residues.

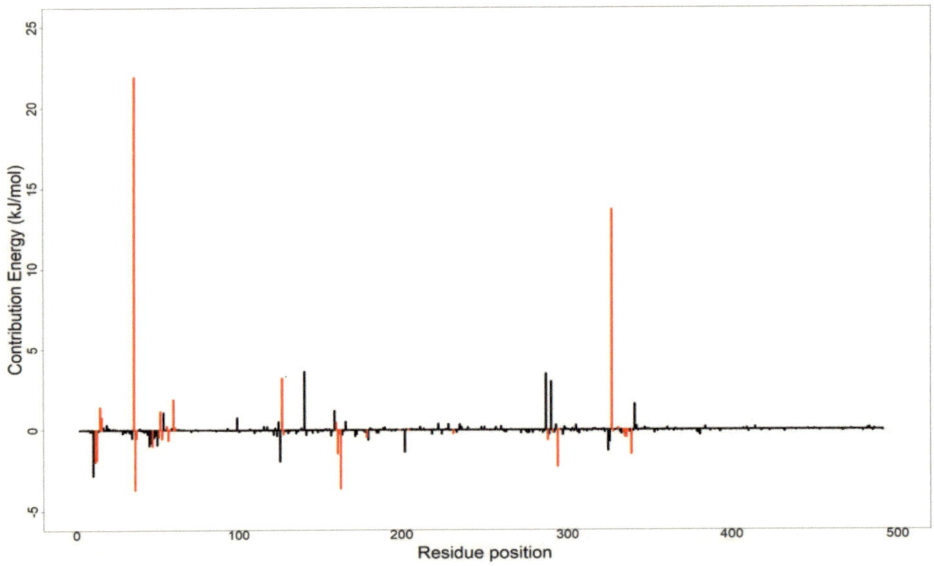

Figure A11.
MM-PBSA plot of the binding free energy decomposition contribution per residue of LmTR*–Colladonin complex. Coded red lines represent surrounding active site amino acid residues.*

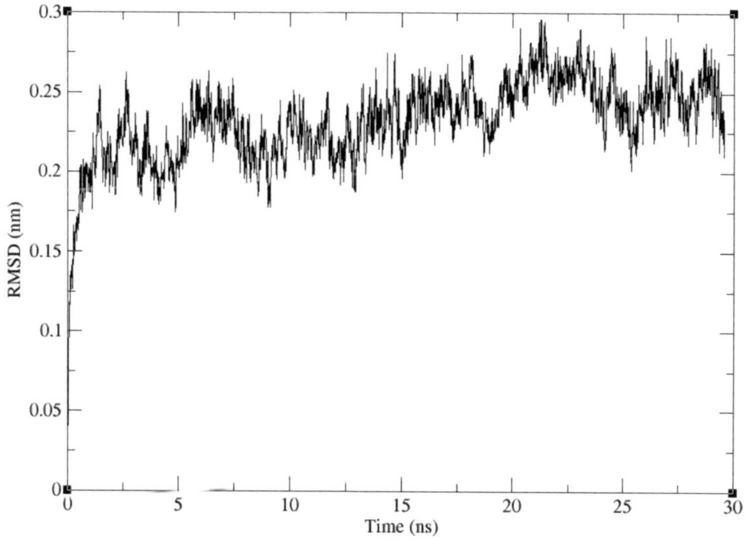

Figure A12.
Shows a graph of RMSD of the backbone of atoms in nm versus time in nanoseconds (ns). This graph is a representation of the average distance of the atoms of the residues at the backbone of the target protein. RMSD of 0.25 Å showed deviation from protein backbone.

Lead compounds	2D structure	IUPAC names
Marmin	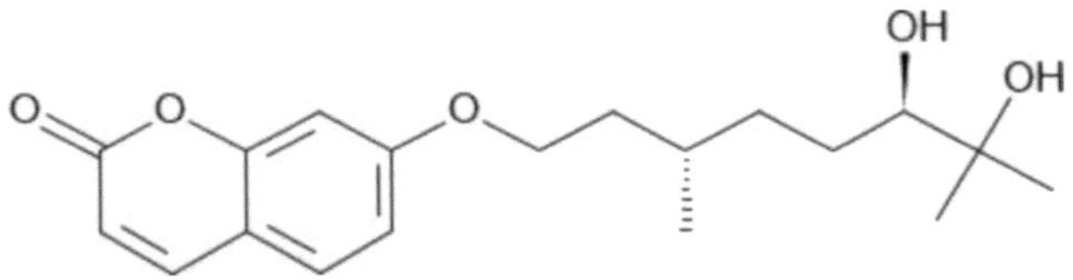	7-[(E,6R)-6,7-dihydroxy-3,7-dimethyloct-2-enoxy]chromen-2-one
Pectachol	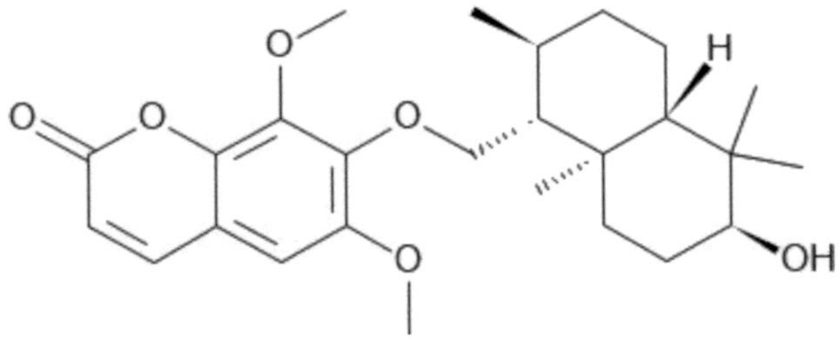	7-[(6-hydroxy-5,5,8*a*-trimethyl-2-methylidene-3,4,4*a*,6,7,8-hexahydro-1*H*-naphthalen-1-yl)methoxy]-6,8-dimethoxychromen-2-one
Colladonin	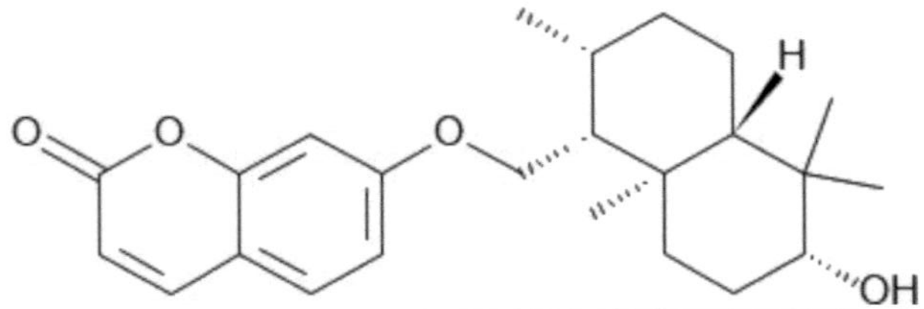	7-[[(4*aS*)-6-hydroxy-5,5,8*a*-trimethyl-2-methylidene-3,4,4*a*,6,7,8-hexahydro-1*H*-naphthalen-1-yl]me thoxy]chromen-2-one
Karatavicinol	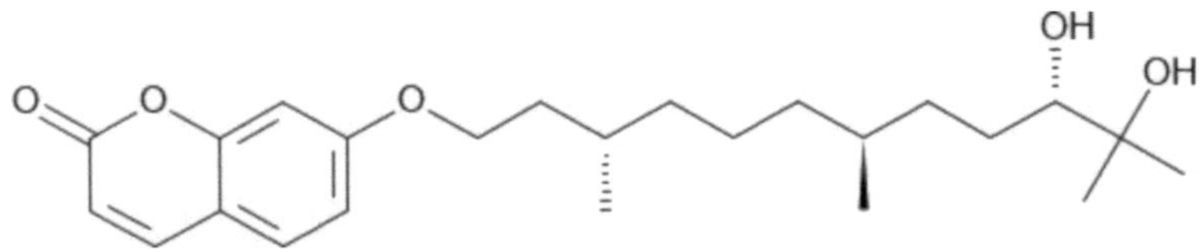	7-[(2E,6E,10S)-10,11-dihydroxy-3,7,11-trimethyldodeca-2,6-dienoxy] chromen-2-one

Table A6.
Structure and IUPAC names of the three novel lead compounds.

A.1 List of abbreviations

ADMET	absorption, distribution, metabolism, excretion and toxicity
AUC	area under curve
CYP	cytochromes P_{450}
DUD-E	directory of useful (docking) decoys-enhanced
GROMACS	GROningen MAchine for Chemical Simulations
HPC	high performance computing
ID	identification
Log P	logarithm of the octan-1-ol/water partition coefficient
MD	molecular dynamics
MM-PBSA	molecular mechanics Poisson Boltzmann surface area
Mw	molecular weight
P-gp	permeability glycoprotein
PASS	prediction of activity spectra for substance
PDB	Protein Data Bank
Rg	radius of gyration
RMSD	root mean square deviation
RMSF	root mean square fluctuation
ROC	receiver operating characteristic
SDF	structure data file
SMILES	simplified molecular input line entry system
UFF	universal force field

Author details

Samuel K. Kwofie[1,2]*, Gabriel B. Kwarko[2], Emmanuel Broni[1,3], Michael B. Adinortey[4] and Michael D. Wilson[3,5]

1 Department of Biomedical Engineering, School of Engineering Sciences, College of Basic and Applied Sciences, University of Ghana, Accra, Ghana

2 West African Centre for Cell Biology of Infectious Pathogens, Department of Biochemistry, Cell and Molecular Biology, College of Basic and Applied Sciences, University of Ghana, Accra, Ghana

3 Department of Parasitology, Noguchi Memorial Institute for Medical Research, University of Ghana, Accra, Ghana

4 Department of Biochemistry, School of Biological Science, University of Cape Coast, Cape Coast, Ghana

5 Department of Medicine, Loyola University Medical Center, Maywood, IL, USA

*Address all correspondence to: skkwofie@ug.edu.gh

References

[1] Murray HW, Berman JD, Davies CR, Saravia NG. Advances in leishmaniasis. Lancet. 2005;**366**(9496):1561-1577

[2] Sundar S, Chakravarty J, Agarwal D, Rai M, Murray HW. Single-dose liposomal amphotericin B for visceral leishmaniasis in India. The New England Journal of Medicine. 2010; **362**(6):504-512

[3] Ghisla S, Massey V. Mechanisms of flavoprotein-catalyzed reactions. European Journal of Biochemistry. 1989; **181**(1):1-17. DOI: 10.1111/j.1432-1033.1989.tb14688.x

[4] Kinnings SL, Liu N, Tonge PJ, Jackson RM, Xie L, Bourne PE. A machine learning-based method to improve docking scoring functions and its application to drug repurposing. Journal of Chemical Information and Modeling. 2011;**51**(5):1195-1197. DOI: 10.1021/ci2001346

[5] Shames SL, Fairlamb AH, Cerami A, Walsh CT. Purification and characterization of trypanothione reductase from *Crithidia fasciculata*, a newly discovered member of the family of disulfide-containing flavoprotein reductases. Biochemistry. 1986;**25**(12): 3519-3526

[6] Krauth-Siegel RL, Enders B, Henderson GB, Fairlamb AH, Schirmer RH. Trypanothione reductase from *Trypanosoma cruzi* purification and characterization of the crystalline enzyme. European Journal of Biochemistry. 1987;**164**(1):123-128

[7] Khan MOF. Trypanothione reductase: A viable chemotherapeutic target for antitrypanosomal and antileishmanial drug design. Drug Target Insights. 2007;**2**: 117739280700200

[8] Beig M, Oellien F, Garoff L, Noack S, Krauth-Siegel RL, Selzer PM. Trypanothione reductase: A target protein for a combined in vitro and in silico screening approach. PLoS Neglected Tropical Diseases. 2015;**9**(6): e0003773. DOI: 10.1371/journal.pntd.0003773

[9] Rodrigues RF, Castro-Pinto D, Echevarria A, Dos Reis CM, Del Cistia CN, Sant'Anna CMR, et al. Investigation of trypanothione reductase inhibitory activity by 1,3,4-thiadiazolium-2-aminide derivatives and molecular docking studies. Bioorganic and Medicinal Chemistry. 2012;**20**(5): 1760-6

[10] Veselovsky AV, Zharkova MS, Poroikov VV, Nicklaus MC. Computer-aided design and discovery of protein–protein interaction inhibitors as agents for anti-HIV therapy. SAR and QSAR in Environmental Research. 2014;**25**(6): 457-471. DOI: 10.1080/1062936X.2014.898689

[11] Taft CA, da Silva VB, da Silva CHT. Current topics in computer-aided drug design. Journal of Pharmaceutical Sciences. 2008;**97**(3):1089-1098

[12] Ehrlich P. Über den jetzigen Stand der Chemotherapie. Berichte der Deutschen Chemischen Gesellschaft. 1909;**42**(1):17-47. DOI: 10.1002/cber.19090420105

[13] Asimul Islam KK. Receptor chemoprint derived pharmacophore model for development of CAIX inhibitors. Journal of Carcinogenesis and Mutagenesis. 2014;**s8**(01):1-9

[14] Chawla B, Madhubala R. Drug targets in leishmania. Journal of Parasitic Diseases. 2010;**34**(1):1-13. DOI: 10.1007/s12639-010-0006-3

[15] Danesh-Bahreini MA, Shokri J, Samiei A, Kamali-Sarvestani E,

Barzegar-Jalali M, Mohammadi-Samani S. Nanovaccine for leishmaniasis: Preparation of chitosan nanoparticles containing leishmania superoxide dismutase and evaluation of its immunogenicity in BALB/c mice. International Journal of Nanomedicine. 2011;**6**:835-842

[16] Sundar S, Singh A. Chemotherapeutics of visceral leishmaniasis: Present and future developments. Parasitology. 2018; **145**(4):481-489

[17] Croft SL, Seifert K, Yardley V. Current scenario of drug development for leishmaniasis. The Indian Journal of Medical Research. 2006;**123**(3):399-410

[18] Sangshetti JN, Kalam Khan FA, Kulkarni AA, Arote R, Patil RH. Antileishmanial drug discovery: Comprehensive review of the last 10 years. RSC Advances. 2015;**5**(41): 32376-32415

[19] Agarwala R, Barrett T, Beck J, Benson DA, Bollin C, Bolton E, et al. Database resources of the National Center for Biotechnology Information. Nucleic Acids Research. 2018;**46**(D1):D8-D13

[20] Pieper U, Webb BM, Dong GQ, Schneidman-Duhovny D, Fan H, Kim SJ, et al. ModBase, a database of annotated comparative protein structure models and associated resources. Nucleic Acids Research. 2014;**42**(D1):D336-D346. DOI: 10.1093/nar/gkt1144

[21] Binkowski TA. CASTp: Computed atlas of surface topography of proteins. Nucleic Acids Research. 2003;**31**(13): 3352-3355. DOI: 10.1093/nar/gkg512

[22] Dundas J, Ouyang Z, Tseng J, Binkowski A, Turpaz Y, Liang J. CASTp: Computed atlas of surface topography of proteins with structural and topographical mapping of functionally annotated residues. Nucleic Acids Research. 2006;**34**:W116-W118

[23] Dallakyan S, Olson AJ. Small-molecule library screening by docking with PyRx. Methods in Molecular Biology. 2015;**1263**:243-250. DOI: 10.1007/978-1-4939-2269-7_19

[24] Padilha EC, Serafim RB, Sarmiento DYR, Santos CF, Santos CBR, Silva CHTP. New PPARα/γ/δ optimal activator rationally designed by computational methods. Journal of the Brazilian Chemical Society. 2016;**27**(9): 1636-1647

[25] DeLano WL. PyMOL: An open-source molecular graphics tool. CCP4 Newsletter on Protein Crystallography. 2002;**40**:82-92

[26] Wiederstein M, Sippl MJ. ProSA-web: Interactive web service for the recognition of errors in three-dimensional structures of proteins. Nucleic Acids Research. 2007;**35**:W407-W410. DOI: 10.1093/nar/gkm290

[27] Eisenberg D, Lüthy R, Bowie JU. [20] VERIFY3D: Assessment of protein models with three-dimensional profiles. Methods in Enzymology. 1997;**277**: 396-404

[28] Laskowski RA, MacArthur MW, Moss DS, Thornton JM. PROCHECK: A program to check the stereochemical quality of protein structures. Journal of Applied Crystallography. 1993;**26**(2): 283-291

[29] Patil R, Das S, Stanley A, Yadav L, Sudhakar A, Varma AK. Optimized hydrophobic interactions and hydrogen bonding at the target-ligand interface leads the pathways of drug-designing. PLoS One. 2010;**5**(8):e12029. DOI: 10.1371/journal.pone.0012029

[30] Van Der Spoel D, Lindahl E, Hess B, Groenhof G, Mark AE, Berendsen HJC. GROMACS: Fast, flexible, and free. Journal of Computational Chemistry. 2005;**26**:1701-1718

[31] Abraham MJ, Murtola T, Schulz R, Páll S, Smith JC, Hess B, et al. GROMACS: High performance molecular simulations through multi-level parallelism from laptops to supercomputers. SoftwareX. 2015;**1–2**:19-25

[32] Wolber G, Langer T. LigandScout: 3-D pharmacophores derived from protein-bound ligands and their use as virtual screening filters. Journal of Chemical Information and Modeling. 2005;**45**(1):160-169. DOI: 10.1021/ci049885e

[33] Bento AP, Gaulton A, Hersey A, Bellis LJ, Chambers J, Davies M, et al. The ChEMBL bioactivity database: An update. Nucleic Acids Research. 2014; **42**(D1):D1083-D1090. DOI: 10.1093/nar/gkt1031

[34] Kim S, Thiessen PA, Bolton EE, Chen J, Fu G, Gindulyte A, et al. PubChem substance and compound databases. Nucleic Acids Research. 2016;**44**(D1):D1202-D1213. DOI: 10.1093/nar/gkv951

[35] Irwin JJ, Shoichet BK. ZINC—A free database of commercially available compounds for virtual screening. Journal of Chemical Information and Modeling. 2005;**45**(1):177-182

[36] Ntie-Kang F, Telukunta KK, Döring K, Simoben CV, Moumbock AFA, Malange YI, et al. NANPDB: A resource for natural products from Northern African sources. Journal of Natural Products. 2017;**80**(7):2067-2076. DOI: 10.1021/acs.jnatprod.7b00283

[37] Mysinger MM, Carchia M, Irwin JJ, Shoichet BK. Directory of useful decoys, enhanced (DUD-E): Better ligands and decoys for better benchmarking. Journal of Medicinal Chemistry. 2012;**55**(14): 6582-6594. DOI: 10.1021/jm300687e

[38] Jiménez-Valverde A. Insights into the area under the receiver operating characteristic curve (AUC) as a discrimination measure in species distribution modelling. Global Ecology and Biogeography. 2012;**21**(4):498-507. DOI: 10.1111/j.1466-8238.2011.00683.x

[39] O'Boyle NM, Banck M, James CA, Morley C, Vandermeersch T, Hutchison GR. Open babel: An open chemical toolbox. Journal of Cheminformatics. 2011;**3**(1):33. DOI: 10.1186/1758-2946-3-33

[40] Goksuluk D, Korkmaz S, Zararsiz G, Karaagaoglu AE. easyROC: An interactive web-tool for ROC curve analysis using R language environment. The R Journal. 2016;**8**(2):213

[41] Heifets A, Lilien RH. LigAlign: Flexible ligand-based active site alignment and analysis. Journal of Molecular Graphics & Modelling. 2010; **29**(1):93-101

[42] Daina A, Michielin O, Zoete V. SwissADME: A free web tool to evaluate pharmacokinetics, drug-likeness and medicinal chemistry friendliness of small molecules. Scientific Reports. 2017;**7**(1):42717

[43] Lipinski CA. Rule of five in 2015 and beyond: Target and ligand structural limitations, ligand chemistry structure and drug discovery project decisions. Advanced Drug Delivery Reviews. 2016; **101**:34-41

[44] Lagunin A, Stepanchikova A, Filimonov D, Poroikov V. PASS: Prediction of activity spectra for biologically active substances. Bioinformatics. 2000;**16**(8):747-748. DOI: 10.1093/bioinformatics/16.8.747

[45] Filimonov DA, Lagunin AA, Gloriozova TA, Rudik AV, Druzhilovskii DS, Pogodin PV, et al. Prediction of the biological activity spectra of organic compounds using the pass online web resource. Chemistry of Heterocyclic Compounds. 2014;**50**(3):

444-457. DOI: 10.1007/s10593-014-1496-1

[46] Kumari R, Kumar R, Lynn A. g_mmpbsa—A GROMACS tool for high-throughput MM-PBSA calculations. Journal of Chemical Information and Modeling. 2014;**54**(7):1951-1962. DOI: 10.1021/ci500020m

[47] Uziela K, Shu N, Wallner B, Elofsson A. ProQ3: Improved model quality assessments using Rosetta energy terms. Scientific Reports. 2016;**6**(1):33509

[48] Shamsara J. Correlation between virtual screening performance and binding site descriptors of protein targets. International Journal of Medicinal Chemistry. 2018;**2018**:1-10

[49] Fu Y, Zhao J, Chen Z. Insights into the molecular mechanisms of protein-ligand interactions by molecular docking and molecular dynamics simulation: A case of oligopeptide binding protein. Computational and Mathematical Methods in Medicine. 2018;**2018**:1-12

[50] Bhakat S. Effect of T68A/N126Y mutations on the conformational and ligand binding landscape of Coxsackievirus B3 3C protease. Molecular BioSystems. 2015;**11**(8):2303-2311

[51] Barthe L, Woodley J, Houin G. Gastrointestinal absorption of drugs: Methods and studies. Fundamental & Clinical Pharmacology. 1999;**13**(2):154-168. DOI: 10.1111/j.1472-8206.1999.tb00334.x

[52] Smith HS. Opioid metabolism. Mayo Clinic Proceedings. 2009;**84**(7):613-624

[53] Lespine A, Ménez C, Bourguinat C, Prichard RK. P-glycoproteins and other multidrug resistance transporters in the pharmacology of anthelmintics: Prospects for reversing transport-dependent anthelmintic resistance. International Journal for Parasitology: Drugs and Drug Resistance. 2012;**2**:58-75

[54] Pardridge WM. Drug transport across the blood–brain barrier. Journal of Cerebral Blood Flow and Metabolism. 2012;**32**(11):1959-1972. DOI: 10.1038/jcbfm.2012.126

[55] Lagunin A, Filimonov D, Poroikov V. Multi-targeted natural products evaluation based on biological activity prediction with PASS. Current Pharmaceutical Design. 2010;**16**(15):1703-1717

[56] Filimonov DA, Druzhilovskiy DS, Lagunin AA, Gloriozova TA, Rudik AV, Dmitriev AV, et al. Computer-aided prediction of biological activity spectra for chemical compounds: Opportunities and limitation. Biomedical Chemistry: Research and Methods. 2018;**1**(1):e00004

[57] Amin A, Tuenter E, Cos P, Maes L, Exarchou V, Apers S, et al. Antiprotozoal and antiglycation activities of sesquiterpene coumarins from ferula narthex exudate. Molecules. 2016;**21**(10):1287

[58] Gliszczyńska A, Brodelius PE. Sesquiterpene coumarins. Phytochemistry Reviews. 2012;**11**(1):77-96. DOI: 10.1007/s11101-011-9220-6

[59] Karplus M, McCammon JA. Molecular dynamics simulations of biomolecules. Nature Structural Biology. 2002;**9**(9):646-652. DOI: 10.1038/nsb0902-646

[60] Hollingsworth SA, Dror RO. Molecular dynamics simulation for all. Neuron. 2018;**99**(6):1129-1143

[61] Cheng X, Ivanov I. Molecular dynamics. Methods in Molecular Biology. 2012;**929**:243-285

[62] Sinha S, Wang SM. Classification of VUS and unclassified variants in BRCA1 BRCT repeats by molecular dynamics simulation. Computational and Structural Biotechnology Journal. 2020; **18**:723-736

[63] Perez A, Morrone JA, Simmerling C, Dill KA. Advances in free-energy-based simulations of protein folding and ligand binding. Current Opinion in Structural Biology. 2016;**36**:25-31

[64] Kwofie SK, Dankwa B, Enninful KS, Adobor C, Broni E, Ntiamoah A, et al. Molecular docking and dynamics simulation studies predict Munc18b as a target of mycolactone: A plausible mechanism for granule exocytosis impairment in buruli ulcer pathogenesis. Toxins. 2019;**11**(3)

[65] Sartori GR, Nascimento AS. Comparative analysis of electrostatic models for ligand docking. Frontiers in Molecular Biosciences. 2019;**6**(52). DOI: 10.3389/fmolb.2019.00052/full

[66] Deng N, Zhang P, Cieplak P, Lai L. Elucidating the energetics of entropically driven protein–ligand association: Calculations of absolute binding free energy and entropy. The Journal of Physical Chemistry. B. 2011; **115**(41):11902-11910. DOI: 10.1021/jp204047b

[67] Fiorentini R, Kremer K, Potestio R. Ligand-protein interactions in lysozyme investigated through a dual-resolution model. Proteins: Structure, Function, and Bioinformatics. 2020;**88**(10): 1351-1360. DOI: 10.1002/prot.25954

[68] Campanera JM, Pouplana R. MMPBSA decomposition of the binding energy throughout a molecular dynamics simulation of amyloid-beta (Aß10−35) aggregation. Molecules. 2010;**15**(4):2730-2748

[69] Genheden S, Ryde U. The MM/PBSA and MM/GBSA methods to estimate ligand-binding affinities. Expert Opinion on Drug Discovery. 2015;**10**(5):449-461. DOI: 10.1517/17460441.2015.1032936

[70] Arango V, Robledo S, Séon-Méniel B, Figadère B, Cardona W, Sáez J, et al. Coumarins from *Galipea panamensis* and their activity against *Leishmania panamensis*. Journal of Natural Products. 2010;**73**(5): 1012-1014. DOI: 10.1021/np100146y

[71] Alam F. Anti-ulcer plants from North-East India—A review. Der Pharmacia Lettre. 2019;**11**(6):73-96

[72] Sajjadi S, Eskandarian A-A, Shokoohinia Y, Yousefi H-A, Mansourian M, Asgarian-Nasab H, et al. Antileishmanial activity of prenylated coumarins isolated from *Ferulago angulata* and *Prangos asperula*. Research in Pharmaceutical Sciences. 2016;**11**(4):324

[73] Ferreira ME, Rojas de Arias A, Yaluff G, de Bilbao NV, Nakayama H, Torres S, et al. Antileishmanial activity of furoquinolines and coumarins from *Helietta apiculata*. Phytomedicine. 2010; **17**(5):375-378

[74] Baiocco P, Colotti G, Franceschini S, Ilari A. Molecular basis of antimony treatment in leishmaniasis. Journal of Medicinal Chemistry. 2009;**52**(8): 2603-2612. DOI: 10.1021/jm900185q

[75] Ravi Kumar G, Jagannadham Medicherla V. Molecular docking based inhibition of trypanothione reductase activity by taxifolin novel target for antileishmanial activity. Journal of Applied Pharmaceutical Science. 2012; **2**(10):133-136

[76] Venkatesan SK, Shukla AK, Dubey VK. Molecular docking studies of selected tricyclic and quinone derivatives on trypanothione reductase of *Leishmania infantum*. Journal of Computational Chemistry. 2010;**31**(13): 2463-2475. DOI: 10.1002/jcc.21538

Chapter 12

Plant-Based Alternative Treatment for Leishmaniasis: A Neglected Tropical Disease

Nargis Shaheen, Chaitenya Verma and Naveeda Akhter Qureshi

Abstract

Leishmaniasis is a third most important vector born disease caused by intracellular parasite belongs to genus *Leishmania*. The leishmaniasis is prevalent in 102 countries/areas worldwide. Approximately, it effected 350 million people worldwide. Leishmaniasis effects developing and undeveloped countries globally. Antileishmanial drugs (pentavalent antimonials, stibogluconate, miltefosine, paramycin, and amphotericin) are most vital tool for curing leishmaniasis. However, none of these drugs is free from side effect including cost, toxicity, drug resistance, administration route, and prolong time, these disadvantages are main obstacle in the *Leishmania* infection eradication. Considering the increasing cases of leishmaniasis and drug resistance there is an urgent need for an effective and novel approach against leishmaniasis. Therefore, many researchers have tried to develop new medicines for the treatment of *Leishmania* infection. In the course of new therapies identification, plant based compounds were found to be an alternative that can be either used directly or with structural modifications. Several plants have been known for ages to be the source of phytochemicals with high values of medicines. These phytochemicals have been extracted by various techniques and have shown efficacy for the curing of several diseases. This chapter study explain various applications based on green approaches drugs for the treatment of leishmaniasis.

Keywords: leishmaniasis, treatment, nanoparticles, alternative, green approach

1. Introduction

1.1 Leishmaniasis

The neglected tropical diseases (NTDs) are a group of about 17 parasitic diseases. The NTDs are prevalent in many tropical and subtropical countries that present the most common illness of the poorest people worldwide [1]. *Leishmania* infection constitutes a foremost public health issue with a rising burden over the last decade and is the second main cause of disease and death [2]. Leishmaniasis is prevalent in 102 countries/areas worldwide [3]. *Leishmania* infection affects approximately 1.5–2 million people, while 350 million are at risk of this pathogen [4, 5]. The causative agent of leishmaniasis is parasite protozoa of the genus *Leishmania* and is transferred via vector sandfly bite belongs to genus *Lutzomyia* and *Phlebotomus* [6].

Three clinical forms of leishmaniasis have been reported concerning parasite location in the infected tissues, that is, visceral leishmaniasis (VL) which is a less common type of leishmaniasis and it causes spleen and liver destruction and causes death if does not receive timely treatment; cutaneous leishmaniasis (CL), which affect only localized skin parts; and mucocutaneous leishmaniasis (MCL), which has the ability of mucus tissue destruction [7, 8]. About 0.7–1.2 million CL and 0.2–0.4 million VL cases are reported annually. Approximately CL cases (90%) are spread across three main areas, that is, (a) Syria, Afghanistan, Saudi Arabia, and Iran; (b) Tunisia and Algeria; and (c) Peru and Brazil [9, 10]. Annual visceral leishmaniasis (VL) cases are estimated to be less than 100,000, down from 400,000 in previous estimates [11], with more than 95% of cases reported to the World Health Organization (WHO) from Brazil, China, Ethiopia, India, Kenya, Nepal, Somalia, and Sudan. Currently, 54 *Leishmania* spp. are known and twenty-one are human's pathogenic [8].

2. Therapeutic approaches and their limitations

Leishmaniasis is one of the most common NTDs, and it comes with a slew of negative and life-threatening consequences, including significant morbidity, early death, and long-term disability. Treatment entails limiting illness spread and utilizing existing criteria, but present medicines, such as chemical pharmaceuticals, need long-term treatment, minimal efficacy, and a slew of hazardous side effects. Only a few prevention strategies are available, despite the fact that no appropriate medications have been produced to prevent the virus, which is widely transmitted among the human population [12]. Some clinically approved medications are discovered among them to treat this endemic condition, that is, meglumine antimoniate (glucatime), sodium stibogluconate (pentostan), amphotericin B, and miltefosine. Excessive use of these chemotherapeutic sources, on the other hand, has been linked to antagonistic consequences [13]. As a result, researchers are looking for natural ways to treat leishmaniasis. Leishmaniasis treatment using chemical-based drugs various pharmacological medications, such as amphotericin B, pentamidine, miltefosine, and paromomycin, have been used in the treatment of leishmaniasis for numerous years. Due to the time-consuming method and high toxicity paired with significant adverse effects, none of the clinically approved medications could be considered as the ultimate source of treatment. Furthermore, the most commonly used medications do not completely eliminate parasites from all afflicted individuals [14]. The applications of several of these drugs, as well as their drawbacks, are explained further below. Pentavalent antimonials can be given via intravenous, intramuscular, and intralymphatic methods, with an optimum dose of 20 mg/kg/day (28–30 days) and a potentiality of 35–95%. This medicine can cause toxicity such as nephrotoxicity, hepatotoxicity, severe cardiotoxicity, and pancreatitis if used excessively [12, 13]. Miltefosine, when given orally, had an inhibitory effect on *Leishmania* growth but also had a negative effect, causing severe infection symptoms such as nephrotoxicity, teratogenicity, vomiting and diarrhea, and hepatotoxicity [15]. Paromomycin, which is also used to treat leishmaniasis, has been documented to have several hazardous side effects during treatment, including severe nephrotoxicity, hepatotoxicity, and ototoxicity [16]. Pentamidine, at a starting dose of 3 mg/kg/day, has the potential to slow *Leishmania* development while also causing significant side effects including as hypotension, hyperglycemia, tachycardia, pancreatic damage, and electrocardiographic abnormalities changes [14]. Existing chemotherapies have a number of drawbacks, including high cost, increased toxicity, and acquired resistance to parasitic strains, as well as other side effects during their prevention mechanism, prompting scientists and medical practitioners to develop a new therapeutic system to treat NTDs. Plant extracts, bioactive chemicals, and secondary metabolites obtained from specific plant species, as well as various types of NPs manufactured using plant extract, have become promising as well as safer preventative medicines in recent decades.

3. Natural methods

Plant-based conventional treatments have been employed in the treatment of infectious diseases since ancient times. Plant extracts and specific bioactive compounds isolated from plants are currently employed as either direct medicinal sources or as herbal medications to treat leishmaniasis and other microbiological infections [17]. Due to their nontoxic, environmentally friendly, and cost-effective features, medicinal plants become more favorable than other chemotherapies. Furthermore, natural chemicals derived from plants are regarded as a safe and effective treatment for leishmaniasis [18].

The root extract *Bidens pilosa* has been reported for antileishmanial potential against promastigotes of *L. amazonensis* with IC = 1.5 μg/ml). The *Eugenia uniflora* oil inhibit the growth of promastigotes and amastigotes of *L. amazonensis* while *Ageratum conyzoides* has been active against amastigots form of *Labrus donovani* [19]. The component of *Casearia sylvestris* and *Melampodium divaricatum* has been reported against *L. amazonensis* with IC50 = 10.7 and 14.0 μg/ml [20]. Furthermore, the active components 1,8-cineole, -pinene, and *p*-cymene from *Protium altsonii* and *P. hebetatum* (*Burseraceae*) showed dose-dependent amastigote inhibition, with IC50 values of 48.4, 37, and 46 g/ml, respectively [21]. The butanol fraction of *K. odoratissima* displayed antileishmanial activities against *L. major* promastigote and amastigote with an IC50 value of 154.1 g/ml [22].

4. Role of plant-based nanoparticles in leishmaniasis treatment

Infectious illness control methods have revolutionized translational sciences, allowing for the development of a better infectious disease control approach. Nanomedicine has showed tremendous promise in the development of very sensitive diagnostic tools with outstanding medication delivery properties. Nanoparticle-conjugated medications have recently been examined as a cost-effective, alternative therapy with improved efficacy. Toxicity, on the other hand, is a significant impediment that must be overcome. Several studies have demonstrated that several metal/metal oxide nanoparticles, as well as the *Leishmania* causative organism, have effective antibacterial effects due to their large surface area and unique characteristics. Nanoparticles made from crude and various solvent-fractionated extracts of medically significant plants are thought to be effective delivery for specific phytoconstituents into cells. Keeping in view the effective antimicrobial activities of silver metal, silver/silver oxide NPs synthesized using a variety of medicinally important plant species, including *Mentha arvensis* L., *Ficus benghalensis*, *Cuminum cyminum*, *Moringa oleifera*, *Silybum marianum*, and *Sechium edule*, at a dosage of 10, 300, 0.5, 246, and 51.88 μg/ml tested against *L. tropica*, *L. donovani*, *L. major*, and *L. donovani*, respectively [23–27]. This condition has also been reported to be prevented utilizing gold and silver bimetallic NPs produced from therapeutically significant plants [28]. However, Au-NPs derived from *Cannabis sativa* had excellent antileishmanial activity against amastigote forms (IC50: 171•00± 2•28 μg/ml) [25]. The flavonoid 7,8-dihydroxyflavone, which is common in plants used to make gold nanoparticles, has also been shown to prevent leishmaniasis [29]. The cytotoxicity of ZnO-NPs against *L. tropica* was likewise observed to be dose-dependent (IC50: 8.30 μg/ml). With an IC50 value of 0.001 mg ml, rod-shaped zinc oxide NPs made from *Lilium ledebourii* tuber extract suppressed the growth of *L. major* [29]. Saleh [30] also found that green TiO_2 nanoparticles were efficient in reducing *L. tropica* toxicity in male rats. Hematite (Fe_2O_3) NPs made from *Rhus punjabensis* extract were found to be effective in the treatment of leishmaniasis [31]. Khalil et al. [32] used aqueous leaf extracts of *Sageretia thea* to make lead oxide NPs (PbO-NPs). PbO-NPs were found to be significantly active in stopping the growth of promastigote and amastigotes forms of *L. tropica*, with IC50 values of 14.7 and 11.95 g/ml, respectively. Plant-mediated iron oxide nanoparticles (*Trigonella foenum-graecum*) have been shown to have considerable inhibitory effects on *L. tropica* [33]. Abbasi et al. [34] also indicated that NiO-NPs made from *Geranium wallichianum* has antileishmanial activity against *L. tropica*.

In addition, the nanostructured drug delivery method has been shown to help with NTDs like leishmaniasis. Furthermore, crude plant extracts and specific phytoconstituents produced from plants that are involved in the preventative mechanism were loaded into the nanostructured drug delivery system and used as a therapeutic source to cure leishmaniasis, as shown below:

- Liposome NPs containing phospholipids are used as a transport system for the delivery of both hydrophilic and lipophilic medicinal medicines [35]. They give superior pharmacokinetic assets as well as target diligence, which is a significant benefit [36]. Through phagocytosis, liposomes can spear macrophages and transport medications directly to their target areas. Various medication formulations, such as AmB colloidal formulations, liposomal AmB, and the AmB lipid network, can significantly reduce the toxicity of traditional pharmaceuticals [20].

- Antileishmanial effects of liposome-encapsulated *Curcuma longa* and *Combretum leprosum* extracts have also been discovered [37, 38].

- The usage of beta-lapachone isolated from the Lapacho tree and encapsulated with lecithin-chitosan NP has been described in the treatment of leishmaniasis [20].

- *Leishmania* has been treated with 8-hydroxyquinoline encapsulated in polymeric micelles [39]. Berberin is an isoquinoline alkaloid derived from medicinal plants that has been shown to have a variety of biologic features, including antileishmanial activity. In VL, a prior study focused on the development of BER-loaded liposomes with the goal of preventing rapid liver metabolism and improving drug selective delivery to diseased organs [40].

According to the literature review, plant-based nanoparticles play an effective function in the treatment of leishmaniasis when compared to other treatments. At a far lower concentration than the required dose of Amp B to cure this condition, phytosynthesized NPs had the same effect on parasite growth suppression. Furthermore, green bimetallic nanoparticles such as Au-Ag, Zn-Ag, and Ti-Ag were produced and successfully used as a medicinal source to treat leishmaniasis [28]. Because of its nontoxic, safe, and efficient vaccine delivery technique, NPs are recommended above other medicinal options to treat this dreadful disease. With the progress of nanosciences, a new way of producing vaccines employing NPs as antigen carriers is now available. Solid lipid nanoparticles may be useful in the development of a leishmanial vaccine [41]. However, no NP-based vaccination is currently available, and further research is required.

5. Restorative mechanism of nanoformulations against leishmaniasis

The protozoan parasite *Leishmania* spp. causes cutaneous and visceral leishmaniasis. Depending on the immune responses induced by the diseased host, several clinical investigations show the development of self-curable to adverse situations [42]. Pentavalent antimonials (such as sodium stibogluconate or meglumine antimoniate) and other antileishmanial medications (amphotericin B, fluconazole, pentamidine, and miltefosine) are the most effective treatments for leishmaniasis. However, undesirable effects, high costs, complicated infusion routes, low cure rates, and rising resistance are all major concerns when it comes to developing more effective leishmaniasis treatments. Furthermore, the efficacy of the medicine employed in treatment differs per leishmanial species [28, 40, 42]. In self-treatment, phagocytes recognize and devour the causative agents, causing *Leishmania* assassination by releasing reactive oxygen species, nitric oxide, and tumor necrosis factors [43]. Following innate immune responses, TH1 immunity activates and produces CD8+, NK, and IFN cells, which kills the *Leishmania* parasites [42]. In sensitive situations, the defense system fails to overcome infections, resulting in erroneous TH2 immune responses as well as antibody responses, which is the main factor in developing new parasite elimination methods. Infected cells' proliferation and viability are inhibited by metal nanoparticles, which is dependent on the NP strength and exposure period [44, 45]. Several in vitro and in vivo data imply that bio-Ag-NPs have leishmanicidal actions via direct (non-inflammatory) or indirect (immunomodulatory) mechanisms [40, 45]. Metal-NPs destroy parasitic cells directly by producing vacuolation within the parasites and disruption to the cellular membrane, without generating immunomodulatory intermediaries such as reactive oxygen species (ROS), nitric oxide (NO), and apoptotic and necrotic factors [45]. Nanoformulations aid site-specific delivery and accumulation of medicines, which is responsible for parasite killing, when *Leishmania* parasites override the oxidative burst inside phagocytic cells and dwell in phagolysosomes [46]. According to Fanti et al. (2018) [45], Ag-NPs are oxidized by acidic conditions within the phagolysosomes following passage through the cellular membranes, and the release of free Ag + ions induces parasite assassination. The indirect strategy, on the other hand, includes inducing immunomodulatory responses at infection sites. Other methods of providing leishmanicidal effects include activating immune response mediators and reducing cell viability and proliferation as a result of metallic nanoparticles. NPs cause a variety of morphological changes, including distorted membrane integrity, cytotoxicity, mitochondrial destruction, cell cycle arrest (G1), increased/decreased ROS and NO production, altered enzymatic activity, and the release of apoptotic or necrotic components [47–49]. As a result of mitochondrial disintegration, ATP production is harmed, which leads to cytotoxic effects and, in turn, impairs infection growth [50]. Furthermore, NP exposure results in a lower parasitic load and a decrease in the trypanothione reductase system, which is an important parasitic enzyme [45].

6. Conclusions

Chemotherapy has become the only option for treating leishmaniasis due to a lack of effective medicines. However, these medications have increased degrees of toxicity, treatment costs, and resistance development against leishmanial parasites, as well as other side effects. Furthermore, due to leishmanial antigen variations and varied immunological responses to the treatment, the efficacy of medicines differs from species to species. Biogenic nanomaterials have been suggested as helpful alternatives to formulate nanovaccines since they are nontoxic, biocompatible, cost effective, and have high targeted drug-loading potentials. Nanoformulations can be used to overcome targeted medication transport hurdles, resulting in increased parasiticidal efficacy. Moreover, plant-derived natural compounds (such as berberine, 7,8-dihydroxyflavone, E-caryophyllene, essential oil constituents, -terpineol, glycosides, tannins, and anthraquinone flavonoids) have been shown to have leishmanicidal activities in various studies, which can further integrate beneficial outcomes. Furthermore, the majority of leishmanicidal investigations revealed only the most basic results, such as determining the influence of test medications (crude extract, extracted bioactive components, essential oil, and purified fraction) on parasite growth. Few of them are able to determine the right formulation as well as the effect on the sandfly promastigote stage (vector). Plants include a range of bioactive chemicals, and the majority of them have been recognized for their medicinal qualities, according to the literature. As a result, standardization may lead to the identification of a specific component that has leishmanicidal properties. Biosynthesized nanoparticles mostly remove infection by triggering the host's immunomodulatory response or, in rare cases, directly by causing parasitic cell vacuolization, resulting in parasite death. Nanovaccines are a relatively new concept in *Leishmania* treatment, and while no vaccine is currently available, research is ongoing to find effective nanovaccines. Although nanotechnology has given hope for better and more successful eradication of neglected tropical diseases, a complete understanding of the molecular mechanisms responsible is still needed.

Conflict of interest

None.

Notes/thanks/other declarations

All authors declare that they have no known competing financial interest or personal relationship that could have appeared to influence the work reported in this chapter.

Author details

Nargis Shaheen[1,2]*, Chaitenya Verma[2] and Naveeda Akhter Qureshi[1]

1 Faculty of Biological Science, Department of Zoology, Quaid-i-Azam University, Islamabad, Pakistan

2 Department of Pathology, College of Medicine, The Ohio State University, Columbus, OH, USA

*Address all correspondence to: nargisshaheen1234@gmail.com; nshaheen@bs.qau.edu.pk

References

[1] World Health Organization (WHO). Control of the Leishmaniases. Report of a Meeting of the WHO Expert Committee on the Control of Leishmaniases. WHO/DOC/949. Geneva: WHO; 2010

[2] Bern C, Maguire JH, Alvar J. Complexities of assessing the disease burden attributable to leishmaniasis. PLoS Neglected Tropical Diseases. 2008;**2**(10):313

[3] Uzun S, Gürel MS, Durdu M, Akyol M, Karaman FB, Aksoy M, et al. Clinical practice guidelines for the diagnosis and treatment of cutaneous leishmaniasis in Turkey. International Journal of Dermatology. 2018;**57**(8): 973-982

[4] Souza A, Marins DSS, Mathias SL, Monteiro LM, Yukuyama MN, Scarim CB, et al. Promising nanotherapy in treating leishmaniasis. International Journal of Pharmaceutics. 2018;**547**:421-431

[5] World Health Organization. Noncommunicable Diseases Country Profiles 2018. Geneva: WHO; 2018

[6] Kamhawi S, Modi GB, Pimenta PFP, Rowton E, Sacks DL. The vectorial competence of *Phlebotomus sergenti* is specific for *Leishmania tropica* and is controlled by species-specific, lipophosphoglycan-mediated midgut attachment. Parasitology. 2000; **121**(1):25-33

[7] Bifeld E, Clos J. The genetics of *Leishmania* virulence. Medical Microbiology and Immunology. 2015;**204**:619-634

[8] Akhoundi M, Kuhls K, Cannet A, Votypka J, Marty P, Delaunay P, et al. A historical overview of the classification, evolution, and dispersion of *Leishmania* parasites and sandflies. PLoS Neglected Tropical Diseases. 2016;**10**(3):e0004349

[9] Alvar J, Vélez ID, Bern C, Herrero M, Desjeux P, Cano J. WHO Leishmaniasis Control Team. Leishmaniasis worldwide and global estimates of its incidence. PLoS One. 2012;**7**(5):e35671

[10] Alvar J, Velez ID, Bern C. Leishmaniasis worldwide and global estimates of its incidence. PLoS One. 2012;**7**:356-371

[11] CDC. Epidemiology and risk factors. Available from: https://www.cdc.gov/parasites/leishmaniasis/epi.html

[12] Gharirvand Eskandari E, Setorki M, Doudi M. Medicinal plants with antileishmanial properties: A review study. Pharmaceutical and Biomedical Research. 2020;**6**(11):1-16

[13] Ghobakhloo N, Motazedian MH, Fardaei M. Expression analysis of multiple genes may involve in antimony resistance among *Leishmania major* clinical isolates from Fars Province, Central Iran. Iranian Journal of Parasitology. 2016;**11**(2):168-176

[14] De Menezes JPB, Guedes CES, Petersen ALdOA, Fraga DBM, Veras PST. Advances in development of new treatment for leishmaniasis. BioMed Research International. 2015;**2015**:1-11

[15] Sundar S, Sinha PK, Rai M, Verma DK, Nawin K, Alam S, et al. Comparison of short-course multidrug treatment with standard therapy for visceral leishmaniasis in India: An open-label, non-inferiority, randomised controlled trial. Lancet. 2011; **377**(9764):477-486

[16] Jhingran A, Chawla B, Saxena S, Barrett MP, Madhubala R. Paromomycin: Uptake and resistance in *Leishmania donovani*. Molecular and Biochemical Parasitology. 2009;**164**:111-117

[17] Oryan A. Plant-derived compounds in treatment of leishmaniasis. Iranian

Journal of Veterinary Research. 2015;**16**(1):1-19

[18] Cheuka P, Mayoka G, Mutai P, Chibale K. The role of natural products in drug discovery and development against neglected tropical diseases. Molecules. 2017;**22**:58

[19] Silveira ES, Castro Rodrigues NLD, Machado NJ, Marciano Fonseca FR, Teixeira MJ, Almeida Moreira Leal LK. Medicinal plants containing coumarin or essential oils from the Brazilian biome may be new option for treating leishmaniasis? Pharmacognosy Reviews. 2021;**14**:53-61

[20] Moreira RRD, SantosDos AG, Carvalho FA, Perego CH, Crevelin EJ, Crotti AEM, et al. Antileishmanial activity of *Melampodium divaricatum* and *Casearia sylvestris* essential oils on *Leishmania amazonensis*. Revista do Instituto de Medicina Tropical de São Paulo. 2019;**61**:e33

[21] Santana RC, Rosados ASS, Mateus MHS, Soares DC, Atella G, Guimaraes AC, et al. *In vitro* leishmanicidal activity of monoterpenes present in two species of protium (Burseraceae) on *Leishmania amazonensis*. Journal of Ethnopharmacology. 2020;**259**:112981

[22] Mirzaei F, Norouzi R, Siyadatpanah A, Mitsuwan W, Nilforoushzadeh M, Maleksabet A, et al. Butanol fraction of *Kelussia odoratissima* Mozaff inhibits the growth of *Leishmania major* promastigote and amastigote. Journal of World's Poultry Research. 2020;**10**:254-259

[23] Baranwal A, Chiranjivi AK, Kumar A, Dubey VK, Chandra P. Design of commercially comparable nanotherapeutic agent against human disease-causing parasite, *Leishmania*. Scientific Reports. 2018;**8**:8814

[24] Bagirova M, Dinparvar S, Allahverdiyev AM, Unal K, Abamor ES, Novruzova M. Investigation of antileshmanial activities of *Cuminum cyminum* based green silver nanoparticles on *L. tropica* promastigotes and amastigotes *in vitro*. Acta Tropica. 2020;**208**:105498

[25] Hameed S, Ali Shah S, Iqbal J, Numan M, Muhammad W, Junaid M, et al. Cannabis sativa-mediated synthesis of gold nanoparticles and their biomedical properties. Bioinspired, Biomimetic and Nanobiomaterials. 2020;**9**:95-102

[26] Javed B, Raja NI, Nadhman A, Mashwani ZUR. Understanding the potential of bio-fabricated non-oxidative silver nanoparticles to eradicate *Leishmania* and plant bacterial pathogens. Applied Nanoscience. 2020;**10**:2057-2067

[27] Ismail HH, Hasoon SA, Saheb EJ. The anti-leishmaniasis activity of green synthesis silver oxide nanoparticles. Annals of Tropical Medicine and Public Health. 2019;**22**:28-38

[28] Alti D, Veeramohan Rao M, Rao DN, Maurya R, Kalangi SK. Gold-silver bimetallic nanoparticles reduced with herbal leaf extracts induce ROS-mediated death in both promastigote and amastigote stages of *Leishmania donovani*. ACS Omega. 2020;**5**: 16238-16245

[29] Prasanna P, Kumar P, Mandal S, Patyal T, Patyal T, Kumar S, et al. Synthesis of 7, 8-dihydroxyflavone functionalized gold nanoparticles and its mechanism of action against *Leishmania donovani*. Research Square. 2020;**16**(21):1-29

[30] Saleh AH. Potential role of titanium dioxide (TiO_2) nanoparticles against the toxicity of *Leishmania tropica* in adult albino male rats. Journal of Global Pharma Technology. 2019;**11**(3):453-457

[31] Naz S, Islam M, Tabassum S, Fernandes NF, Carcache de Blanco EJ,

Zia M. Green synthesis of hematite (α-Fe_2O_3) nanoparticles using *Rhus punjabensis* extract and their biomedical prospect in pathogenic diseases and cancer. Journal of Molecular Structure. 2019;**1185**:1-7

[32] Khalil AT, Ovais M, Ullah I, Ali M, Jan SA, Shinwari ZK, et al. Bioinspired synthesis of pure massicot phase lead oxide nanoparticles and assessment of their biocompatibility, cytotoxicity and *in-vitro* biological properties. Arabian Journal of Chemistry. 2020;**13**:916-931

[33] Ain QU, Islam A, Nadhman A, Yasinzai M. Comparative analysis of chemically and biologically synthesized iron oxide nanoparticles against *Leishmania tropica*. bioRxiv 2019

[34] Abbasi BA, Iqbal J, Mahmood T, Ahmad R, Kanwal S, Afridi S. Plant-mediated synthesis of nickel oxide nanoparticles (NiO) via *Geranium wallichianum*: Characterization and different biological applications. Materials Research Express. 2019;**6**: 0850a7

[35] Momeni A, Rasoolian M, Momeni A, Navaei A, Emami S, Shaker Z, et al. Development of liposomes loaded with anti-leishmanial drugs for the treatment of cutaneous leishmaniasis. Journal of Liposome Research. 2013;**23**:134-144

[36] Kaye P, Scott P. Leishmaniasis: Complexity at the host-pathogen interface. Nature Reviews. Microbiology. 2011;**9**:604-615

[37] Aditya NP, Chimote G, Gunalan K, Banerjee R, Patankar S, Madhusudhan B. Curcuminoids-loaded liposomes in combination with arteether protects against *Plasmodium berghei* infection in mice. Experimental Parasitology. 2012;**131**:292-299

[38] Barros NB, Migliaccio V, Facundo VA, Ciancaglini P, Stábeli RG, Nicolete R, et al. Liposomal-lupane system as alternative chemotherapy against cutaneous leishmaniasis: Macrophage as target cell. Experimental Parasitology. 2013;**135**:337-343

[39] Duarte MC, Lagedos LMRR, Lage DP, Martins VT, Carvalho AMRS, Roatt BM, et al. Treatment of murine visceral leishmaniasis using an 8-hydroxyquinoline-containing polymeric micelle system. Parasitology International. 2016;**65**:728-736

[40] Calvo A, Moreno E, Larrea E, Sanmartin C, Irache JM, Espuelas S. Berberine-loaded liposomes for the treatment of *Leishmania infantum*-infected Balb/c mice. Pharmaceutics. 2020;**12**:858

[41] Saljoughian N, Zahedifard F, Doroud D, Doustdari F, Vasei M, Papadopoulou B, et al. Cationic solid-lipid nanoparticles are as efficient as electroporation in DNA vaccination against visceral leishmaniasis in mice. Parasite Immunology. 2013;**35**:397-408

[42] Noormehr H, Zavaran Hosseini A, Soudi S, Beyzay F. Enhancement of Th1 immune response against *Leishmania* cysteine peptidase A, B by PLGA nanoparticle. International Immunopharmacology. 2018;**59**:97-105

[43] Olekhnovitch R, Ryffel B, Müller AJ, Bousso P. Collective nitric oxide production provides tissue-wide immunity during *Leishmania* infection. The Journal of Clinical Investigation. 2014;**124**:1711-1722

[44] Rosas-Hernandez H, Jimenez-Badillo S, Martinez-Cuevas PP, Gracia-Espino E, Terrones H, Terrones M, et al. Effects of 45-nm silver nanoparticles on coronary endothelial cells and isolated rat aortic rings. Toxicology Letters. 2009;**191**:305-313

[45] Fanti JR, Tomiotto-Pellissier F, Miranda-Sapla MM, Cataneo AHD,

Andrade CGTJ, Panis C, et al. Biogenic silver nanoparticles inducing *Leishmania amazonensis* promastigote and amastigote death *in vitro*. Acta Tropica. 2018;**178**:46-54

[46] Shoaib Sarwar H, Varikuti S, Farhan Sohail M, Sarwar M, Akhtar S, Satoskar AR, et al. Oral delivery and enhanced efficacy of antimonal drug through macrophage-guided multifunctional nanocargoes against visceral leishmaniasis. European Journal of Pharmaceutics and Biopharmaceutics. 2020;**152**:307-317

[47] Park E-J, Yi J, Kim Y, Choi K, Park K. Silver nanoparticles induce cytotoxicity by a Trojan-horse type mechanism. Toxicology In Vitro. 2010;**24**:872-878

[48] Kruszewski M, Brzoska K, Brunborg G, Asare N, Dobrzynska M, Dušinská M, et al. Toxicity of silver nanomaterials in higher eukaryotes. Advances in Molecular Toxicology. 2011;**5**:179-218

[49] Zahir AA, Chauhan IS, Bagavan A, Kamaraj C, Elango G, Shankar J, et al. Green synthesis of silver and titanium dioxide nanoparticles using *Euphorbia prostrata* extract shows shift from apoptosis to G0/G1Arrest followed by necrotic cell death in *Leishmania donovani*. Antimicrobial Agents and Chemotherapy. 2015;**59**:4782-4799

[50] AshaRani PV, Low Kah Mun G, Hande MP, Valiyaveettil S. Cytotoxicity and genotoxicity of silver nanoparticles in human cells. ACS Nano. 2009;**3**: 279-290